ADULT AURAL REHABILITATION

Impairment of hearing such as to reduce the quality of, and pleasure in communication affects about one fifth of the adult population. Yet only about one tenth of these make effective use of a hearing aid to overcome the handicap arising from defective hearing. The majority attempt to cope without help, often becoming progressively more isolated. Stigma; misunderstanding of the handicap and its effects; misconceptions about the role, benefits and limitations of hearing aids; and inappropriate amplification with inadequate instruction and guidance are all factors in the under-recognition and under-treatment of hearing loss.

This book has the objectives of seeking to rectify these aberrant attitudes with their unfortunate outcome, and creating a more positive approach to effectively assisting the hearing-impaired adult. Hearing aids (for most persons benefit far more from a pair of hearing aids than from one only), are regarded as the primary tools for providing assistance in hearing. However, to make the tools effective, informational and supportive counselling, not only to hearing-impaired people themselves, but often to those close to them, is absolutely vital. The technical and personal aspects of individualized hearing aid provision are considered in both theoretical and practical terms. Advice is given as to how and when counselling may be provided for both parties. The role of other forms of communication enhancement such as speechreading and assistive listening devices is also considered, as is the part played by amplification in the treatment of tinnitus. Written from an international perspective, the book is aimed principally at professionals in audiology (i.e. audiological scientists, physiological measurement technicians and hearing therapists), but will also interest doctors, speech therapists and others, particularly those working with elderly patients or clients.

ADULT AURAL REHABILITATION

EDITED BY

Denzil N. Brooks

Audiological Scientist
Withington Hospital
Manchester

SPRINGER-SCIENCE+BUSINESS MEDIA, B.V.

Originally published by Chapman and Hall Ltd in 1989
Softcover reprint of the hardcover 1st edition 1989

Typeset in Palatino 10/12 by Photoprint, Torquay, Devon

ISBN 0 412 33290 6

British Library Cataloguing in Publication Data

Adult aural rehabilitation.
1. Hearing aids
I. Brooks, Denzil N. (Denzil Noel), *1930–*
617.8'9

ISBN 978-0-412-33290-6   ISBN 978-1-4899-3452-9 (eBook)
DOI 10.1007/978-1-4899-3452-9

CONTENTS

Contents

Contents

CONTRIBUTORS

Susan Bellman MA, MB, BChir,
FRCSI, DLO
Hospital for Sick Children
Great Ormond Street
London

Denzil N. Brooks PhD
Regional Audiology Unit
Withington Hospital
Manchester

Denis Byrne PhD
National Acoustic Laboratories
Chatswood
New South Wales, Australia

Valerie Cleaver PhD
Institute of Sound and Vibration
University of Southampton

Anthony Corcoran MSc
Royal Victoria Hospital
Westbourne
Bournemouth

Karen Pedley MSc
Regional Audiology Unit
Withington Hospital
Manchester

Geoff Plant BA, TTCTD, TPTC
National Acoustic Laboratories
Chatswood
New South Wales, Australia

David Preves PhD
Argosy Electronics Inc.
Edina
Minneapolis 55435, USA

PREFACE

'Man's need for communication with his fellow man is possibly his greatest need and the fulfilment of his other needs and desires is largely dependent upon, or at the last greatly facilitated by, his ability to satisfy this basic one.'

Louise Tracy

Defective hearing disrupts human communication. It gives rise to anxiety, frustration, stress, isolation, loss of self-esteem, even loss of livelihood for the individual with a reduced capacity to receive and interpret sound. Because we live in families and communities, the effects of hearing loss are not restricted to the impaired individual. Those who associate with that person, especially those who are very close, are affected and prone to many of the same emotions and stresses.

From the earliest times man has sought for remedies for hearing loss. Incantations, infusions, cuppings and bleedings, all have been advocated and, with the rare, serendipitous exception, have been equally ineffective. The only real assistance for countless generations was to cup the hand behind the ear and ask the speaker to raise their voice.

Over the last century or so, we have seen the development of electrically powered hearing aids. Initially these were unsightly and bulky. Wearing even a single hearing aid was burdensome; to wear two would be near impossible. The early aids were of limited assistance, especially to those with *sensorineural* loss, and from this arose the belief that help was only possible for those with *conductive* losses. Even when hearing aids with much better performance became available, the myth that 'nerve deafness' could not be helped persisted. Additionally, the stigma associated with wearing a hearing aid deterred many persons from seeking early help. Hence, by the time an aid was obtained, the capacity to benefit without additional help and support had considerably diminished. As a result of these factors, the stereotype of the hearing aid as a rather ineffective crutch for the impaired ear was reinforced.

The thesis of this book is that the improvements that have taken place in the design, manufacture and fitting of hearing aids are such that amplification is now the primary and most effective form of assistance to the hearing impaired. Hearing aids (one for each defective ear), carefully prescribed according to the degree and nature of the hearing loss, sensitively and knowledgeably supplied, and supported by empathetic counselling will efficiently and effectively meet the majority of the needs, not only of those with diminished hearing ability, but also of those near and dear to them. It must be stressed that attention has to be given to all the aspects identified. Hearing aids supplied without careful matching to individual need or without appropriate counselling are as unlikely to be used wisely and well, as would randomly selected false teeth given to an edentulous individual.

The aim of the book is to provide practical guidance on the rehabilitation of the hearing-impaired adult based on an appreciation of the many factors that contribute to that person's handicap. Chapters 1 and 2 review the epidemiology of hearing impairment and the history of man's attempts to reduce the handicap arising from a deficient auditory input. Chapter 3 is concerned with the assessment of benefit brought about by amplification and the role of rehabilitation in increasing that benefit.

Denis Byrne (Chapter 4) has long supported the philosophy of predetermining and providing hearing-aid performance based on measurement of the individual's actual hearing capacity. His chapter details the development and practical application of this technique.

The attitude to hearing loss and hearing aids, both of the hearing-impaired individual and of those close to that person, can have a substantial bearing on the success or failure of a hearing-aid fitting. The factors that contribute to attitude are analysed in Chapter 5, but stress is laid on the fact that it is the whole person and not just the combination of attitudes that matters. The mechanics of fitting a hearing aid are discussed in Chapter 6. Inevitably, much of the text will be a reiteration of old and well-tried techniques, but it is hoped that even for the experienced clinician there may be some useful tips, especially in helping the growing number of elderly persons with hearing impairment.

For the confirmed binauralist, Chapter 7 may have little to offer, but for the many who still think of fitting a single hearing aid it will, hopefully, offer new insights and inspiration.

Be the fitting monaural or binaural, be the patient young or old, some counselling is essential if eventual success is to be achieved in overcoming the handicap of hearing loss. Perhaps the biggest single reason for failure to manage and successfully utilize a hearing aid in the past has been the failure to recognize the absolutely vital role of counselling. In Chapter 8 it is suggested that an understanding of the effects of hearing loss, modification of aberrant attitudes and preparation for amplification should, in the majority of individuals, be brought about before the hearing aid is supplied.

'No man is an island' said Donne, and Karen Pedley (Chapter 9) highlights the ways in which relationships with family, friends and others can affect every aspect of the life of the hearing-impaired person. Their role in the rehabilitation of the new hearing-aid user is also considered.

Every potential aid user has an individual set of problems, but for some there are special difficulties due to, for example, another handicap such as blindness. Valerie Cleaver (Chapter 10) explores these areas of special difficulty, bringing insight and suggesting practical means of enhancing benefit. Jointly with the editor (Chapter 11) Dr Cleaver looks at some of the additional or alternative methods of enhancing communication.

Although the hearing aid is the major tool for assisting the hearing-impaired person, there are circumstances and situations in which more dedicated systems can be beneficial. Geoff Plant (Chapter 12) provides a sound theoretical framework as well as a review of these assistive listening and communication devices.

It has been said that every hearing-impaired person has head noises, although not all are troubled or distressed by them. The converse is not true. Not every person with 'normal' hearing is free of tinnitus, and may find the unwelcome guest an almost intolerable burden. Tony Corcoran (Chapter 13) succinctly covers the very wide field of causation, effect and treatment of tinnitus, including the role of the hearing aid and its relative, the tinnitus masker.

Some causes of hearing loss are avoidable, intense noise probably being the best known. Dr Bellman (Chapter 14) takes a cradle-to-grave look at causes of hearing loss that might be eliminated or diminished. Medicine and education both have a part to play in reducing the prevalence of deafness in future generations.

David Preves (Chapter 15) looks at some of the current limitations of hearing aids and gives us a glimpse into the future. Microelectronics has made vast strides in the last decade and hearing aids have been major beneficiaries. There seems to be real hope for improving the capacity of hearing aids to sift speech from noise, and for minimizing acoustic feedback, two of the commonest causes of complaint with present technology.

I am immensely grateful to my colleagues and friends for their substantive contributions to this book. For the rest I must take responsibility. My interest in this area of work was heightened in 1972 by the award of a Winston Churchill Travelling Fellowship that enabled me to travel to Europe and Scandinavia and see the best of the services in those countries. I am indebted to that organization for the wealth of experience gained, this being the foundation for the services developed in South Manchester.

I am indebted to many colleagues for help and support, but two deserve special mention. Mr N.W. Gill was the initial inspiration for my studies in rehabilitative audiology, and Miss Dorothy Johnson, Hearing Therapist, has contributed enormously to the development of the counselling programme. I am indebted to them both for their wisdom and friendship.

To my wife Barbara, I am especially grateful for the patience and understanding shown over the months of preoccupation.

1

THE ADULT
HEARING-IMPAIRED

Denzil Brooks

'My most precious gift, my hearing has deteriorated very much.' So wrote Beethoven as a young man of 28. We might feel that as a composer he had a somewhat exaggerated view of the importance of hearing, but closer examination reveals that his judgement had less to do with music than with his role in society. His severe hearing loss did not prevent him from writing his magnificent Ninth Symphony with its inspiring chorale based on Schiller's 'Ode to Joy', but it did make him shun society and avoid the embarrassment of social intercourse. In his famous 'Heiligenstadt Testament' he wrote:

O my fellow men, who consider me, or describe me as unfriendly, stubborn or misanthropic, how greatly do you wrong me because you do not know the secret reason why I appear to you to be so. I have been forced to accept the prospect of a permanent infirmity. Though endowed with a passionate and lively temperament and even fond of the distractions offered by society, at an early age I was forced to seclude myself and live in solitude. I could not bring myself to say to people 'Speak up, I am deaf'. For me there can be no relaxation in human society, no refined conversations, no mutual confidences. I must live like an outcast and creep into society only as often as sheer necessity demands.

Beethoven perceived his defective hearing as a disability. It restricted his social activity and forced withdrawal on him. He was not only handicapped in terms of human communication but also in relation to his music. Although he could still 'hear' within himself, his ability to play the piano was severely diminished. His friends commented that all his playing was loud. The subtleties of dynamic interpretation were no longer audible to him. Orchestral conducting also became impossible due to his inability to hear either tonal quality or tempo.

In using Beethoven as an example of an individual with diminished hearing, the terms 'impairment', 'disability' and 'handicap' have all been used. These words are sometimes used as if interchangeable, but in fact each should be used specifically. Before proceeding to further examination of the nature and extent of hearing loss in adults, it is important to clarify the meaning and scope of these terms.

(a) Hearing impairment

The World Health Organization (WHO) defines impairment as any loss or abnormality of psychological, physiological or anatomic structure or function. The conventional methods for assessing hearing impairment are pure-tone or speech audiometry with deviations of greater than 10 dB from the defined normal value(s) being regarded as 'outside normal limits'. Degree of impairment is measured as the difference between the individual's threshold of hearing and the defined norm. The same hearing impairment may affect different individuals in different ways depending on their lifestyles. The reduced ability to function in a normal manner constitutes disability.

(b) Hearing disability

Disability (WHO) is defined as any restriction or lack of ability (resulting from an impairment) in performing an activity in the manner or within the range considered normal for a human being. Being unable through hearing impairment to participate in a family conversation disables the individual, but the disablement may be minimized or eliminated by the provision of suitable help – such as a hearing aid. In a rather noisier situation, for example, when at a party or in a public bar, the same degree of hearing loss may be much more disabling and the reduction in difficulty brought about by the aid may be less. There may remain some handicap despite the use of amplification.

(c) Hearing handicap

The WHO defines handicap as a disadvantage for a given individual, resulting from an impairment or disability, that limits or prevents the fulfilment of a role that is normal (depending on age, sex and social or cultural factors) for that individual. Quantifying handicap is, in consequence, a complex task dependent on the interaction of a number of factors. The communication needs, perceived or real, of the individual and of those close to that person – the 'significant others' – will be of major importance. Age, 'attitudinal' rather than chronological, will have a substantial bearing. Handicap will depend on environment, perceptions about hearing impairment as a handicap, personal experiences with others having hearing loss with or without some form of assistance such as a hearing aid and on personality. A hearing impairment that may effectively cripple one individual may be written off as inconsequential by another. Likewise, hearing handicap may be assessed by an outsider as having a certain degree of severity, and by the individual concerned as being of quite different magnitude. In consequence there are no universally accepted standards for determining the degree of hearing handicap. As will be seen later, there are several possible assessment tools, each with its own advantages and limitations.

1.1 THE CHANGING PATTERN OF HEARING LOSS

In England a couple of generations ago, running ears were commonplace both in adults and children. Many required mastoid surgery – a fearsome operation. Severe loss of hearing was a not infrequent result of the disease or its treatment. Occasionally, life itself was endangered. For the more fortunate the consequences might be no more than a permanent perforation of the tympanic membranes, or a scarred membrane with, perhaps, middle-ear adhesions that considerably reduced the efficiency of the middle ear.

The high prevalence of middle-ear disease was, to some degree a reflection of the poor social conditions. Poverty and deprivation, crowded and insanitary housing, poor standards of nutrition and health care, all combined to weaken resistance and render the young especially vulnerable to middle-ear infections. Hinchcliffe (1972) has shown how the prevalence of perforated eardrums as a cause of hearing loss and as an outcome of otitis media relate to an index of poverty, the inverse of the gross national product. Many other studies illustrate the high prevalence of ear disease in poorer communities today, with inevitable consequences in terms of reduced hearing.

With improvements in housing, hygiene and health care and with the introduction of antibiotics, the chronic discharging ear has become a rarity in Western society. The pattern of ear disease and associated hearing loss has dramatically altered over the last half century. The radical mastoid operation is almost unknown. Nevertheless, there are still many elderly persons whose hearing is deficient as a result of aural problems in childhood. The numbers are diminishing with the passage of time and in the future, there should be considerably less hearing loss manifest in the elderly resulting from childhood disease.

A review of data relating to candidates for hearing aids in the UK National Health Service will help to illustrate the changes that have taken place. In 1953, 46% of new applicants were diagnosed as having a purely conductive loss and 27% a sensorineural loss (Figure 1.1). By the

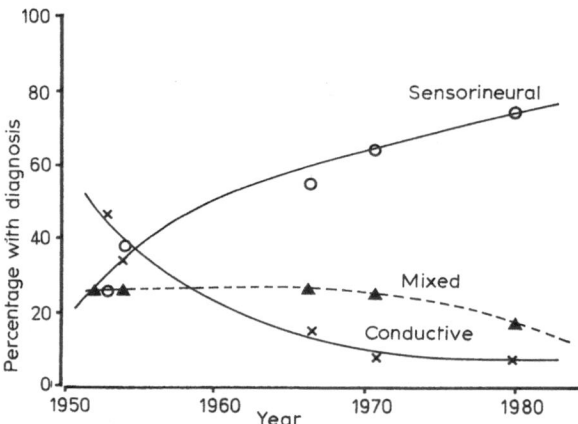

Figure 1.1 Review of data for patients diagnosed as requiring hearing aids, 1950–85. ×, conductive hearing loss; ▲ mixed loss; ○ sensorineural loss.

1980s only 8% were diagnosed as having conductive loss, with 75% having sensorineural hearing loss.

However, in some of the elderly the diagnosis may be based less on otological or audiological grounds than on the age of the patient. Many of those described as having 'old-age' deafness (presbycusis) may, on closer examination, be seen to have sequelae to middle-ear disease half a century ago. In a study in Manchester (Brooks, 1979) candidates for hearing aids in whom the diagnosis was presbycusis were tested with pure-tone audiometry and acoustic admittance measurement. In two-thirds the hearing loss was indicated as of a purely sensorineural nature typical of presbycusis. In the remaining third, there was significant middle-ear involvement. The majority of the group indicating past middle-ear disease could clearly recollect having earaches, visits to clinics and bouts of hearing loss as children. By contrast, very few of those with the uncontaminated sensorineural hearing loss could recollect anything suggesting childhood middle-ear problems.

Within the next 30 years or so the majority of those manifesting middle-ear disease from childhood will have died. Presumably the prevalence of conductive loss arising from middle-ear disease will then almost disappear. Conductive hearing loss due to otosclerosis will, in all probability, still exist, though there is some suspicion that prevalence may be declining due to fluoridation of water supplies.

There are other factors that change the pattern of hearing loss over time. Sequelae to infectious diseases have become less common. Two or three generations ago, measles and scarlet fever were significant causes of defective hearing. Today, probably due to the higher standards of general health, these diseases now only rarely affect hearing. Meningitis still remains a potential hazard, but less so than in the past. It is to be expected and hoped that the amount of hearing loss due to high levels of noise should diminish in the future. In some industries (e.g. steel rolling and weaving) automation and robotics have substantially reduced the number of persons at hazard.

Unfortunately, there are new factors appearing. Deafness due to cytomegalovirus in neonates is a cause for concern. Some commonly used drugs are ototoxic. Streptomycin is probably the best known, but the list of such drugs is now very long. Sometimes there may be no alternative. If life is threatened, desperate measures may need to be taken. At other times awareness of the potential hazards from these drugs is vital.

1.2 PREVALENCE OF HEARING DISORDERS

(a) Subjectively assessed hearing loss

Early studies in the UK were based either on self-assessment in response to such questions as, 'Do you suffer from deafness?', or by interviewer assessment. Wilkins (1948) examined a stratified random sample of the population and found less than 2% of the population aged 25–34 years reporting hearing difficulty. The percentage rose to around 27% in the over 75s. Somewhat higher figures were obtained in a national survey of 367 000 persons over the age of 65 where over 30% were assessed as having difficulty in hearing (Townsend and Wedderburn, 1965). Using data from the US Health Survey, the Metropolitan Life Insurance Company (1976) estimated the prevalence of hearing loss as almost 40% in the over 75s, the rate halving approximately with each decrease in age of ten years. Milne (1976) found higher rates, especially in the more aged. His findings suggested a prevalence of 35% in the 62 to 69 year age range; 42% in the 70 to 79 year age range and 54% in the 80 to 90 year olds. Similar prevalence rates were found by Gilhome-Herbst and Humphrey (1981) who interviewed 253 elderly persons aged over 70 registered with an Inner London group practice. In response to the question, 'Do you think you are at all deaf?', nearly 40% of those in their 70s responded positively. In the 80 to 84 year olds, the positive response rose to 54% and in the over 85s to 69%. Davis (1983) reported on the National Survey of Hearing carried out for the Medical Research Council. One question employed to subjectively assess hearing impairment related to difficulty in hearing someone talking in a normal voice. In the 17 to 24 year age range only about 1% had such difficulty, but the percentage rose with increasing age to around 15% in those over 75.

These data on the elderly tend to be rather widely dispersed because different questions have been asked in assessing prevalence of hearing impairment, and as discussed later (p. 8) this may substantially affect responses.

(b) Objectively assessed hearing loss

Pure-tone audiometry is the conventional technique for objectively assessing hearing impairment. The range of normality for clinical purposes is usually regarded as within 10 dB of the threshold of hearing, which is based on measurements obtained on otologically healthy young adults. However, to adopt a criterion for impaired hearing of any loss greater than 10 dB would result in a very large proportion of the adult population failing. A level that reflects difficulty in social communication should be more apposite than a statistically derived cut-off point.

Education authorities and those responsible for the health of school-children have, until within the last few years, accepted close to 30 dB as the level for onset of handicapping hearing loss. Evidence is now growing that hearing losses as small as 15 dB can, in some children, result in significant retardation in language acquisition and educational progress, at least in the short term. However, this is for children who are still learning language, whereas the adult population have already acquired that skill, and therefore a more liberal criterion is probably more appropriate. Overall, a level of about 25 dB across the speech frequencies appears to be a reasonable compromise for the onset of significantly socially handicapping hearing impairment in the adult individual.

Gilhome-Herbst and Humphrey (1981) in their studies on the elderly, evaluated hearing impairment by pure-tone audiometry as well as by self-assessment. Several other studies have employed audiometry specifically with the elderly (Alpiner, 1963; Chafee, 1967; Martin and Peckford, 1978; Hart, 1980; Milne, 1980), the first four being assessments of residents in homes for the elderly. All six studies showed rates of hearing impairment increasing with age at an accelerating rate.

More recently, Davis (1983) published data indicating that in the 51–60 year age range, 23% have hearing poorer than 25 dBHL (averaged over 0.5, 1, 2, and 4 kHz). In the age range 61–70 years this rises to 34% and in the subjects over 71 years of age to 74%. Figure 1.2 presents data from several studies showing the rates of hearing impairment by self-assessment and by audiometric evaluation as a function of age. The difference between the two lines represents the gap between subjective and objective assessment, admitted and measured hearing impairment when the latter is defined as being greater than 25 dB over the speech range. It might be argued that the subjective data represent the true onset of social difficulty, and that the audiometric threshold is, in consequence, set at too sensitive a level. The arguments in favour of the 25 dB criterion have been set out above, and accord with the experience of involved professionals. It is suggested that there are other reasons for the difference between objective and subjective assessments, and these are considered below.

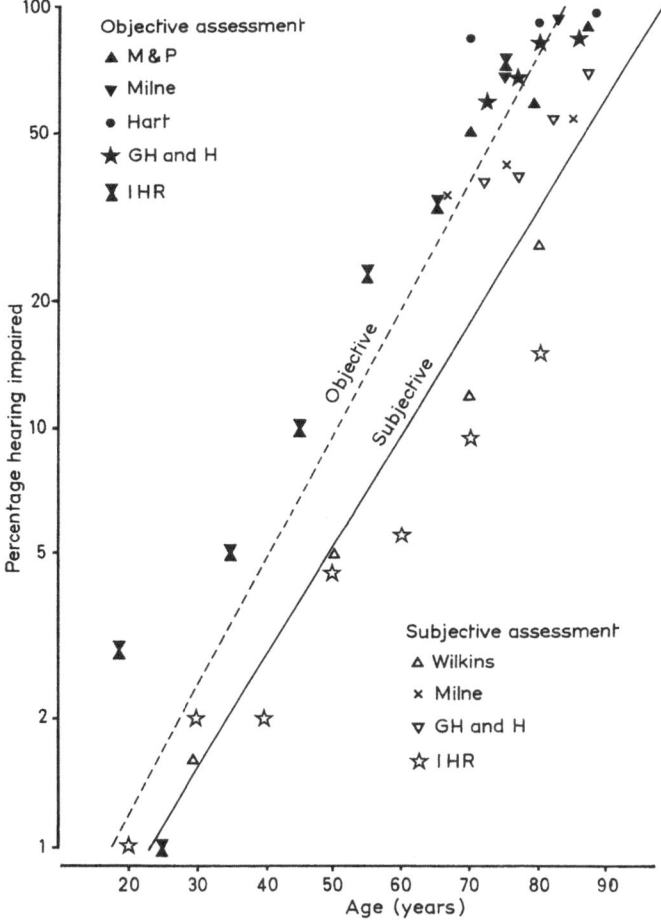

Figure 1.2 Data showing rates of hearing impairment by self-assessment and audiometric evaluation as a function of age. (Note: A logarithmic scale for prevalence has been used.)

Semantic misunderstanding

The study of Gilhome-Herbst and Humphrey (1981) is probably fairly typical of the approach employed in seeking for self-assessment of hearing difficulties. Participants were asked, 'Do you think you are at all deaf?' Because of the connotations of the word 'deaf' it is possible that many who were aware of some degree of hearing impairment would not admit to this in response to this question. In an unpublished study at Manchester Regional Audiology Unit, 400 hearing-aid candidates with average thresholds of 50 dB were asked to select the term that best described their hearing loss from a choice of three: 'hearing impaired', 'hard of hearing' and 'deaf'. Less than 4% described themselves as 'deaf', and these were not specifically those with the greatest audiometric losses, but tended rather to be individuals who found hearing loss to be particularly burdensome. The responses of the remaining 96% were almost equally divided between the other two terms. Many an elderly person will, with a little persuasion, accept that hearing is below normal, a little impaired, but will bridle at any suggestion that they are deaf.

Lack of awareness

There are many individuals, of all ages, who indicate some degree of hearing impairment on audiometry but who deny having any experiences indicating diminished hearing. Among the more elderly, especially those living alone and with few social contacts, there may be a genuine lack of awareness that hearing is diminished. Person-to-person communication may be limited to only one or two people in a week, for example, the home help and the milkman, with conversation limited to discussing the weather or the cost of living. Shopping is done at a supermarket where there is no problem involved in asking about costs. Radio and TV volume may be higher, but this goes unrecognized unless the neighbours complain. Possibly, due to poor sight, the hard-of-hearing individual sits close to the screen and hence to the loudspeaker, remaining unaware of the compensation for hearing loss made thereby. In such situations the individual may quite honestly not realize that hearing is defective.

In the study by Milne (1976) into hearing loss in 487 persons over the age of 62, two questions were asked relative to hearing. These were: 'Do you suffer from deafness?', and 'Are you hard of hearing?' Replies to either were coded as 'subjective deafness present'. In women aged 70 or over, nearly 20% of those responding negatively to the questions had hearing sensitivity below 30 dB at 1000 Hz (at 4000 Hz nearly 58% had sensitivity below 30 dB). Subjectively, a high proportion of the elderly were, therefore, unaware of their hearing impairment.

Acceptance of hearing loss as normal

With increasing age there is a tendency to accept less-acute hearing as an inevitable occurrence, a normal concomitant of aging. In the Manchester Audiology Clinic study referred to previously on p. 8, hearing-aid candidates who were mostly of pensionable age were asked two questions: (1) 'Do you think your hearing is absolutely normal?', (2) 'Do you think your hearing is normal for your age?' Only 1% of the subjects said 'yes' to the first question, but 24% thought their hearing was normal for their age. Merluzzi and Hinchcliffe (1973) reported the onset of just noticeable hearing impairment as a function of age. This was 10 dB or less for persons under the age of 45 years, but at 60 years of age it was approximately 20 dB, at 70 it rose to 30 dB and by the age of 80 to around 45 dB. A similar finding was reported by Lutman, Brown and Coles (1987) who subjectively assessed degree of disability/handicap as a function of increasing age with hearing loss held constant. The authors attributed the lower disability/handicap rating in the elderly to the expectation of many such subjects that some degree of disability/ handicap was inevitable and a normal expectation as a result of the aging process, independent of the hearing loss. The perceived handicap due specifically to hearing loss is therefore reduced by the amount accorded to aging.

It seems reasonable to hypothesize, therefore, that the upper line in Figure 1.2 provides a measure of the population with hearing level below the criterion adopted, and hence the number potentially in need of hearing rehabilitation. The lower line indicates the number of persons who recognize that impairment. The gap between the lines suggests that there is considerable scope for attitude modification, not only among the hearing impaired themselves, but also in the population at large. There is a need to reduce the stigma associated with 'deafness', to heighten awareness of what can be done nowadays to assist those with hearing loss and to encourage the hearing impaired to seek for help rather than accepting hearing loss as an inevitable and unalleviable condition accompanying the aging process.

1.3 PREVALENCE AND DEGREE OF HEARING LOSS

The consideration of prevalence has, up to this point, been concerned with all hearing losses greater than specified criterion level, but has not taken any account of the degree of severity. In terms of service provision it is important to have information about degree, as rehabilitation needs tend to increase with increasing severity of loss. Those with mild degrees of hearing impairment may be completely satisfied and fully rehabilitated by means of a correctly fitted and supplied hearing aid of moderate gain and power output. With increasing degree of hearing loss, more gain and power are required of the aids, but expectations about the degree of reduction in handicap may have to be scaled down. Other forms of assistive strategy need to be considered.

Rahko *et al.* (1985) measured the hearing thresholds for pure tones of a carefully selected, representative group of 369 Finnish inhabitants aged 65 years. Taking the average over the range 500 to 2000 Hz, the number of persons with hearing impairment approximately halved with each increase in criterion level of 10 dB over the range from 15–55 dB. Plomp (1977) arrived at the same pattern of distribution of hearing loss by degree from data based on studies in the USA.

For the UK, with a population approaching 60 million, these data suggest around 2 million persons will have losses between 45 and 64 dB, the region where hearing aids are most beneficial. About a further half million will have losses of the order of 65 to 84 dB, requiring aids of greater gain, power and sophistication. They will probably need extra help in coping with amplification and additional forms of assistance. More than 100 000 persons will have hearing loss of greater severity than 85 dB and many of these will require considerable help in dealing with the handicap arising from this degree of impairment.

At the other end of the spectrum, some 3 million persons will have hearing levels between 35 and 44 dB and around 5 million between 25 and 35 dB. In total these data indicate about 8 million persons with mild hearing loss, 2 million with moderate loss and over half a million with severe loss (Newton, 1986). Many of the individuals with hearing losses between 30 and 44 dB could be assisted by suitable forms of amplification (not necessarily hearing aids, but such devices as TV amplifiers, etc.) and by instruction in coping strategies and hearing tactics. Over the last few years there has been a noticeable and encouraging growth in the number of candidates for help in this area of mild hearing loss.

1.4 PREVALENCE AND TYPE OF LOSS

In looking at the changing pattern of hearing loss, it was noted that over the last 30 years there has been a very substantial decline in the prevalence of conductive hearing loss arising from middle-ear disease in childhood, a trend that should continue for some years yet until this probably becomes insignificant as a factor in adult hearing impairment. However, even if middle-ear disease, noise and other avoidable causes of hearing loss could be completely eliminated, there would remain a substantial number of elderly persons with hearing loss not specifically attributable to any disease or noxious influence. With increased longevity, the number of aged persons with hearing loss due to no other cause than aging can be expected to increase.

1.5 PRESBYCUSIS

Presbycusis is the term used to describe the progressive elevation in hearing threshold that occurs with aging. The term was coined by Zwaardemaker (1894) who carried out one of the first systematic investigations into changes in hearing sensitivity with age and who pointed out the essentially high-frequency nature of the loss. Presbycusis can be considered from a number of standpoints.

(a) Sensitivity

The first major audiometric study of hearing acuity as a function of age was made by Bunch in 1929. He tested 353 hospital admissions aged between 20 and 70 years and documented diminishing sensitivity in the frequencies above 500 Hz as age increased. Since that time there have been many studies, some on totally unselected populations, others on carefully screened populations in which those manifesting, or having a history of, otological disease or noise-induced hearing loss were excluded. Robinson and Sutton (1979) critically evaluated the available data for subjects ranging in age from six to 80 years. Taking the hearing level at 18 years of age as the standard, they demonstrated that median hearing level H at age N could be best predicted by the formula $H = a(N-18)^2$, where a is a coefficient dependent on the frequency of the stimulus and the sex of the individual. Below 1000 Hz, the coefficient a is the same for both sexes. Above, it is greater for males than females, the difference being maximal at 4000 Hz. The pattern then is of hearing loss increasing at an accelerating pace with age, the loss being greater for males than females, especially in the higher frequencies.

(b) Perception of speech

It has long been suggested that in addition to the reduction in sensitivity with increasing age, there is progressive difficulty in discrimination of speech. Considerable research effort has been expended in seeking to determine whether the deficiency in speech discrimination is entirely due to the reduction in sensitivity or whether there are additional factors that cause disproportionate difficulty with speech comprehension. When speech testing is carried out in conditions that impose additional stress on the listener, for example, in the presence of competing noise, in reverberant conditions or with speed of presentation of speech artificially increased, then the performance of elderly adults deteriorates more rapidly than that of young adults with comparative degrees of hearing loss. Gaeth (1948) described this effect as 'phonemic regression'. Jerger (1973) analysed the speech performance versus intensity functions for 4095 testable ears of 2162 persons aged from six to 89 years. He was able to hold degree of hearing loss constant and plot maximum speech discrimination score as a function of age. For the subjects with very small degrees of hearing loss there was little deterioration seen as a function of age, but with increasing loss, poorer performance with increasing age was clearly evident. The conclusion drawn from this was in accord with other studies; suggesting that with aging there is a progressive deterioration of central processing in addition to the peripheral loss of sensitivity.

However, determining the real decrement in performance in elderly individuals is fraught with difficulty and many of the studies can be criticized methodologically. As Marshall (1981) points out relative to the Jerger (1973) study, it is probable that with increasing age the hearing loss would be progressively more severe in the higher frequencies, whereas the average loss was calculated over the mid-range (500–2000 Hz) frequencies.

In two studies where hearing losses were audiometrically matched for two groups, one young and one elderly, no differences were found in speech discrimination. Quoting from Marshall (1981) 'The heterogeneity of results may be attributable to a heterogeneity of pathological conditions that result in a conglomerate of subgroups who have only one thing in common – age.' This leads to the third factor to be considered with regard to presbycusis – pathology.

(c) Pathological basis of presbycusis

Schuknecht (1955) stated that presbycusis is the cochlear manifestation of a diffuse process that involves all the body tissues. In the light of the discussion in the previous section perhaps one might amend this to include the whole of the auditory tract rather than limiting presbycusis to the cochlea. Within the cochlea, four patterns of pathology have been proposed as probably contributors to presbycusis:

1. *Sensory.* The hair cells degenerate and finally atrophy. There may be secondary atrophy of the supporting cells. The basal end of the cochlea is most likely to be affected and the hearing loss is manifested in the audiogram as an abrupt high-frequency loss.
2. *Neuronal.* Atrophy of spiral ganglion cells disproportionate to the hair

cell degeneration. This may result in insignificant loss as measured by pure-tone threshold audiometry, but substantial loss of discriminatory ability.

3. *Metabolic.* Progressive degeneration of the stria vascularis has been shown to occur frequently in older persons. The stria vascularis is thought to be the source of endolymph and hence, to some extent, responsible for the DC potential across the organ of Corti. Reduction of the potential will diminish the transduction capacity of the hair cells with consequent reduction in cochlear sensitivity. In some individuals there may be a positive family history of early-onset hearing loss of a progressive nature (Lowell and Paparella, 1977). In such cases speech discrimination may remain at a high level.

4. *Mechanical.* Most tissues lose elasticity in advanced age. The basilar and other membranes of the inner ear are probably no exception to this general process. Audiometrically this might be expected to produce a hearing loss which by definition is sensorineural, but by effect is primarily conductive. However, changes in the dynamics of the cochlea might be expected to have effects additional to simple loss of sensitivity.

Additional to the cochlear contributions to presbycusis, a number of retro-cochlear causes have been suggested. These include narrowing of the internal auditory meatus exerting pressure on the auditory nerve, neuronal degeneration in the ascending auditory tract and neuronal atrophy in the cortical regions associated with audition.

(d) Treatment

Whereas the majority of conductive hearing losses are amenable either to medical or surgical treatment, the opposite is unfortunately the case with sensorineural hearing loss. In a small percentage of individuals where the hearing impairment can be identified as secondary to some treatable medical condition, then appropriate treatment might arrest or even reverse the hearing loss. There has been much publicity about cochlear implants as a 'cure' for deafness. Even with the most generous estimates the percentage of subjects suitable for this type of surgery is minute. It is appropriate only to those who are beyond the range of conventional treatments. At the present stage of technology, expectation from even a multi-channel implant must, for the majority of those receiving this form of treatment, be limited.

The identification of four possible contributory factors in presbycusis has not, so far, been progressed to the practical diagnostic level. Tests to identify each component and attribute or apportion hearing loss to that component do not yet exist. If such tests are devised in the future and shown to be accurate, then differential diagnosis might lead the way to treatments for arresting or reversing deteriorating hearing. Metabolic presbycusis, for example, might conceivably be reversed or delayed by improving the microcirculation of the stria vascularis. At present, however, this remains wishful thinking. Presbycusis is, in medical or surgical terms, incurable. Consequently, treatment must concentrate on alleviating the handicap, or minimizing the difficulties brought about by deteriorating hearing. Unquestionably the most effective form of assistance today is personal amplification with hearing aids. Additional to this there are a number of assistive strategies and devices. Lipreading (speechreading) is a skill acquired naturally by most hearing-impaired persons. Tuition to polish that skill can, for some individuals, be extremely helpful, for others less so. The role of speechreading is considered in more detail in Chapter 11. Dedicated television and radio amplifiers are a boon to many hearing-impaired individuals living with less hearing-impaired relatives. Telephone assistive devices likewise can transform a highly stressful situation into one of real pleasure. These and other methods of mitigating the effects of hearing loss are discussed in Chapter 12. However, the greatest benefit over the widest range of situations is provided by correctly selected and supplied personal hearing aids.

1.6 HEARING AIDS

Considering both the advantages and disadvantages of amplification, a reasonable criterion for recommending use of a hearing aid might be an average hearing loss of 30 dB across the speech frequencies. If that be so, there are some 8 million persons in the UK who should be benefiting from a hearing aid. Yet the number in use is thought to be only about one and a quarter million or about one-sixth of those who might benefit. Penetration rates are much the same in Scandinavia, and possibly somewhat lower in the USA (Skadegard, 1982).

Why is the take-up rate so low? Some of the reasons will be discussed at greater length in the succeeding chapter, but there is little doubt that hearing aids have had a poor image in the past, especially hearing aids supplied to the elderly. Usually the decision to obtain help through amplification is delayed for many years. In consequence, those obtaining aids are less adaptable, less dextrous, less motivated and less able to cope with the task of hearing-aid orientation. Performance tends to be well below optimum, and the hearing aid (not the user, or the system, or the lack of instruction) is blamed. The perception of those associated with the hearing-impaired individual – family, friends, peer group, doctor – is that the aid is ineffective. Thus when others recognize that their hearing is failing, they reject the concept of early assistance with amplification because it has been seen as providing little benefit. A vicious spiral of delay – poor performance; poor image leading to further delay has been created – and the hearing aid is blamed.

There might have been some measure of justification for this attitude in the past. The early carbon and valve aids were of poor quality, but modern hearing aids, when properly fitted with adequate instruction and counselling, can give considerable assistance to the majority of those with hearing loss. To a large extent the modern aid is to hearing impairment what spectacles are to visual impairment or false teeth to the edentulous. It is the author's view that the hearing aid, carefully selected and supplied with appropriate counselling, is the primary tool for helping the hearing impaired and that with earlier referral, and hence younger, more adaptable, dextrous and eager subjects the vicious spiral can be broken.

1.7 HEARING AIDS AND THE ELDERLY – SPECIAL CONSIDERATIONS

Hearing is by no means the only faculty that is likely to be impaired with advancing age. Vision, mobility, dexterity, mental agility and general health and wellbeing all tend to deteriorate with the passage of time. Each can react with hearing impairment or have a bearing on the efficacy of treatment. A brief look only at the special needs of the elderly will be made here as the subject will be considered in greater depth in Chapter 10.

The visually handicapped do not usually have more than normal difficulty in inserting the earmould as this procedure does not involve vision to any significant degree, but they may have other initial manipulation problems, especially in such tasks as changing the battery. Unhurried instruction, patient explanation and the establishment of good routines can help with these tasks and ease the learning process.

Diseases such as arthritis may severely limit the range and extent of an elderly person's movements. The constraint on physical activity reduces the opportunities for activities such as visiting friends, clubs, concerts or theatres, so greater importance is attached to hearing the family news, local gossip and doings of friends. Hearing loss makes this more stressful. Enjoyment decreases leading to further withdrawal. A downward spiral is created that can easily lead to total isolation. Rheumatism and arthritis in the hands make manual activity slow and painful. A lifetime of manual work can result in horny skin. Small movements are difficult to make and small objects are difficult to feel. One of the inevitable consequences of miniaturization in hearing aids is that the controls have become smaller, frequently requiring a considerable degree of skill to manipulate. In such cases instruments with more readily adjustable controls should be selected or steps taken to minimize the need for adjustment. If the environment is acoustically stable, that is, if sound levels do not fluctuate widely, then a fixed gain control may be the answer. If there is a spouse or carer who can give help, a clearly marked gain control may be beneficial, enabling the helper to adjust the volume control to the desirable level.

Mental agility and speed of acquiring new skills diminish with advancing years. Hence the process of supplying a hearing aid to an elderly person has to be paced quite differently from the process with a younger subject. Instruction may need to be spread over several sessions, imparting only the information relevant to the stage of learning and avoiding overloading the individual with a mass of detail.

General health may affect the prognosis for hearing-aid success. The demands of treatment for a malignancy or some other major ailment may be so dominant that the problems of hearing loss pale into insignificance. The patient who already has a major disability may find it hard either to accept a further disability, or to become actively involved in the treatment of that disability. A person awaiting an operation for cataract may be unable to cope with the problems of learning to use a hearing aid, subconsciously expecting that with the restoration of good vision the hearing problem will diminish. Some individuals are unable to divide internal coping resources between two (or more) problems.

Whatever the additional handicaps, the approach to maximizing benefit must be through evaluating each person's individual needs and then tailoring the assistance to those needs. It is vital to recognize that the elderly hearing-impaired are not a class apart. They are otherwise normal persons whose hearing has deteriorated. Their hopes, expectations, perceptions and attitudes were similar to those of the rest of their society until modified by the encroachment of hearing loss.

REFERENCES

Alpiner, J. (1963) Audiological problems of the aged. *Geriatrics* **18**, 19–26.
Brooks, D.N. (1979) Hearing aid candidates – some relevant features. *Brit. J. Audiol.*, **13**, 81–4.
Bunch, C.C. (1929) Age variations in auditory acuity. *Arch. Otolaryngol.* **9**, 625–36.
Chafee, C. (1967) Rehabilitation needs of nursing home patients: a report of a survey. *Rehabilitation Literature*, **28**, 377–82.
Davis, A.C. (1983) Hearing disorders in the population: first phase findings of the MRC National Study of Hearing. In *Hearing science and hearing disorders* (eds M.E. Lutman and M.P. Haggard), Academic Press, London.

Gaeth, J.H. (1948) A study of phonemic regression in relation to hearing loss. Phd thesis, Northwestern Univ, Chicago.

Gilhome-Herbst, K. and Humphrey, C. (1981) Prevalence of hearing impairment in the elderly living at home. *J. Royal Coll. of General Practitioners*, **31**, 155–60.

Hart, F.S. (1980) *The hearing of residents in homes for the elderly – South Glamorgan*. University Hospital South Wales.

Hinchcliffe, R. (1972) Epidemiological aspects of otitis media. In *Otitis media* (eds A. Glorig and K.S. Gerwin), Chas. C. Thomas, Springfield, Illinois.

Jerger, J. (1973) Audiological findings in aging. *Adv. Otorhinolaryngol.*, **20**, 115–24.

Lowell, S.H. and Paparella, M.M. (1977) Presbycusis: what is it? *Laryngoscope*, 1710–17.

Lutman, M.E., Brown, E.J. and Coles, R.R.A. (1987) Self-reported disability and handicap in the population in relation to pure-tone threshold, age, sex and type of hearing loss. *Brit. J. Audiol.*, **21**, 45–58.

Marshall, L. (1981) Auditory processing in aging listeners. *J. Speech Hear. Dis.*, **46**, 226–40.

Martin, D. and Peckford, R. (1978) Hearing impairment in homes for the elderly. *Social Work Service*, **17**, 52–62.

Merluzzi, F. and Hinchcliffe, R. (1973) Threshold of auditory handicap. *Audiology*, **12**, 65–9.

Metropolitan Life Insurance Company. Hearing Impairments in the United States. *Metropolitan Life Insurance Statistics*, **57**, 7–9.

Milne, J.S. (1976) Hearing loss related to some signs and symptoms in old people. *Brit. J. Audiol.*, **10**, 65–73.

Milne, J.S. (1980) Cited by Gilhome-Herbst, K. in *Medicine in old age, hearing and balance* (ed. R. Hinchcliffe), Churchill Livingstone, Edinburgh, Ch. VIII: Psycho-social consequences of disorders of hearing in the elderly.

Newton, A. (1986) Quotation from speech. Reported in *Soundbarrier*, **11**, 3.

Plomp, R. (1977) Auditory impairment and the limited benefit of hearing aids. *J. Acoust. Soc. Amer.*, **63**, 533–49.

Rahko, T., Kallio, V., Kataja, M., Fagerstrom, K. and Karma, P. (1985) Prevalence of handicapping hearing loss in an aging population. *Ann. Otol. Rhinol. Laryngol.*, **94**, 140–4.

Robinson, D.W. and Sutton, G.J. (1979) Age effect in hearing – a comparative analysis of published threshold data. *Audiology*, **18**, 320–34.

Schuknecht, H.F. (1955) Presbycusis. *Laryngoscope*, **65**, 402–19.

Skadegard, J. (1982) Hearing aid markets and trends in Western Europe. *Hear. Aid J.* **35**, (10), 19–24.

Townsend, P. and Wedderburn, D. (1965) The aged in the welfare state. Occasional papers in social administration, No. 14, G. Bell and Sons Ltd, London.

Wilkins, L.T. (1948) The social survey, No. 92. Survey of prevalence of deafness in the population of England, Scotland and Wales. Central Office of Information, London.

Zwaardemaker, H. (1894) The range of hearing at various ages. *Zeitschrift. Psychol.*, **7**, 10–28.

2

THE HISTORICAL SETTING

Denzil Brooks

In Chapter 1 the proposition was advanced that the most appropriate help for the hearing impaired at the present time is amplification, carefully tailored to individual need and supported with adequate counselling. A consideration of the historical development of hearing aids is relevant because thereby light can be thrown on a number of current attitudes and problems. Two aspects will be considered, one relating to the development of the instruments for assisting hearing and the other to the development of service provision. These two strands will be reviewed independently although, in fact, they are closely interwoven.

2.1 THE DEVELOPMENT OF THE HEARING AID

From time immemorial the hearing-impaired individual has obtained benefit from a hand cupped behind the ear. By this means increase in sensitivity of 15 to 20 dB in the mid- to upper-frequency range can be attained with, additionally, some degree of suppression of sounds from the rear (Barr-Hamilton, 1983). The natural successor to the cupped hand was the ear trumpet. The first such devices were probably made from the horns of animals or from a rolled-up leaf (Berger, 1984). By the seventeenth century ear trumpets were being produced in metal, usually brass or copper, but for the wealthier clients with hearing impairment, such as Queen Victoria, silver was employed. By their very nature ear trumpets tend to be rather obtrusive. Soldiers deafened in World War I who used the ear trumpets provided for them were known as 'Tin Ear Joes'. However, human nature is such that many ingenious efforts were made to disguise the instruments. Small horns were attached to the tops of walking sticks that might then be held discreetly and somewhat casually against the ear. Larger versions were concealed within a top hat, the mouth of the horn being placed behind the front of the hat, which was made of black silk rather than the more usual felt. For ladies, and perhaps men with wigs, small folded horns or auricles were produced that could be worn closely against the side of the head. For domestic environments, a cornucopia on the table might be used as a collector, with the sound channelled to the impaired ear through a small tube. False flower vases were designed to have the same role of a sound collector. Perhaps the ultimate ear trumpet was the acoustic throne made for King Goa VII of Portugal. The two arms were carved into the form of lions' heads with open mouths. Within the body of the chair tubing conveyed the sound from these collectors to the earpiece, which the king inserted into his ear. What emerges from this brief consideration of acoustical hearing aids is the desire, from the earliest times and through all levels of society, to hide as much as possible the presence of hearing impairment. This principle of concealment will be seen as a constant factor in the history of the hearing aid.

(a) Electrical hearing aids

Towards the end of the nineteenth century the first electrically powered hearing aids began to appear. These were the so-called carbon aids. The early models had three essential components – a source of electrical energy, a microphone and a telephone or earphone – the current from the battery through the telephone being modulated by the microphone. Gain was limited and the frequency response was peaky. Inherent noise levels were high partly due to adventitious movement of the granules of carbon in the microphone and partly to the carbon dust that inevitably developed from the agitation and breakdown of the granules.

In the early 1920s the maximum gain was increased with the introduction of the carbon amplifier or booster. When wearing a carbon microphone, users had to be careful not to lean too far forward or backwards as this cut out the sound. The same problem could occur with the carbon amplifier when sitting down if, as was frequently the case, the booster was worn strapped to the leg. Different combinations of microphones and telephones were possible and hence, the first attempts at selection of performance according to subjective choice were made. According to Berger (1984) the Radioear Corporation, in 1935, introduced the first such 'master hearing aid' known as the Selex-a-phone.

Due to the bulkiness of the microphones and batteries, there was little real possibility of disguising a carbon hearing aid, although the literature produced by some of the companies would suggest that if worn accord-ing to their instructions, the instrument could be made completely invisible. Unfortunately, this meant wearing the microphone unit beneath at least one layer of clothing, with adverse effects on the performance.

The invention of the thermionic valve or vacuum tube in 1906 led to major advances in hearing aids, both from the technological and cosmetic standpoints. At first thermionic valves were bulky, costly and fragile but by the early 1920s, size and cost had been reduced and life expectancy greatly increased. In 1923 the Marconi Company in England produced a cabinet-model hearing aid and in America, the Western Electric Company produced the 10A, a binaural aid in a large cabinet weighing 220 lbs (Berger, 1984). In 1936, Littler reviewed the then available hearing aids. Gains of over 40 dB in the mid-frequencies were available on some models, and frequency responses were considerably less peaky with the introduction of the crystal microphone.

The Amplivox Company is usually credited with introducing, in 1935, the first truly wearable electronic hearing aid, a multi-pack instrument weighing in at about 1200 gms. Over the next few years, several companies produced valve aids that could be worn on the person. Enormous ingenuity was displayed by manufacturers and users alike in disguising the various component parts. Special garments were devised for concealing the amplifier and battery pack. Microphones were produced that could be affixed to the clothing in the guise of a piece of jewellery – a brooch or a flower cluster for the ladies, or a tie pin for the men. The receiver worn at the ear could, for the ladies, be made to appear as a rather large earring (with a small tube to convey the sound into the ear canal). Some users, usually female, crocheted miniature covers for the receiver, using silk or wool of the same shade as the hair. Others even collected hair cuttings after visiting the hairdresser and glued these to the outer surface of the receiver, combing them into the hair style. The cord connecting the receiver to the amplifier was taken under the hairline to the back of the neck where it was then pinned prior to descending over the shoulder to the aid. For men there was little chance of such camouflage as the prevailing hairstyle was the rather severe 'short back and sides', which provided no scope for concealment. To make the receiver less obvious, it was worn underneath the shirt collar and connected to a skeleton earmould through a length of transparent tubing.

(b) The transistor

A most significant advance in hearing-aid technology came with the invention of the transistor in December 1947. Not only was this very considerably smaller than the smallest valves, it was also much more efficient, requiring no wasteful filament heater. Hearing-aid manufacturers were quick to exploit the cosmetic potential of the transistor. Aids were designed into eye-glasses – the so-called library frames. They were made to look like fountain pens or hair slides, these being obtainable in different shades to match the hair colour. Quite rapidly a consensus was reached that the most appropriate place for a hearing aid was at, or just behind the ear.

The dramatic reduction in amplifier size was matched by improved power-supply technology. For more than half a century, the dry battery based on the Leclanché cell had been used as the power source for small electrical appliances, including hearing aids. Alternatives did exist, but it required the impetus of war to speed development of power supplies that were more efficient in terms of power/weight ratio. The Ruben or mercury cell has a capacity per unit volume three to six times that of the Leclanché cell. It also has a much flatter discharge characteristic, the voltage remaining at approximately 1.3 volts over the whole life of the cell, whereas the voltage generated by a Leclanché cell diminishes from about 1.5 volts to a practicable minimum of about 1 volt as the cell discharges. More recently, the zinc–air cell, with its still greater capacity per unit volume and lower potential toxicity if swallowed by a curious child, has taken an increasing share of the market.

As with the amplifier components and power sources, transducers were reduced in size. Moving-coil and moving-iron microphones were introduced and developed. These could be miniaturized on a compatible scale with the transistors but had some drawbacks. High-frequency response was limited and there was a tendency to magnetic and mechanical or vibrational feedback between the output and input transducers. The former was largely overcome in postaural aids by locating the output transducer horizontally at the top of the aid and the microphone vertically at the base. Mechanical coupling between input and output was reduced by mounting the transducers on soft suspensions in sealed compartments.

In the 1960s the crystal (or piezo-electric) microphone made a comeback. The fragile crystals of Rochelle salt were replaced by ceramic materials with piezo-electric properties. The problem of high output impedance was overcome by mounting a field effect transistor within the microphone housing. The ceramic microphone had a wide-frequency response, was relatively robust, and was less prone to magnetic feedback. Its main drawback was vibrational sensitivity.

The standard of excellence in microphone technology has, for a long time, been the condenser microphone. However, the need for a high polarizing voltage eliminated them as practical devices for hearing aids. The introduction of synthetic materials, which could be permanently polarized led to the development of the electret microphone, which has now become virtually standard in hearing-aid design. The electret has a wide-frequency response, is robust and almost completely insensitive to vibration or magnetic interference, and can be made extremely small while retaining good sensitivity. It is highly compatible with transistor technology.

Output transducers and other hearing-aid components have gone through a similar evolution. Standards of quality have improved while size has been reduced. Hearing aids are now available that have very smooth frequency responses extending up to 8000 Hz with the capacity for considerable electronic modification to allow the response to be tailored to individual requirement. Output power can be adjusted to suit the tolerance levels of the wearer and many aids have the facility of direct input, enabling the user to couple directly to the high-quality signals from TV, phonograph or other suitable source.

Microprocessor technology is now being applied to improve intelligibility in noisy situations. A more extensive consideration of these noise-reduction systems is provided by Dr Preves in Chapter 14.

By the late 1950s, hearing aids that could be worn at or in the ear were being produced. Miniaturization has continued and now a growing proportion of aids are being made that are contained entirely within the ear canal.

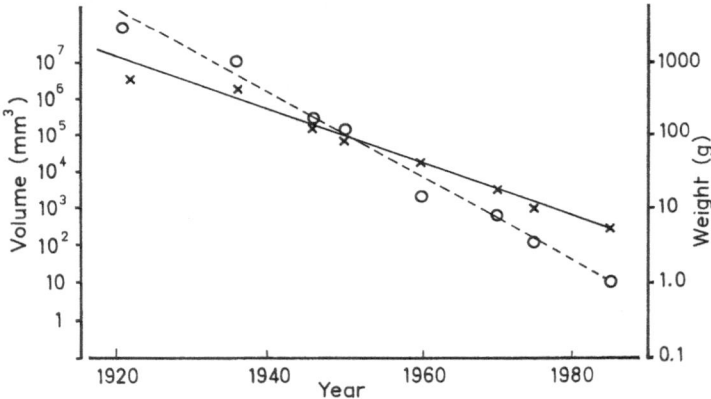

Figure 2.1 The diminishing volume and weight of hearing-aid models in the period 1920–80. ◯, weight; ×, volume.

As this review illustrates, there has been a steady reduction in the size of hearing aids over the last 60 years. Figure 2.1 illustrates graphically this progression. The volume (crosses) in cubic millimetres and weight (circles) in grams of representative aids is plotted against time. In 1921 the Vactuphone, an aid employing a single triode valve, was described in the *Volta Review*. The dimensions of the aid, in centimetres was about 18 × 18 × 10, or just over 3 000 000 cubic mm. At 7 lbs in weight it was considerably lighter than some of the aids that followed it, the record surely being held by the Western Electric 10A at 220 lbs (Berger, 1984). By 1950, when valve technology was at its highest level of development, a typical four-valve aid had dimensions of 8 × 6 × 2 cms and a weight of 180 gms. Today an in-the-canal aid may be as little as 8 mm in diameter and 8 mm in length, weighing less than one gram.

What emerges yet again from this review of hearing-aid development is the consistent and insistent pressure to make hearing aids less noticeable. Manufacturers make hearing aids smaller because consumer demand is primarily for hearing aids that cannot be seen. It is a tribute to the industry that concurrent with these dramatic achievements in size reduction, there has been no reduction – indeed in the majority of areas an improvement – in quality and in versatility.

2.2 THE DEVELOPMENT OF SERVICE PROVISION

The first-known manufacturer of hearing aids for sale is William Bull of London who in the latter half of the seventeenth century advertised: 'All sorts of Trumpetts and Kettle Drums, ffrench Hornes, Speaking Trumpetts, Hearing Hornes for Deafe people & all Sorts of powder flasks and allso Wind Gunes made and minded by William Bull Trumpett Maker to his Maiestie.' Over the next 200 years or so many ear trumpets were produced and sold by small companies, but the beginnings of modern commercial aid production and marketing can probably be regarded as commencing with the carbon hearing aid. Quantity-production methods, travelling salesmen and unrestrained advertising pushed up sales despite the poor quality of reproduction. The introduction of the thermionic valve further boosted sales in Europe and in the United States, although from its inception, the hearing aid has the distinction of being the most expensive of the commonly employed prostheses.

World War II gave rise to new attitudes towards the care of the disabled. In Europe, the concept of socialized medicine was developed and this has had a profound effect on the treatment of the hearing impaired. In the next section, some of the different approaches to service provision for adults with defective hearing will be reviewed.

(a) England

Around a century after William Bull, the business of F.C. Rein was established (ca. 1800). This was the company that made the acoustic throne for King Goa VII of Portugal and whose showroom was rather grandly titled 'The Paradise for the Deaf'. Gradually a number of other companies were established for the manufacture and sale of aids to hearing that were initially purely acoustical. By the 1930s carbon and valve aids were readily available to those who could afford them. It is estimated that by 1940 there were 50 000 valve aids and 10 000 carbon aids in use in England (Balbi, 1944).

In 1941 a UK Government committee was established to consider the rehabilitation and resettlement of disabled persons and among its recommendations in 1943 was one that stated that 'something should be done to make deaf (sic) persons more fit to play their part as useful members of the community'. A year later a Committee on Electro-acoustics was established by the Medical Research Council, charged with advising the Council, and through them, the government, upon 'design, performance and application of electro-acoustic equipment used in the investigation and alleviation of deafness, and to institute such fundamental investigations as may be considered necessary in this connection'. A major objective that this committee set itself was 'determining the characteristics of a hearing aid that will be of service to the majority of deaf people' not only in electro-acoustical terms, but also of such construction that it could be 'manufactured and supplied to the public at reasonable cost'. Using speech as the test material, 228 hearing-impaired subjects were tested and the findings suggested that the objective of meeting the needs of the majority of the aidable hearing-impaired could be achieved with a hearing-aid having two alternative choices of frequency response. Both rose at the rate of 12 dB per octave up to 750 Hz. One then remained flat over the higher frequencies, the other continued to rise at 6 dB per octave. This recommendation formed the basis of the performance specification for the first Medresco (an acronym derived from MEDical RESearch COuncil) hearing aid.

The introduction of the Medresco aid was a landmark in more ways than one. It was the first aid produced to a specification derived by a panel of scientists whose recommendations were based on large-scale clinical trials. It was the first hearing aid to be produced at the behest of a government for distribution on a widespread basis. It was the first aid intended for free distribution, free that is, in immediate cost terms to the recipient, the cost being borne by the entire community through statutory health insurance and taxation.

There was obvious concern in the private sector that widespread availability of a 'free' hearing aid would destroy the market for commercial sales. For many reasons this fear proved to be unfounded. The demand for hearing aids was dramatically increased, but hospitals and clinics were unable to cope. Waiting lists for the Medresco were as much as three to four years, and potential users looked to the private sector for quicker service. In the commercial sector, innovation was much swifter and there was greater recognition of the cosmetic aspects of hearing-aid design.

In 1960, a decade or so after the first head-worn aids appeared, a transistorized Medresco was introduced. This was a body-worn type about the size of a packet of ten cigarettes with a single fixed-frequency response rising at about 8 dB per octave from 250–3500 Hz. As many as 50% of all persons obtaining hearing aids at this time purchased them privately, a clear indication of the low acceptability of the Medresco.

Unfortunately, in their desire to obtain a larger share of the market, some companies resorted to tactics that were ethically unacceptable. Claims were made in advertisements that were not only unsupportable, but palpably untrue. A tactic known as 'switch selling' was employed by some companies where an extremely low-cost hearing aid was widely advertised. When the salesman called following the interest expressed by the client, the 'cheap' aid was demonstrated. It was designed to be cosmetically and acoustically unacceptable, and when the customer expressed abhorrence, a much more acceptable and efficient model was demonstrated – at considerably greater cost! The reputation of the whole industry was tarnished by such activities and to curb the excesses of the unscrupulous minority, legislation was proposed. After a number of unsuccessful attempts, a bill was passed in Parliament in 1968 establishing a Hearing Aid Council, a body supported by the industry and representing both suppliers and consumers. The Council established minimum qualifications for hearing-aid dispensers and introduced a Code of Practice.

After mounting public pressure, in July 1973, the Minister of Health, Sir Keith Joseph, announced that a wide range of head-worn hearing-aids would gradually be phased into the National Health Service programme. These had to meet stringent electro-acoustic specifications and supply contracts were awarded on a 'best-buy' basis. Provision was also made for departments issuing hearing aids to obtain models outside the contract ranges where this was deemed necessary.

Sir Keith also indicated the Government's intention to improve quality of care in line with the statement by Michael Reed in 1949 when he said 'the patient must be handled by somebody who understood the problems of the deaf, and who by his training and, if possible, experience would be capable of teaching the patient to use his aid, helping him in his difficulties and generally acting as counsellor and friend.' The service to the hearing impaired provided by the NHS has improved substantially in the last decade with better hearing aids, more and better trained staff and availability of help with assistive listening devices.

Alongside the NHS there remains a healthy and flourishing private sector. A substantial proportion of the aids purchased in this domain are in-the-ear (ITE) or in-the-canal (ITC) instruments that are not available through the State provision. Relationships between the public and private sectors have been troubled in the past, but at least, on the professional level, there is now a degree of harmony due to the introduction of a Hearing Aid Audiology Group within the professional umbrella organization, the British Society of Audiology.

(b) Denmark

Denmark introduced a state-operated hearing-aid supply service in 1951. Two Acts provided the legislative framework for State provision of hearing aids. The first, in 1950, related principally to children. The second, in 1951, extended the National Insurance Act to give provision of hearing aids free of direct cost. Technical specifications were produced for hearing aids and tenders invited from manufacturers for bulk supply of approved instruments. This policy has continued, with specifications being drawn up by a panel consisting of experts in audiology and acoustics, directors of the hearing centres and representatives of the Ministry of Social Affairs. This scheme encourages healthy competition between the major Danish hearing-aid companies, and allows for regular updating of specifications as technology improves and understanding of the needs of the hearing impaired advances. Furthermore, because the centres issuing the hearing aids in the early days of the service meticulously checked that every instrument supplied met the electro-acoustical specifications and refused to accept any that fell below the high standards demanded, quality control was raised to new levels. In the long term this was beneficial to the Danish consumers and manufacturers alike. Danish aids are now synonymous with quality.

The philosophy of binaural amplification was promoted in Denmark, a great deal of the credit for this going to Dr Ole Bentzen of Aarhus. Initially, there were difficulties in obtaining official sanction for the free provision of two aids, but a fortuitous incident involving a bilaterally hearing-impaired politician brought about the necessary legislation and approval.

From the inception of the audiological service in Denmark it was realized that to achieve effective rehabilitation, much more was required than merely diagnosing hearing loss and providing suitable amplification. A comprehensive rehabilitation programme was designed to help potential hearing-aid users in understanding the nature and effects of hearing loss and to ensure that everyone received adequate training in the use of hearing aids and other devices to improve communication and in hearing tactics. This training course caters for the needs of 80–95% of new patients. For a minority, extra help may be given in the form of hearing training, lipreading, speech remediation or a form of signed communication. For those with extreme difficulty, such as the suddenly totally deafened, referral may be made to the State Hearing Institute at Fredericia, a residential facility providing personal support at a time of crisis and intensive training in communication strategies.

(c) Sweden

Sweden also accepted the philosophy of State provision, the government passing an act in 1954 to establish services largely based on the Danish model. In 1955, grants were authorized to cover a large part of the cost of hearing aids to the individual. These grants were increased in 1962 to a level that covered the majority of available aids and in 1968, the ceiling on grant level was removed and approval given for the fitting of two aids where deemed appropriate. As in Denmark, tenders were invited for bulk supply of aids from international manufacturers and stringent quality controls were introduced and enforced. Hearing aids are issued according to a recommendation based on the Australian National Acoustic Laboratories formula with reduced total gain.

A unique feature of the Swedish system is the 'free' provision of additional accessories to assist the hearing impaired. Many hearing-impaired persons have difficulty hearing their door or telephone bell. Others, perhaps because they live in a flat or with relatives with normal hearing, are unable or unwilling to turn up the volume on the television or radio. It may not be possible to eliminate these problems simply by providing a hearing aid. There are alternative devices designed to assist with every one of the situations outlined. On average, patients in Sweden receive three extra devices such as a TV amplifier, a telephone listening system and an audio-visual alarm clock or a signalling device for callers at the door (Lundborg et al., 1971).

Aural rehabilitation services were introduced using teachers with additional training, and now there are numerous rehabilitation courses at the universities. Group instruction is increasingly being performed by audiology assistants supported by hearing therapists. It is proposed to take services more into the community in the future rather than concentrating resources in the hospitals. Liaison with other involved authorities such as social welfare departments is being fostered.

As in Denmark, a residential facility is provided for adults with severe communication problems, particularly where this affects their employment. This is situated in Uppsala and provides vocational training courses of twelve months' duration. Shorter courses are also provided at Stockholm and Gothenburg.

Research into hearing disorders and their alleviation was encouraged and the Karolinska Institute has a justly deserved international fame for its publications in the sphere of hearing and hearing impairment.

(d) Other European countries

In most other European countries the cost of hearing-aids provision is funded only in part by the State or through some system of health insurance. The amount allowed may be dependent on the type and degree of the hearing loss, greater financial support being provided for an individual with severe sensorineural hearing loss requiring a high-power aid with compression than for a person with a 'simple' conductive hearing loss. The provision tends to be through accredited dealers working in liaison with the professional staff at the hospital ENT departments. Formalized rehabilitation programmes are less common than in countries where State involvement is high.

(e) Australia

In 1948 the government of Australia recognized the need to find ways of assisting the large numbers of ex-servicemen deafened during World War II and also the large number of children born deaf as a result of rubella epidemics in 1939 and 1941. The National Acoustic Laboratories (NAL) were established in 1948 to examine the use of hearing aids by the hearing impaired and to study the effects of noise on man. Because information on these subjects was sparse, NAL established its own methods of operation, generated its own comprehensive research and development programmes, and have achieved a worldwide recognition for leadership in these areas.

Due to the high cost of importing hearing aids and the limited performance of the aids that were available, NAL set up its own design and production facilities. A wide range of aids is now produced to cater for the needs of the majority of the hearing-impaired. A small number of specialized aids are imported to meet the needs of the minority.

The NAL Hearing Service now operates the second largest hearing-aid programme in the world – second only to the British NHS programme. Services include assessment of hearing, selection and fitting of appropriate systems to assist in communication, aftercare to maximize benefit and free maintenance and batteries. There are centres in 40 major towns and cities around Australia providing the services to those eligible, that is, persons under 21 years of age, the majority of pensioners and armed services personnel.

The service commitment is backed up, as indicated above, by a large research and development programme. Of particular note is the Hearing Aid Selection protocol developed by Byrne and colleagues (Chapter 4).

(f) The United States

The development of the hearing-aid industry in the United States can be traced back to Miller Reece Hutchison. According to Berger (1984), Hutchison, in partnership with James H. Wilson founded the Akouphone Company in about 1898. A table-model carbon aid was marketed at a price of $400. Within a few years other companies entered the market and many tens of thousands of carbon aids were sold. Watson and Tolan (1949) estimated that some 50 000 were still in use in the USA in 1944.

From the late 1930s the carbon aids slowly gave way to thermionic valve instruments and sales rose steadily. Many new manufacturers entered the field with the expectation of making substantial quick profits. Many failed. In one 5-year period, out of 100 manufacturers at the beginning only 15 were still in business at the end.

In 1948 the Hearing Aid Association was formed with one of its objectives being the maintenance of good ethical practice. In 1952 a subgroup of members who had established their competence by examination formed the Society of Hearing Aid Audiologists. This gradually took over the role of the parent organization and in 1965 became the National Hearing Aid Society (NHAS). A continuing role of this organization has been the training of those involved in dispensing aids and it is estimated that over 8000 persons have completed some form of NHAS training.

For many years, hearing-aid sales continued to rise, but in the mid-1970s there was a slowing down, no doubt due partly to the spate of investigations into trade practices. Another factor adding to the uncertainty related to the many proposals for Medicare coverage of hearing aids or for National Health Insurance with possible hearing aid benefits. A further factor has been the change in policy of the American Speech–Language Hearing Association (ASHA). Historically, ASHA adopted a hands-off approach to dispensing hearing aids. Audiologists endeavoured, on the basis of pure-tone and speech tests, to decide the amplification characteristics for the individual, possibly even to the extent of specifying a particular model of aid, but the delivery of the hearing-aid was delegated to a hearing-aid dispenser. In 1978 the Code of Ethics was revised to permit dispensing by clinical audiologists under specified conditions. Current estimates (Margolis, 1987) would suggest that around 50% of ASHA-certified audiologists are now dispensing hearing aids.

Sales of hearing aids rose dramatically when it became public knowledge that President Reagan was wearing an in-the-ear hearing aid, and the trend towards higher sales has continued.

2.3 DIFFERENT SYSTEMS – DIFFERENT VALUES

The system of hearing-aid supply in the UK has many roots. It was instituted at the birth of socialized medicine, a philosophy based on the concept of the healthy giving support to the sick and disabled. The aid provided was designed on the basis of a fixed-frequency response chosen to suit the majority, both the aid and the support services being developed at a time of financial constraint in the immediate post-war years. For reasons that are now obscure due to the passage of time, it was decided that supply should be based entirely on the hospital service.

One result was that in the short term very many persons who otherwise could not have afforded help were provided with amplification. Demand was greatly stimulated and acceptance of hearing aids gradually increased. A less-happy consequence was that in the public sector hearing-aid design ossified. Progress lagged far behind the private sector. Nevertheless, in 1970 the rate of supply of hearing aids in the UK was one of the highest in the world, though quantity was not matched by quality.

Since the government initiatives of 1973, there has been a very considerable improvement in all aspects of service provision. The range of NHS aids has improved. Quality is of at least as high a standard as for commercially dispensed aids. There are more and better trained staff and more extensive rehabilitative provision. Alongside the National Health Service, the private sector continues to flourish, providing a competitive spur to the state scheme.

The system of provision of hearing aids in the United States is at the opposite end of the spectrum. Until very recently, government involvement has been minimal, its only role being to ensure basic standards of competence through licensing. The majority of hearing aids have been supplied through trained dispensers at the market price. Despite the high standard of living and the relative affluence of many elderly persons, cost does deter the less wealthy from obtaining help. Franks and Beckmann (1985) surveyed 100 persons aged 65 years or older in eastern Washington. The item ranked highest for rejecting the possible help of a hearing-aid was cost. In a survey of 1600 normal hearing adults conducted by the Gallup Organisation (1980), the second highest reason for not obtaining a hearing aid in the event of having a hearing problem was expense. This cost barrier is reflected in the fact that the overall rate of supply in the USA in 1970 was less than that of the UK despite the average per capita income being more than double (Bentzen and Courtois, 1973). Some degree of rehabilitation may be provided by the hearing-aid dispenser or, to a growing extent, by audiologists, but availability and extent vary widely across the country.

On the credit side, manufacturers, audiologists and researchers in the United States have been responsible for much technical progress. The pace of miniaturization has been dramatic, with reduction in size being matched with improvement in quality of performance. Along with this there has been development in other aspects of aid function such as acoustic tuning, feedback-limiting systems, signal-from-noise-enhancing circuits and digital, programmable aids.

Denmark followed the British system of providing hearing aids at no direct cost to the individual, but stimulated the hearing-aid industry by involving manufacturers in the negotiations about technical requirements, quality control and costs. From the beginning, services were developed to support the issue of hearing-aids. Danish rehabilitation services were a model for other countries to observe, and then to seek to emulate. In 1970 Denmark had the highest per capita rate of hearing-aid supply, and probably the highest rate of binaural issue.

In Sweden, as in Denmark, the hearing-aid service progressed towards supplying hearing aids without direct cost to the needy. An additional thrust was towards technological support. Special devices to help with telephone, radio and TV listening; alerting devices for the home or to assist in waking in the morning and other communication aids were provided as deemed necessary.

In Australia the National Acoustic Laboratories have carried out a systematic programme of research into theoretical aspects of hearing-aid fitting, and the majority of hearing aids supplied through the scheme of governmental financial support are now selected according to a defined protocol. Utilization of aids has increased since the implementation of the new formula-based scheme.

It can be seen that the different systems developed in different countries have strengths and weaknesses that affect take-up and utilization. Over the last few years there has been much exchange of ideas between countries and an erosion of the differences. There is now general acceptance that to merely provide a hearing-impaired person with an amplifying system is unsatisfactory. The issue of a hearing aid must be accompanied by a measure of rehabilitation structured to the individual needs of the potential user. There is growing recognition that amplification characteristics should be tailored to the pattern of the hearing loss rather than to employing one or two basic frequency responses and expecting the individual to learn to live within these constraints. What is not universally agreed as yet is the formulation of the desirable characteristic for any given hearing configuration, but the differences between protocols are diminishing. It seems unlikely that any one formula will ever be completely acceptable to all professionals and to all hearing-impaired individuals, and it is probably as well that this is so. As long as differences exist there will be a striving for better techniques, and this can only be to the betterment of those with hearing loss.

REFERENCES

Balbi, C.M.R. (1944) A basis for prediction of the performance of hearing aids. *J. Inst. Elect. Eng.*, **91**, 79.

Barr-Hamilton, R.M. (1983) The cupped hand as an aid to hearing. *Brit. J. Audiol.* **17**, 27–30.

Bentzen, O. and Courtois, J. (1973) Statistical analysis of the problem for the deaf and hard of hearing in the world of 1970. *Scand. Audiol.* **2**, 17–26.

Berger, K.W. (1984) *The hearing aid. Its operation and development*, 3rd edn, National Hearing Aid Soc., Livonia, Mich.

Franks, J.R. and Beckman, N.J. (1985) Rejection of hearing aids: attitude of a geriatric sample. *Ear Hear.* **6**, 161–6.

Gallup Organisation (1980) A survey concerning hearing problems and hearing aids in the United States, Princeton, N.J.

Lundborg, T., Linzander, S., Lindstrom, B., Sward, I. and Fransson, A. (1971) Special devices for the hearing handicapped patient. *Nordisk Audiologi.* **3/4**, 96–132.

Margolis, R.H. (1987) Hearing instrument dispensing in university clinic. *Hear. Instrum.*, **38**, (10) 38–9, 67.

Watson, L.A. and Tolan, T. (1949) *Hearing tests and hearing instruments*. Williams and Wilkins Co., Baltimore, p. 425.

3

HEARING AIDS: POSSESSION, USE, BENEFIT AND THE ROLE OF REHABILITATION

Denzil Brooks

The low rate of take-up of hearing aids in the UK, Scandinavia and the USA was noted in Chapter 1. In the less well-developed parts of the world the possession of hearing aids is very much lower still. In considering the scope and value of rehabilitation based on hearing aids it is instructive to look at the reasons underlying the differential rates of supply, and also the differential degrees of use among those who possess hearing aids because the act of obtaining a hearing-aid does not necessarily imply that that instrument will be used. Factors that inhibit or enhance hearing-aid use will be examined, as will the means of assessing benefit obtained through amplification.

3.1 COMPARATIVE INTERNATIONAL HEARING-AID TAKE-UP RATES

The rate of take-up of hearing aids in any society will depend on a number of factors, such as the actual need within the community, perceived need, availability of relevant and helpful advice, availability of hearing aids, this further depending on cost (if any), and ability and willingness to pay.

1. Actual need

The same degree of hearing impairment will create different degrees of need in different individuals in different societies. In a small village community in a Third-World country where field cultivation is the primary occupation, a hearing loss of 30 dB, or even 50 dB, may well be of little consequence. In the extended family or close-knit village community everyone is aware of the individual with hearing difficulty. Communication is primarily concerned with the essentials of life rather than with social or business activities. Compensation is a matter of routine. By contrast, in a heavily communication-dependent Western city a similar degree of loss may be near catastrophic. It may create severe problems in employment and may drastically reduce the pleasures and benefits of social life, which may be an essential concomitant of the business activity. Need, therefore, is highly relevant to take-up. The more communication-orientated the society, the greater the need for efficient hearing.

2. *Perceived need*

Figure 1.2 (p. 7) illustrated that perceived need does not correlate directly with degree of hearing impairment. Threshold of impairment may be defined audiologically as at a level of 30 db averaged over the speech frequencies, but onset of disability will depend on the life style of the individual and their readiness to accept some degree of handicap rather than to seek help. The need perceived by the individual with hearing loss may be very different from the need perceived by the family, who find it stressful talking to that person; or by the neighbours who are inconvenienced by over-loud television and radio; or by the family doctor who possibly sees hearing loss as merely a slight inconvenience that is inevitable, an irremediable accompaniment to old age; or by the professional audiologist who sees it as a potential cause of isolation and loss of enjoyment in life. The professional may also see this possible lack of awareness of need as a challenge. Should public consciousness of the potentially handicapping effects of hearing impairment be raised by a programme of education? This question recurs when we consider the next factor relevant to possession of hearing aids.

3. *Availability of good and relevant advice*

Assuming need for assistance has been perceived by the individual with hearing impairment, or by the spouse, family or other person(s) having a significant degree of influence, the next step is to seek for advice. In the majority of instances, it will be to the medical profession that the seeker turns. Alternatively, help may be sought from a hearing-aid dealer. Ideally the advice given by that person should be to first obtain a medical opinion. In the UK, the Hearing Aid Council Code of Practice sets out a number of conditions for which medical advice is mandatory – the discharging ear; a sudden onset hearing loss; a loss accompanied by vertigo, etc. In the USA, medical clearance is required, but this can be waived if the hearing-aid candidate so desires. Assuming medical advice is sought, will that advice be correct, helpful and based on current knowledge? Regrettably, the evidence in the UK is that advice from doctors and even ear specialists is often both inaccurate and unhelpful. A number of studies (Harris, 1962; Brooks, 1979; Humphrey, Gilhome-Herbst and Faruqi, 1981) show that of those hearing-impaired persons seeking for assistance from their family doctor, less than two-fifths are referred on for practical help with a hearing aid. Three-fifths or so are put off from seeking further help by such remarks as 'What do you expect at your age?' or 'An aid won't help – you have nerve deafness'. The latter remark indicates that many doctors are unaware of the improvements that have taken place in hearing-aid performance. It is reasonable to assume that attitudes of doctors are similar in many other countries and highlights the urgent need to bring to the attention of front-line medical staff the fact that nowadays, amplification can substantially assist the great majority of the hearing impaired.

4. Availability of hearing aids

In the industrialized countries, hearing aids are readily available, either through State channels, or by private purchase. In many less well-developed parts of the world, it may be nearly impossible to find a source of supply. For example, in West Africa there is no State provision and few, if any, private dealers. The consequence is that the rate of acquisition of aids in 1980 was only 40 per million of population compared with over 6000 per million in Denmark.

5. Ability and willingness to pay

Cost is undoubtedly a significant factor in the decision as to whether or not to obtain amplification. The highest take-up rates occur in those countries that provide aids at no direct cost to the hearing impaired. In 1981, when Skadegard (1982) reviewed the state of the industry, Denmark had the highest consumption of aids at 6.9 per 1000, closely followed by Iceland with a rate of 6.0 per 1000 and the UK with a rate of 5.1 per 1000. The UK rate was higher than that of the USA (4.0 per 1000), despite the fact that the per capita income in the UK was only about half of that of the USA.

From the foregoing considerations it can be seen that national rates of take-up of hearing aids have many contributory and interwoven factors. The overall situation is that the more affluent a society is, the higher the rate of hearing-aid possession – a reversal of the situation regarding prevalence of hearing loss. The extent of technological development and wealth creation is the major determinant of possession. Stephens (1977) demonstrated that per capita, GNP accounted for 88% of the total variance in hearing-aid possession. Interrelated with this, countries supplying aids without direct cost have, in general, higher rates of possession than those where the individual has to bear the whole cost.

3.2 INDIVIDUAL USE AND BENEFIT MEASURES

Turning now to the individual, how can the effectiveness of the system in rehabilitating the hearing impaired be assessed? Use, benefit and satisfaction are possible measures. Amount of daily use is the most frequently employed measure as it is not only a relatively easy parameter to assess, but also seems, logically, to relate to the value of the aid to the user. It is unlikely that an individual will consistently wear a hearing-aid if there is no benefit or satisfaction from its use. Unfortunately, the converse is not necessarily true. Under-use of amplification may be due to many factors other than lack of benefit or satisfaction. Nevertheless, as a convenient group measure the amount of daily use has proved to be the most popular tool. Use may be the amount of time that the aid is said to be used on a daily basis, or it may be the amount of time actually used, the two quantities not always being the same.

Benefit is defined by Oja and Schow (1984) as the improvement in some measure in the aided condition as compared to the unaided condition. They observe that to be relevant to real life, the measure(s) employed should sample various situations representative of those in which the individual is likely to be using the aid. It is difficult, therefore, in assessing the benefit of hearing-aid amplification, to employ a schema giving a single numerical value whereby individuals or systems can be compared. Benefit is multifaceted.

Satisfaction can only be assessed subjectively. For this reason there has been a degree of scepticism about the value of such a measure. However, as it does reflect the feelings of the user, it should be accorded some measure of acceptance.

(a) Amount of use

One of the earliest published surveys of hearing-aid use appears to be that of Gray and Cartwright (1951). This was carried out in the UK only a few years after the introduction of the large and obtrusive two-pack Medresco aid, when the prime objective was to reduce waiting lists and supply aids to those in need with the greatest possible expedition.

Priority was given to the younger, working population such that 59% of those supplied with aids were under the age of 60 years. No attempt was made to provide regular reassessment or counselling, although the need for this was accepted in principle.

The researchers interviewed 989 subjects representative of the total population supplied. Use was higher among the employed than the retired or the non-employed. It was maximal in the middle age groups and thereafter declined with increasing age. Median daily use was about 3.5 hours, but almost one in seven stated that they did not use the aid at all. The majority indicated that they found the aid beneficial. Despite the cumbersome and unattractive nature of the dual-pack, body-worn instruments, around three-quarters of those using them indicated that their ability to distinguish sounds was better with the aid than without.

Usage in the UK did not appear to increase significantly after the introduction of the monopack transistor body aid, probably due to the change in nature of hearing-aid applicants, the trend being towards older persons with sensorineural hearing loss. Brooks (1972) reviewed 195 patients supplied with Medresco aids approximately two months after receipt, 99 by interview and 96 by questionnaire. Just over 30% of those seen and substantially more (57%) of those not seen claimed to be using the aid on a regular basis. It is probable that more accurate answers were obtained in the face-to-face situation than from the postal questionnaire. Some subjects at interview admitted that they used the aid only occasionally, but that for those limited situations it was invaluable. Yet they did not like to admit to such low level of use. Unless the interviewer checked very carefully and firmly, there was a tendency to inflate the amount of daily use to give a better impression. Another reason for the apparent exaggeration of daily use level is that the elderly often do not grasp the principles of mathematical averaging. If asked to estimate 'average daily use', they tend to discount days when the aid is not worn and base the estimate only on the 'good days' when the aid is worn for longer periods. This is less likely when data is obtained by an interviewer who can evaluate use on a day-by-day basis. Twelve per cent of those interviewed and 6% of those not interviewed admitted to not using the aid at all. The most commonly advanced reason for rejecting the aid was cosmetic.

Much higher use rates in Denmark were reported by Ewertsen (1974) in a review of 1006 subjects: 90% were apparently using the aid extensively; 4% said they used it only rarely and 6% stated that it was not used at all. Two factors contributing to this higher-use rate were thought to be (1) the availability of more socially acceptable behind-the-ear hearing aids, and (2) the extensive counselling given to support the use of the hearing-aid. It was noted in the previous chapter that almost from its inception, the Danish hearing-aid service laid substantial emphasis on the need for rehabilitation over and above the provision of a hearing aid. The change to behind-the-ear aids in the UK certainly brought about markedly increased acceptance and use.

Haggard, Foster and Iredale (1981) monitored use over an 18-month period in 54 postaural hearing patients of whom 45 were first-time users. Daily amount of use was assessed by exchanging the individual's aid for a few days with a specially modified aid containing a chemical E-cell (this being a device connected to the on–off switch that registers time in terms of electrical charge). Twenty-three subjects dropped out of the study and hence the data may be biased towards more co-operative and healthier persons with a better attitude to hearing-aid use. The mean daily use period assessed objectively was six hours, and this correlated well with the subjectively assessed use, although there was evidence of a small degree of exaggeration among those using the aid for only small amounts of time. The subjects in this study did receive a measure of post-issue assistance, and this might also have tended to improve acceptance and use.

In an effort to evaluate the role of counselling in hearing-aid use Brooks (1981) assessed use in two groups of first-time, postaural, hearing-aid users over a period of one year. The groups, each containing 36 persons, were matched for sex, age, hearing loss and living situation, that is, with spouse, family, or alone. The average age of 69 years and hearing loss of 49 dB was typical of new applicants for hearing aids through the National Health Service.

One group received extensive counselling to support the use of the hearing-aid, the other group received the aid with only basic instruction such as is routine in most NHS clinics. The amount of daily use was assessed both objectively and subjectively. Objective assessment was by means of monitored use of zinc–air cells, the change in weight of which on discharge can be accurately related to current drawn, and hence to hours of use. Subjective assessment was by questionnaire and interview at the end of the twelve-month period. Daily use was more than double compared to use made of body-worn aids. Exaggeration of the amount of use almost disappeared, probably because the need to overstate use had gone. Most individuals were using the aids on a regular or semi-regular basis.

In the non-counselled subjects, 16 (44%) used the aid more than four hours per day and seven (19%) were observed not to be using their aids at all. Of the counselled subjects, 21 (58%) used the aid more than four hours per day and only one did not use the aid at all. Mean daily use for the non-counselled patients was 3.8 hours and for those receiving counselling, 5.3 hours. This is close to the 6.0 hours per day found in the

Haggard *et al.* (1981) study where, as noted, there was some element of self-selection in the participating subjects.

Two points emerge from these studies. Firstly, head-worn aids are used considerably more than body-worn models, and this is predominantly due to their greater cosmetic acceptability. Secondly, use increases when counselling is provided. Ward (1980) suggests that as little as one hour of post-issue guidance can substantially improve use, further time spent producing diminishing returns pro rata in terms of daily use (although there may be benefits in other aspects of communication-handicap reduction). Stephens (1977) cites a number of studies in Europe that confirm higher levels of use in subjects receiving rehabilitation in addition to the provision of the hearing-aid. A further benefit arising from the provision of rehabilitation is suggested by the same author. Some studies have indicated a trend to lower use with increasing age, but in those countries where rehabilitation is a routine part of the hearing-aid provision, no such fall-off with increasing age is noted. Support for this suggestion comes from the study by Surr, Schuchman and Montgomery (1979) who found a substantial decrease in use in the more elderly. They comment: 'The younger individuals in our clinic received, more consistently, the longer training programme.'

Further light on the role of counselling comes from two studies of under-use and dis-use of hearing aids. Kapteyn (1977b) found three reasons for poor use, the first relating to the earmould. The unpleasantness of loud sounds was second and handling difficulties ranked third. It was also observed that poor use was associated with longer-than-normal adaptation to the instrument. Brooks (1985) reviewed 437 NHS patients around two years after issue and evaluated reasons for non-use (N = 55) and under-use (N = 30). Difficulty in inserting the individual earmould was the most common cause of poor or non-use, and this was especially a problem in elderly individuals who lived alone and therefore had no relative to help. The next largest cause for poor use related to noise. Such comments as: 'It amplifies everything' or 'Background noises are too loud', were common. Poor health and advanced age alone or in combination were next in rank as contributing to under-use of hearing aids. Only three out of the total number of 437 gave lack of benefit as their main reason for not using the aid.

Upfold and Wilson (1980) reported that the most common reasons for not using an aid were that it was a nuisance, or uncomfortable, suggesting poor earmould quality or inaccurate insertion, or because of the appearance of the aid. Noisiness and lack of benefit were other reasons cited for non-use.

Berger *et al.* (1982) reviewed 358 subjects issued with hearing aids fitted by the authors using a very structured approach. Almost half the reported problems reported related to noise. This included groups of people talking, non-speech noise and sudden, unexpected noises. Earmould problems ranked second, accounting for one-fifth of the difficulties experienced, and other handling problems such as manipulating the switches and volume control ranked third. However, to put things in context, the authors also report that almost two-thirds of those reviewed described the aid as providing a lot of help and only about 7% found the aids of little benefit, these being mainly elderly persons with more severe hearing losses.

Hickson, Hamilton and Orange (1986) found two factors that were significantly related to use in their study of 135 adults issued with aids at the National Acoustic Laboratory in Brisbane. The first was attitude of the potential user. Those with negative attitudes fared less well than those with a positive outlook. The second related to the client's ability to handle the instrument.

Although there is not a consensus among the authors quoted and the papers reviewed as to the rank order of difficulties contributing to hearing-aid under-use, there is general agreement as to the principal factors. These relate to the earmould, noise, attitude and handling skills. The majority of presenting problems can be viewed as amenable to counselling to some degree. As Upfold and Wilson (1980) state:

Persons who did not use an aid because it was a nuisance, or uncomfortable, or of poor appearance, or did not help or was noisy, must be seen as reporting that insufficient care, attention or skill (or combination of these) were applied to aid selection and/or fitting.

Support for this statement comes from the previously quoted study of postaural aid users in Manchester (Brooks, 1985). Of the 437 subjects reviewed, 288 had been supplied with the aid without any counselling other than that given at the single visit to hospital when the aid was supplied. When reviewed, 44 were not using the aid. The remaining 149 persons had received guidance both before and after the issue of the aid and of these, 11 were not using their aids. The difference in rate of non-use was significant at the 5% level ($\chi^2 = 5.6$:1df).

In summary, the amount of daily use made of the hearing aid appears to be a valuable tool for assessing the merits of different aids and delivery systems. Levels of use suggest that behind-the-ear hearing aids are more acceptable than body-aids, and there is growing evidence that in-the-ear hearing aids have even greater acceptability (Griffing, 1976). Use data suggest also that counselling is necessary for many, possibly all, potential hearing-aid users. Without good advice before as well as after provision of the aid, optimum results will not be achieved. The elderly, who currently form the largest group requiring amplification, are especially in need of help in achieving the right attitude to a hearing aid and obtaining the best benefit from it.

3.3 BENEFIT MEASURES

It was stated previously that benefit is multifaceted. In consequence, a number of different techniques have been employed to try to quantify this elusive quality. In that the most obvious aspect of hearing impairment is loss of sensitivity, a measure of the gain achieved by the hearing aid can be taken as a first approach to measuring benefit.

Improvement in speech discrimination has greater face validity, but as with measurement of aided gain, there is frequently a wide gap between laboratory tests and real-life situations. Questionnaires that probe a wide range of situations perhaps come nearest to assessing improvement in communication ability, but problems arise in trying to devise adequately sensitive questionnaires that are relevant to a wide range of different life styles.

(a) Aided threshold gain

Aided threshold gain is a long-established measure of 'benefit'. Underlying the measurement is the assumption that there is an optimal gain at each frequency that depends in some specific manner on the degree of hearing loss at that frequency. Benefit is then seen as closeness of approach to the theoretical target. As a measure of benefit, the technique has a number of drawbacks. Firstly, there is as yet no universal agreement on how much gain is required for a specific loss, nor even that such a quantity can be defined for individual application. Secondly, different methods of assessing gain for the same aid on the same individual can give widely different values. Thirdly, responses to pure-tone stimuli may not relate well to the more relevant sounds of life such as speech. Fourthly, aided gain is a threshold measure and hence not directly related to everyday listening where sounds tend to be in the middle of the auditory intensity range.

Aided threshold measurement can be of great value to the professional who is seeking to assess what a specific hearing aid is doing on a specific ear. As a measure of benefit related to communication in the living world, it is a poor tool and in terms of assessing the value of rehabilitation procedures, it has no practical application.

(b) Improvement in speech perception

Improvement in speech discrimination has been a traditional measure of aided benefit at least since the pioneering work of Carhart (1946a,b). However, in 1960, Shore, Bilger and Hirsh demonstrated that measures of speech discrimination and speech-reception threshold had low test–retest reliability. Small changes in score could not be regarded as significant but were an inevitable outcome of the nature of the test material. With the high quality of performance attainable with modern hearing aids, and with candidates for amplification generally having smaller degrees of hearing loss and minimal discrimination loss, these basic speech tests are of little value.

In 1968 Jerger said:

On the problem of measuring speech understanding the only solution I see is to start all over from scratch. I would declare a national day of burning, an orgy of destruction in which every monosyllabic word list, every quadrilateral of rhyming consonants is consigned to a giant bonfire. . . . Then in the cold light of the fire's dying embers we would all sit down at a large table, clinicians, researchers and therapists and try to hammer out the essence of this thing we call understanding of speech.

One of the major problems of the majority of current speech tests is that they are unrelated to real life listening conditions. Speech presented in the absence of background noise is unrepresentative of normal human communication. Test conditions can be made more taxing, for example, by using a low signal-to-noise ratio and sentences of some complexity. In this manner a more realistic measure of benefit might be obtainable, but there are inherent problems in such an approach. If the task is made too difficult, the subject can easily become discouraged and produce scores no longer representative of the true hearing ability. With the elderly, who form the bulk of the population seeking help through amplification, poor concentration and reduced memory span may arbitrarily reduce scores. An approach to this problem adopted by Jerger is the use of synthetic sentences (Speaks and Jerger, 1965). These consist of words combined according to specified rules based on transitional probabilities. They are essentially meaningless, but have the structure of meaningful sentences. The testee does not have to reproduce the sentence by a feat of memory, but only to identify, in the presence of competing noise, which it is from a closed set of ten. As a test, this is closer to reality than many other speech tests, the test material being close to conversational dialogue and the responses required being to identify rather than to reproduce the content faultlessly.

The use of 'synthetic sentence identification' (SSI) is more time-consuming than the use of word lists in terms of the amount of numerical data obtained (if that be a reasonable target). It is arguable that a smaller amount of relevant information is more valuable than a mass of data of dubious relevance. The SSI test has been employed in rank-ordering hearing aids, the rankings correlating well with other specific parameters of aid performance. However, in terms of assessing the benefits of rehabilitation, the test is as yet unproven.

In sum, conventional speech testing probably tells us very little about the effectiveness of a fitting protocol or a rehabilitative programme for the majority of subjects.

(c) Reduction of hearing handicap

The term hearing handicap refers to the disadvantage imposed on an individual by impairment of his hearing. Similar degrees of hearing loss will produce quite different amounts of handicap in different individuals. A relatively small hearing loss may provide little handicap to an independent, self-contained elderly person living with a thoughtful and caring family. The same degree of loss might be crippling to an executive who depends critically on obtaining accurate information at board meetings and by telephone. These examples indicate that handicap, while related to degree of hearing impairment, is also determined by a number of other factors not directly related to hearing, such as occupational status, relationships with significant others, personality (itself a complex of many factors), socioeconomic status, health status and situational communication demands. Hearing sensitivity accounts for less than 50% of the variability in hearing handicap or, conversely, the major part of the variability is contributed by one or more of the above factors (and probably others not identified here). Reduction of hearing handicap would seem to be an especially appropriate measure of the effectiveness of rehabilitation procedures as it is handicap, rather than impairment, that determines the quality of life for the individual with hearing loss.

Over the last 20 or more years, a number of questionnaires have been devised to try to measure the degree of handicap imposed by hearing loss in the individual. Not all of these have been devised with the purpose of assessing effectiveness of rehabilitation. For example, the Hearing Measurement Scale (Noble and Atherley, 1970) was developed as a tool for assessing the handicap brought about by noise-induced hearing loss, the authors strongly contesting the idea that handicap could be reliably estimated from pure-tone measurements of hearing levels. Other researchers have suggested that a modified version of the Hearing Measurement Scale might be used for elderly adults with presbycusis, but the original tool has not been validated for this purpose. The modification required would probably be substantial, as the original test was devised for persons in employment, and the majority of the elderly with hearing loss are retired. The patterns of relevant activity for the two groups are quite different.

The Hearing Handicap Scale (HHS) of High, Fairbanks and Glorig (1964) was the first scale to be widely employed for self-assessment of the complex effects brought about by hearing impairment. The questions were mainly related to difficulty in specified situations and did not significantly tackle the psychological and emotional aspects of hearing handicap. As such, it provides only a limited measure of hearing handicap (Weinstein, 1984) and may be inappropriate for use with the elderly due to the scope of the questions and the type of response required. Tannahill (1979) used the HHS to assess benefit from amplification with a group of adults with mild to moderate sensorineural hearing loss by administering the test before and four weeks after supplying the aid. There appeared to be a significant reduction in handicap.

The Social Hearing Handicap Index (SHHI) of Ewertsen and Birk-Nielsen (1973) similarly concentrated on situational aspects of hearing. There was, as might therefore be expected, good correlation between scores on the SHHI and degree of hearing loss. In other words, it was more a measure of hearing impairment than of hearing handicap.

The Hearing Performance Inventory (HPI) was developed by Giolas, Owens, Lamb and Schubert (1979) to assess hearing performance in problem areas experienced in everyday listening. It is a measure of the respondents' perceptions of how they perform, rather than a direct measure of hearing handicap. Originally it contained 158 questions and would undoubtedly have taxed the concentration of many typical elderly hearing-impaired persons. In later versions, the number of questions has been reduced to 90. Owens and Fujikawa (1980) used the HPI to assess benefit derived from hearing aids in a group of subjects with severe to profound hearing loss. Users reported improved abilities to communicate, the degree of improvement being greater in the less-severely impaired individuals.

Further scales have been developed for use specifically with the elderly (Weinstein and Ventry, 1982) but the aim has been more that of determining the most appropriate form of counselling rather than assessing benefit in terms of reduced handicap. Much further work is necessary before handicap scales are adequately validated for assessing benefit from amplification and rehabilitation.

3.4 USER SATISFACTION

Appreciation of the hearing-aid supplied was employed by Kapteyn

(1977a,c) in a study of 155 persons questioned six months after issue of a hearing aid. A ten-point scale was used on which ten indicated an appreciation rating of 'excellent', shading through a score of five for 'middling' to one where the aid was rated as 'useless'. The average score was between seven (rather good) and eight (good).

In a study in Manchester, 300 subjects issued at three different centres were asked after a period of four months to rate their satisfaction on a ten-point scale similar to that used by Kapteyn. Only 15 failed to complete this task, and of the 285 who did respond, 198 (69%) gave scores of eight to ten. Only 19 (7%) indicated satisfactions of three or below. There was no significant difference between those who had and those who had not received counselling, although, as previously noted, there was a substantial difference in the amount of use and the number of non-users between the two groups.

These data suggest that the use of a satisfaction score as an index of benefit has a number of limitations. The pattern of responses is very highly skewed towards the upper end of the scale. This may reflect a genuine degree of satisfaction with the instrument or it may indicate a desire on the part of the respondent to seek to please the interviewer. Even if the response is a genuine reflection of feeling, this may not accurately represent the benefit. If expectation is low, then a marginal improvement in hearing ability may result in a relatively high satisfaction, and vice versa.

3.5 USE, BENEFIT AND SATISFACTION: RELATIONSHIPS

In his analysis of data Kapteyn (1977a) found good correlations between satisfaction with the aid and benefit in terms of understanding in various situations. Daily use also correlated significantly with satisfaction. Gerber and Fisher (1979) in a study of 30 hearing-aid users also found a high correlation between use and a measure that they defined as satisfaction. However, 'satisfaction' in this study was not sought from the subject, but derived from the ability to hear with the aid as compared with the ability to hear without the aid. As such, it more closely corresponds to the definition of benefit proposed by Oja and Schow (1984).

Haggard *et al.* (1981) use a forced-choice speech test to assess benefit and found only a small improvement (+ 9.4%) in scores in the aided over the unaided position. Many users, however, reported satisfaction with the aids, and the average daily use was around six hours. This argues for a closer correlation between satisfaction and use than either of these two measures with benefit. Oja and Schow (1984) found low correlations between all three measures in their study and suggest that the three measures are largely unrelated.

The inconsistency of these findings suggests that much depends on how satisfaction and benefit are defined. Arguably, use is the most reliable measure at the present time for assessing the success of a hearing-aid fitting.

REFERENCES

Berger, K.W., Abel, D.B., Hagberg, E.N., Puzz, L.A., Varavvas, D.M. and Weldale, F.J. (1982) Successes and problems of hearing aid users. *Hear. Aid J.*, **35**, (11), 26–30.

Brooks, D.N. (1972) The use and disuse of Medresco hearing aids. *Sound*, **6**, 80–5.

Brooks, D.N. (1979) G.P. attitudes to those seeking hearing aids, unpublished study.

Brooks, D.N. (1981) Use of postaural aids by National Health Service patients. *Brit. J. Audiol.*, **15**, 79–86.

Brooks, D.N. (1985) Factors relating to the underuse of postaural hearing aids. *Brit. J. Audiol.*, **19**, 211–17.

Carhart, R. (1946a) Selection of hearing aids. *Arch. Otolaryngol.*, **44**, 1–18.

Carhart, R. (1946b) Tests for selection of hearing aids. *Laryngoscope*, **56**, 780–94.

Ewertsen, H.W. (1974) The use of hearing aids (always, often, rarely, never). *Scand. Audiol.*, **3**, 173–6.

Ewertsen, H.W. and Birk-Nielsen, H. (1973) Social Hearing Handicap Index: social handicap in relation to hearing impairment. *Audiology*, **12**, 180–7.

Gerber, S.E. and Fisher, L.B. (1979) Prediction of hearing-aid users' satisfaction. *J. Amer. Aud. Soc.*, **5**, 35–40.

Giolas, T.G., Owens, E., Lamb, S.H. and Schubert, E.D. (1979) The Hearing Performance Inventory. *J. Speech Hear. Dis.*, **44**, 169–95.

Gray, P.G. and Cartwright, A. (1951) *The Medresco hearing-aid*. Central Office of Information, London.

Griffing, T.S. (1976) Cosmetic appeal and ITE aids. *Hear. Aid J.*, **29**, (12), 11, 25.

Haggard, M.P., Foster, J.R. and Iredale, F.E. (1981) Use and benefit of postaural aids in sensory hearing loss. *Scand. Audiol.*, **10**, 45–52.

Harris, A.I. (1962) *Health and welfare of older people in Lewisham* Central Office of Information, London.

Hickson, L., Hamilton, L. and Orange, S.P. (1986) Factors associated with hearing aid use. *Aust. J. Audiol.*, **8**, 37–41.

High, W.S., Fairbanks, C. and Glorig, A. (1946) Scale of self-assessment of hearing handicap. *J. Speech Hear. Dis.*, **29**, 215–30.

Humphrey, C., Gilhome-Herbst, K. and Faruqi, S. (1981) Some characteristics of the hearing-impaired elderly who do not present themselves for rehabilitation. *Brit. J. Audiol.* **15**, 25–30.

Jerger, J. (1968) Research-present status and needs. In Proceedings of the

Institute of Aural Rehabilitation (ed. J.G. Alpiner), Univ. of Denver Program in Communication Disorders, Denver, Colo.

Kapteyn, T.S. (1977a) Satisfaction with fitted hearing aids. I. Analysis of technical information. *Scand. Audiol.*, **6**, 147–56.

Kapteyn, T.S. (1977b) Satisfaction with fitted hearing aids. II. Investigation into the incidence of psycho-social factors. *Scand. Audiol.*, **6**, 171–8.

Kapteyn, T.S. (1977c) Factors in the appreciation of a prosthetic appliance. *Audiology*, **16**, 446–52.

Noble, W.G. and Atherley, G.R.C. (1970) The hearing measurement scale: a questionnaire for the assessment of auditory disability. *J. Aud. Res.*, **10**, 193–214.

Oja, G.L. and Schow, R.L. (1984) Hearing-aid evaluation based on measures of benefit, use and satisfaction. *Ear Hear.*, **5**, 77–86.

Owens, E. and Fujikawa, A. (1980) The hearing performance inventory and hearing-aid use in profound hearing loss. *J. Speech Hear. Dis.*, **23**, 470–9.

Shore, I., Bilger, R. and Hirsh, I. (1960) Hearing-aid evaluation: reliability of repeated measurements. *J. Speech Hear. Dis.*, **25**, 152–70.

Skadegard, J. (1982) Hearing aid markets and trends in Western Europe. *Hear. Aid J.* **35**, (10), 19–24.

Speaks, C. and Jerger, J. (1965) A method for measurement of speech identification in the presence of background noise. *J. Speech Hear. Res.*, **8**, 185–94.

Stephens, S.D.G. (1977) Hearing-aid use by adults: a survey of surveys. *Clin. Otolaryngol.* **2**, 385–402.

Surr, R.K., Schuchman, G.I. and Montgomery, A.A. (1979) Factors influencing use of hearing aids. *Hear. Instrum.*, **30**, 19–21, 48.

Tannahill, J. (1979) The hearing handicap scale as a measure of hearing-aid benefit. *J. Speech Hear. Dis.*, **44**, 91–9.

Upfold, L.J. and Wilson, D.A. (1980) Hearing-aid distribution and use in Australia. The Australian bureau of statistics 1978 survey. *Aust. J. Audiol.*, **2**, 31–36.

Ward, P.R. (1980) Treatment of elderly adults with impaired hearing: resources, outcome and efficiency. *J. Epidem. and Community Health*, **34**, 65–8.

Weinstein, B. (1984) A review of hearing handicap scales. *Audiology (A journal for continuing education)* **9**, 91–109.

Weinstein, B.E. and Ventry, I.M. (1982) Assessing hearing handicap in the elderly. *Hear. Aid J.*, **35**, (2), 17–20.

4

TECHNICAL ASPECTS OF HEARING AIDS

Denis Byrne

Modern hearing aids provide a wide range of performance options. By choosing different hearing aids, settings or earmould and coupling systems, the gain, frequency response and maximum power output can be varied substantially. Thus, individualized fitting of hearing aids is possible provided that we can determine the most suitable performance characteristics for each client.

The hearing-aid selection process consists of four stages. These are:

1. determining the required amplification characteristics for the individual;
2. selecting a hearing-aid/earmould/coupling combination that will provide the required performance;
3. verifying that the required performance has been provided in the individual ear;
4. evaluating aided hearing and hence the effectiveness of the aid fitting.

This chapter will deal with these stages in turn except that some preliminary considerations will also be discussed.

4.1 PRELIMINARY CONSIDERATIONS

Before choosing amplification characteristics we need to decide: (a) who to fit; (b) which ear (or ears) to fit; (c) what type of aid to fit.

(a) Hearing-aid candidacy

The likelihood of a person receiving benefit from a hearing-aid depends on attitudinal, environmental and audiological factors. Although the client's initial attitude is one of the better predictors of hearing-aid usage (Hickson, Hamilton and Orange, 1986), attitude (unless extremely negative) is unlikely to be decisive in determining whether a hearing aid will be fitted. Environment is significant because benefit is doubtful if a hearing-aid is expected to be used only in noisy conditions. However, close enquiry will show that many clients who complain only about hearing-aid difficulties in noise, also have problems under other conditions where a hearing-aid would be helpful. The most common audiological criterion for determining hearing-aid candidacy is degree of hearing loss. The older textbooks suggest that a hearing aid is not required unless the three-frequency average (500, 1000 and 2000 Hz) hearing level, in the better ear, is at least 30 dB HTL (this on the old American (ASA) standard), i.e. 40 dB HTL on the current international (ISO) standard. However, with the development of newer hearing aids and improved fitting methods, smaller and smaller degrees of hearing loss, including some unilateral cases, are being fitted. For example, the use of open earmoulds often produces successful fittings for clients having normal hearing up to 500 Hz or even 1000 Hz. There are probably few cases where we should advise against hearing-aid fitting if the client reports significant hearing difficulties and is motivated to try a hearing aid. Exceptions would include severe unilateral hearing losses and clients with normal hearing up to 2000 Hz and who typically have difficulty hearing only in noise. Despite some suggestions to the contrary, low scores on speech-discrimination tests are not a reliable contraindication for hearing-aid fitting.

(b i) Which ear should be aided (better or poorer)

When deciding which ear to fit there are three options: the better ear, the poorer ear, or both ears. Although the last option (binaural fitting) is often the best choice, let us first assume a monaural fitting and examine the arguments for choosing between the better and poorer ears.

The older textbooks (e.g. Watson and Tolan, 1949; Davis and Silverman, 1964) suggest that the choice should be based primarily on the severity of the hearing losses in each ear. In keeping with this, the procedure of the National Acoustic Laboratories (NAL), and probably those of many other establishments in the 1950s and 1960s was to add together the 500, 1000 and 2000 Hz hearing levels of both ears. If the total was less than 120, then the poorer ear should be fitted; if it equalled or exceeded 120 dB, then the better ear should be fitted.

The principle embodied in these and similar rules is that the better ear should not be fitted if it has enough hearing to be useful when unaided. On the other hand, it will usually be more effective to fit the better ear if neither ear has useful unaided hearing. Also, the better must be fitted if the aided hearing of the poorer ear would still be less than unaided hearing in the better ear.

Recent literature gives prominence to such factors as speech discrimination and dynamic range, e.g. Berger, Hagberg and Rane (1977), Ross (1978). However, there is no evidence that a moderate interaural difference in either or both of these factors (usually favouring the better ear) is more important than the reasons for choosing the other (usually poorer) ear on the basis of severity of hearing loss. In fact, in a recent study (Swan, Browning and Gatehouse, 1987; Swan and Gatehouse, 1987) it was found that most moderately hearing-impaired clients (of those who had any preference) preferred to use a hearing-aid in the poorer ear, although most had superior aided speech-discrimination scores in the better ear.

In summary, the evidence for choosing one ear rather than the other is essentially anecdotal except for the Swan *et al.*, 1987 study. That study tends to refute the modern tendency to choose the better ear in the majority of moderately hearing-impaired cases. I suggest that the NAL rule (stated earlier) is still a good starting point for choosing which ear to fit. There would, however, be many exceptions, particularly if it is intended to use ITE hearing aids that permit only limited gain without acoustic feedback.

(b ii) Binaural versus monaural fitting

There is abundant evidence that binaural hearing is superior to monaural hearing and that binaural hearing-aid fitting is advantageous for many hearing-impaired clients (Libby, 1980). However, there are many unresolved questions about which clients should be fitted binaurally. When making this decision, the factors that seem most relevant are: degree of hearing loss; interaural symmetry; client attitude; and client needs. These and other factors are considered in Chapter 7.

Binaural fitting should be considered for all candidates. It appears to be desirable for most severely hearing-impaired clients and for a significant proportion (perhaps 50%) of the less severely impaired. For clients with only mild or moderate hearing losses, the desirability of binaural fitting will depend largely on the client's need and attitude and, in many cases, it may be appropriate for the client to use a binaural fitting in some situations and a monaural fitting in others.

(c) Choice of aid styles

Hearing-aid styles fall into three broad categories: body-worn, behind-the-ear (BTE) and in-the-ear (ITE). Within each category there are various types and models. For example, in-the-canal (ITC) aids can be distinguished from ITE aids and both types are available in custom-made or modular form. The specific choice of model may be influenced by practical considerations related to the client's needs, his capacity to manage different models, and his preferences. The choice may also be influenced by the dispensing system that, in some instances, may make it inefficient to use certain types of aids (e.g. custom ITEs). For the great majority of clients, ear-level aids (BTE and ITE) are preferable to body-worn models. As well as being cosmetically more acceptable, they usually have a more suitable real-ear frequency response, particularly at the high frequencies (Byrne, 1983). ITE aids are becoming increasingly popular and may have some advantages in terms of better vertical plane localization and increased real-ear gain around 2–4 kHz. However, claims that far less gain is needed with an ITE aid compared with a BTE aid are unjustified and may be related to the fact that ITE earmoulds typically have longer ear canals (Hodgson and Wernick, 1985). ITE aids have some disadvantages in terms of greater susceptibility to acoustic feedback and less extensive fitter and user controls. At present there are unresolved questions in choosing between a BTE and an ITE for a client with a mild or moderate hearing loss.

4.2 PRESCRIBING THE REQUIRED AMPI IFICATION

(a) Is selective amplification necessary?

There are three basic amplification parameters to be considered when selecting a hearing-aid for each client. These are: gain (the amount of amplification), frequency response (the relative gain at different frequencies) and maximum power output (the maximum level that the aid is capable of producing). It has always been recognized that gain and maximum power output (MPO) need to be individually selected, but the need for frequency-response selection has been contentious. Following the classic 'Harvard' (Davis *et al.*, 1947) and 'Medresco' (Radley, Bragg, Dadson *et al.*, 1947) studies, it was widely believed that a single frequency-response characteristic was appropriate for most, or all clients. This view is no longer common and several recent studies have shown the advantages of selective amplification (for a review see Byrne, 1983). Further confirmation comes from research at NAL that indicates that only a moderate range of frequency-response characteristics is required to fit a large range of audiogram configurations (Byrne, 1986a,b; Byrne and Murray, 1986).

(b) Gain–selection principles

Hearing-impaired persons require speech to be amplified to a level where it can be understood. Gain is required to compensate for the reduced loudness of speech as perceived by a hearing-impaired individual compared with a normal hearing person. The general principle in prescribing gain is to provide sufficient to raise a typical speech input (i.e. a moderate speech level) from a normal-hearing person's preferred listening level (PLL) to that of the hearing-impaired individual.

Various methods have been proposed for implementing the above gain–selection principle. One is to measure the client's most comfortable listening level (MCL) and to provide gain equal to the difference between this MCL and the normal MCL. Although this would appear logical, the values obtained for MCL can vary considerably depending on measurement methods and from time to time (Christen and Byrne, 1980). MCL is, therefore, a method of estimating PLL rather than a direct method of measuring it. An alternative is to estimate PLL (or, more specifically, the gain required to amplify speech to PLL) from HTL. This is possible because it has been shown that, for sensorineural hearing losses, the gain used by experienced hearing-aid wearers increases at about half the rate the HTL increases (for a review , see Byrne, 1983). Advantages of using HTL measurements are that they are more reliable than MCL and more readily obtainable in some cases (e.g. young children). A third approach to calculating gain requirements is to estimate PLL to be mid-way (or some other point) between HTL and loudness discomfort level (LDL).

(c) Frequency-response selection principles

Several principles need to be considered when prescribing frequency response (Byrne, 1983; Haggard, 1983). One is that, in general, the potential for understanding speech is proportional to the amount of the speech signal that is audible, averaged over a range of about 200 Hz to 5000 Hz. According to the Articulation Index (ANSI, 1969) the maximum contribution of each frequency band of speech will be reached when the speech peak levels are 30 dB above threshold. This suggests that speech intelligibility would be maximized if the frequency response was selected so that the speech peaks in all frequency bands were delivered at 30 dB SL or a higher level. However, this will nearly always result in a sound level that is unacceptably high. This will induce the aid-wearer to turn down the volume control (i.e. reduce gain at all frequencies) to obtain his/her preferred listening level. The crux of frequency-response selection is, therefore, to provide the maximum amount of signal *after* the hearing-aid volume control has been adjusted to a comfortable listening level. This will be achieved if all frequency bands of speech, taken separately, are amplified to PLL or to equal loudness at a comfortable level (Skinner, 1980; Lippmann, Braida and Durlach, 1981; Byrne, 1986b). This principle provides the rationale for several current hearing-aid selection procedures (e.g. Skinner, Pascoe, Miller and Popelka, 1982; Byrne and Dillon, 1986).

Another basic concept is the need to fit an amplified speech signal into the dynamic range of hearing. This is usually defined as the range between HTL and LDL. This concept would imply that the peaks of speech can be amplified up to LDL. However, PLLs are such that the speech peaks can, in fact, only be amplified to a level between one-third and two-thirds of the way up to LDL (Byrne and Cotton, 1987). In other words, the amplified speech signal must be fitted into the lower half, or two-thirds, of the dynamic range. To fit speech within the dynamic range, we must consider the spectrum of the unamplified speech signal as well as the client's threshold and LDL curves. Because speech has most energy in the low frequencies, it is necessary to give a significant amount of mid-frequency and high-frequency emphasis even for clients with a flat audiogram. Finally, masking phenomena are significant, at least theoretically, to frequency-response selection. In general, it is desirable to avoid too much relative gain at the lower frequencies because high-level, low-frequency sounds may mask higher frequency sounds occurring simultaneously, or almost simultaneously. However, it appears that there is little, if any, risk of masking associated with procedures that amplify all frequency bands of speech to PLL.

(d) Gain- and frequency-response procedures

Numerous procedures have been proposed for prescribing the gain and frequency response of a hearing aid (for reviews see Lybarger, 1978; Braida, Durlach, Lipmann, et al., 1979; Byrne, 1983). Nearly all such procedures can be classified into three types: MCL, HTL and 'bisection'. In MCL procedures the guiding principles are to compensate for differences between normal MCL and the hearing-impaired individual's MCL, at each frequency (e.g. Crouch and Pendry, 1975) or to amplify each frequency band of speech to MCL, but possibly to include adjustments for other factors (e.g. Skinner et al., 1982).

The earliest HTL procedure is audiogram 'mirroring'. This is fallacious, mainly because it compensates for inter-frequency differences in threshold curves, whereas the corresponding differences in MCL curves are often much smaller (Byrne, 1983). Most HTL procedures are based on the half-gain rule (Lybarger, 1944), the idea being that gain should be approximately half of HTL. When the half-gain rule is applied at each frequency, differences in audiogram slopes are compensated for by half as much difference in frequency-response slopes. That is, frequency response is varied according to a 'half-slope' rule. Examples of half-gain formulae include Lybarger (1955), Byrne and Tonisson (1976), Berger *et al.* (1977), McCandless and Lyregaard (1983) and Byrne and Dillon (1986). Three of these use a half-slope rule but the Byrne and Dillon formula uses a one-third-slope rule and Lybarger uses a one-quarter-slope rule.

Bisection procedures are, typically, based on the curve defined by the points halfway between HTL and LDL (i.e. halfway through the effective dynamic range) at each frequency (e.g. Wallenfels, 1967). A recent example is based on bisecting HTL and the upper limit of comfortable loudness, a point that is typically about 13 dB below LDL (Cox, 1983).

The feasibility of using HTL, MCL or bisection methods for prescribing gain and frequency response depends on the degree to which the measurements in question can predict PLLs and, particularly, interfrequency differences in PLLs. Recent research (Byrne and Murray, 1985; Byrne and Cotton, 1987) suggests that all three methods are inherently capable of a similar, and acceptable, degree of accuracy. Individual formulae of a particular type may, however, vary greatly (Byrne, 1987a). It is probable, in fact, that there are good and poor formulae of all three types.

One procedure (NAL method) will be described in somewhat more detail to illustrate the practical application of gain- and frequency-response selection.

(e) NAL Hearing-aid selection procedures

1. Development

The first NAL hearing-aid selection procedure (Byrne and Tonisson, 1976) was based on an approximately half-gain (46%) rule and a half-slope rule. It included adjustments for the interfrequency differences in the speech spectrum and in the 60 phon equal-loudness contour. The aim of the procedure was to prescribe frequency response in such a manner that all frequency bands of speech would contribute equally to the loudness of the signal, thereby providing a maximally useful speech signal after the hearing-aid volume control had been set for comfortable listening.

An important and (at that time) novel feature of the procedure was that gain and frequency response were prescribed in terms of real-ear performance (REP), typically measured by aided threshold testing. The procedure involved initially selecting an aid that would be likely to provide the desired REP, measuring REP with the selected aid and then altering the aid, if necessary, to correct for any significant discrepancies between the desired and obtained REP.

The rationale of the Byrne and Tonisson procedure was confirmed by research (Byrne, 1986a,b) which, however, also showed that the procedure did not achieve its aim consistently. Analysis indicated that the aim could be achieved by a modified set of formulae (Byrne and Dillon, 1986), which are shown in Table 4.1.

Table 4.1 Formulae for calculating real-ear gain and coupler-measured gain (maximum volume control setting) for BTE, ITE and body-worn aids according to the revised NAL procedure (Byrne and Dillon, 1986).

Gain at each frequency = X + Y + Z where:
   X = 0.05 (HTL [0.5 kHz] + HTL [1 kHz] + HTL [2 kHz])
   Y = 0.31 × HTL at the frequency of interest
   Z = a frequency-dependent constant as shown below:

Frequency	Real-ear gain (all aid types)	2cc coupler gain BTE	ITE	Body-worn
250 Hz	−17	1	−1	−4
500 Hz	−8	9	9	2
750 Hz	−3	12	13	8
1000 Hz	+1	16	16	13
1500 Hz	+1	13	14	22
2000 Hz	−1	15	14	25
3000 Hz	−2	22	15	26
4000 Hz	−2	18	13	17
6000 Hz	−2	12	4	−

The basic formula prescribes the required real-ear gain at each frequency derived from HTL. The other formulae show the coupler-measured gain that is most likely to provide the required real-ear gain for BTE, ITE and body-worn hearing aids.

2. Validation

The new procedure was validated by comparing the effectiveness of its prescriptions with a systematic series of variations in frequency response (Byrne and Cotton, in press). Specifically it was found that the prescribed frequency was nearly always judged to be more intelligible than, or equally as intelligible as, any other response. However, in about

25% of cases some other frequency response was judged to be more pleasant. To detect such cases, an evaluation procedure has been devised to supplement the use of the formula (Byrne, 1987b).

3. *Applying the NAL procedure*

The essential steps are:

1. Calculate the required coupler-measured gain and frequency response using the formula appropriate to the type of aid.
2. Fit and then test the real-ear performance (REP) as worn.
3. Calculate the required real-ear gain and frequency response and compare these values with the values obtained by REP testing.
4. If the obtained and required values do not agree closely, modify the aid system (if possible) to achieve a better match.

It should be noted that frequency response is much more important than gain, and variations in the latter of up to ± 15 dB are to be expected. However, small differences in frequency-response shape often lead to significant differences in the perceived intelligibility and/or pleasantness of speech, so it is desirable to match the attained response as closely as is possible to the target using the available technology.

(f) Selection of maximum power output

The general principles in selecting maximum power output (MPO) are (1) that MPO should be sufficiently high to permit an adequate level of signal to be delivered and (2) that MPO should be sufficiently low to prevent any sounds being amplified to an uncomfortable level. The consequences of setting MPO too high are that the client will be exposed to uncomfortably loud sounds and this may induce him (or her) to reject the aid, to limit its use, or to use an undesirably low volume setting to minimise the risk of sounds being amplified to an uncomfortable level. The consequences of selecting an MPO that is too low are that the client may not hear speech satisfactorily or that speech, particularly the client's own voice, may be distorted because the hearing aid may be frequently driven into saturation.

MPO selection involves (1) calculating the minimum level that is adequate, (2) calculating the maximum level that is acceptable, (3) determining a level that meets both of these requirements or, if that is not possible, determining the best compromise between the two requirements. Logically, MPO should be prescribed at several frequencies because discomfort may be experienced if MPO is too low at any frequency and the hearing aid's effectiveness may be reduced if MPO is too low at any frequency. This may require a compromise because the MPO adjustment in current hearing aids only changes the overall level (i.e. the level at all frequencies). However, the facility to shape the MPO curve (without changing the frequency-response curve) is technically feasible (Dillon and Macrae, 1984) and hopefully it will be included in future hearing aids.

Various MPO selection procedures largely based on similar principles have been suggested (for a review see Skinner, 1988). The following is an interim NAL procedure. First, the minimum desirable level (MDL) is calculated at several frequencies, usually 0.25, 0.5, 1, 2, 3, and 4 kHz, this being hearing threshold (in dB SPL) plus 35 dB. The rationale of this procedure is that, for maximum speech intelligibility the speech peaks must be at least 30 dB above threshold. Next, the maximum acceptable level (MAL) is calculated as 5 dB below LDL at each frequency. After these calculations MPO is prescribed as follows:

1. if MDL and MAL agree (i.e. if the dynamic range is exactly 40 dB), then this is the level prescribed for MPO;
2. if the dynamic range is less than 40 dB, MPO is equal to LDL (in fact, if the dynamic range is less than 30 dB, a level slightly exceeding LDL may be tried to see whether it is acceptable;
3. if MAL exceeds MDL, any level between them may be satisfactory.

However, it is also desirable that the client's voice, which is more intense than most other hearing-aid inputs, does not saturate the aid. Therefore it is usually preferable to select a level closer to MAL and MDL may not always be sufficient to prevent the client's own voice from saturating the aid.

The threshold and LDL measurements may be made either with pure tones or narrow bands of noise. However, after prescribing MPO on the basis of narrow-band stimuli it is necessary to check that broad-band stimuli such as speech cannot be amplified to an uncomfortable level (Walker, Dillon, Byrne and Christen, 1984). If any discomfort occurs, the overall MPO should be reduced slightly.

It is important that the desired relationship between MPO and LDL, and between MPO and HTL be obtained in the individual ear. This can be achieved by making the threshold and LDL measurements with an audiometer coupled to a hearing-aid earphone and the client's own earmould. This type of arrangement has been described in several recent publications (e.g. Cox, 1983; Dillon, Chew and Deans, 1984; Hawkins, 1984). The audiometer with the hearing-aid earphone is calibrated in a 2 cc coupler in the same way that a hearing-aid's output is measured.

(g) Other hearing-aid performance parameters

Directional microphones
These are less sensitive than omnidirectional microphones to sounds

coming from behind the hearing-aid wearer. This provides an improvement in signal-to-noise ratio that is maximal in anechoic conditions and minimal in reverberant conditions. Overall, directional microphones should offer a modest but worthwhile advantage in certain listening conditions and should have no disadvantages in others.

Compression in hearing aids

The use of compression is a complex and controversial subject (for review and analysis see Walker and Dillon, 1982). Compression limiting (i.e. having a high threshold for the onset of compression coupled with a high compression ratio) is widely regarded as superior to peak clipping because far less distortion occurs when the hearing aid is saturated. However, the value of syllabic compression, which is activated by moderate as well as high inputs, is doubtful. Research results have been mostly negative both for single-channel and multi-channel systems (Braida *et al.*, 1979; Walker and Dillon, 1982) although there are some exceptions (e.g. Laurence, Moore and Glasberg, 1983). More sophisticated compression systems are exemplified in some of the new 'automatic signal processing' (ASP) hearing aids. In these aids, the frequency response automatically reacts to the frequency distribution in the input, seeking to optimize the signal/noise ratio. This technology remains to be fully evaluated.

4.3 ACHIEVING THE PRESCRIBED AMPLIFICATION

Hearing-aid selection involves calculating the required amplification and selecting a hearing-aid system that can provide it. This second step consists of choosing a hearing-aid model, the control settings, the type of earmould and other aspects of the acoustic coupling system ('plumbing') such as the earhook and filters. If we consider every combination of hearing-aid × setting × earmould × plumbing as a hearing-aid fitting option, the number of options is extremely large. We need, therefore, a comprehensive set of performance data on all fitting options and a systematic approach to selecting the most suitable option for each client.

(a) Hearing-aid performance variations: electrical

To provide a good range of options with current hearing aids, it will probably be necessary to have from three to ten models in each of the major aid types (BTE, ITE, body-worn). This assumes that it is intended to use all three types, that each model is relatively flexible in its performance options and that there is little duplication of performance between models.

Performance data on each model are available from the manufacturer but should be checked by measurements conducted in the clinic. As well as the basic gain and MPO (saturation sound pressure level, or SSPL 90) curves, it is desirable to measure each setting of the fitter-adjustable controls. Most hearing aids (but excluding some ITE models) have at least two controls. The relatively standard controls are a tone control (bass-cut) and an MPO control. Performance data for two such controls are shown in Figure 4.1.

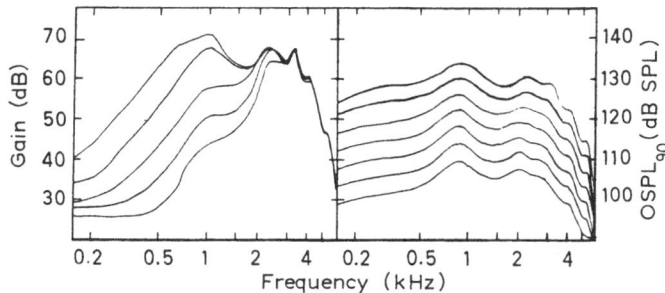

Figure 4.1 Tone control settings (bass-cut) and MPO settings of a BTE hearing aid (Phonak PPC 2 with 300 ohm attenuator).

The controls shown in Figure 4.1 are five-position and seven-position switches, which are convenient for the hearing-aid fitter. If the controls are continuously variable trim pots, the curves on the data sheets may only show the maximum and minimum positions. Unless the range of variation is small, it may be useful to identify and measure at least one intermediate position. If more than two controls are provided, they will probably include one or more of the following: a high-cut tone control (useful but seldom provided); a gain control; one or more controls for choosing between peak clipping and compression or for varying compression characteristics. In custom ITE aids, performance variations are achieved by choosing different components when assembling a hearing aid. With body-worn aids the hearing-aid fitter may have a choice of earphones that provide some variation in performance.

Overall, the choice of different hearing-aid models and settings provides a wide selection of gain and MPO levels (but not MPO shaping), and a wide variation in bass-cut, operating below about 2 kHz.

(b) Acoustical modification of hearing-aid performance

The real-ear performance of a hearing aid depends considerably on the acoustical coupling between the aid and the ear. The choice of different types of earmoulds and, to a lesser extent, different acoustical filters and earhooks, provides a wide range of fitting options. Information on earmould variations is available in Cox (1979), Libby, Johnson and Longwell (1981), Killion (1982), Libby (1982) and Dillon (1985). The effects of some useful modifications are shown in Table 4.2. Modifications 1–4 of Table 4.2 reduce the low-frequency output by various amounts depending on the size of the vent. Venting also removes the occlusion effect, which tends to make the client's own voice sound loud and booming, and it allows unamplified sound to pass into the ear unimpeded and undistorted. For these reasons, it is generally desirable to use venting provided that acoustic feedback is not incurred and provided that the required frequency response can be achieved.

Table 4.2 Effects of some comon earmould modifications (relative to gain with a standard, occluding earmould with 2 mm tubing).

Modification	Frequency (kHz)								
	0.25	0.5	0.75	1	1.5	2	3	4	6
1. 2 mm Vent	−7	−1	0	0	0	1	1	1	2
2. Long open mould	−17	−10	−5	−3	0	2	2	1	1
3. Short open mould	−27	−22	−17	−13	−7	0	0	0	−1
4. Tube fitting	−26	−20	−14	−12	−8	0	2	0	0
5. 6C10 reverse horn	0	2	2	−2	−1	−5	−10	−12	−17
6. 6C5 reverse	0	1	0	0	0	0	−4	−6	−11
7. Libby horn, 3 mm	−1	−2	−2	−2	1	0	6	8	2
8. Libby horn	−1	−2	−3	−3	0	−2	6	10	6

Modifications 5–8 of Table 4.2 affect mainly the high frequencies (above 1.5 kHz). The horn earmoulds (see Killion, 1982; Libby, 1982) increase the high-frequency output, whereas the reverse horn earmoulds (Killion, 1982) have the opposite effect. Horn earmoulds are very useful as it is often difficult to achieve sufficient gain and MPO at frequencies above 2 kHz. Reverse horns are also useful, particularly as few hearing aids provide high-cut controls. It is possible to obtain further fitting options by combining low-frequency and high-frequency modifications. However, some combinations (e.g. a large vent and a horn earmould) may not be possible.

Hearing aids may be fitted with different types of acoustic filters (damping elements), usually placed within the earhook. Figure 4.2 shows the gain and SSPL 90 curves of a BTE hearing aid with no filter and with two different types of filters. Filters provide only a modest variation in fitting options because they affect only a narrow range of frequencies and because nearly all hearing aids should be fitted with the mid-frequency peak reduced or eliminated.

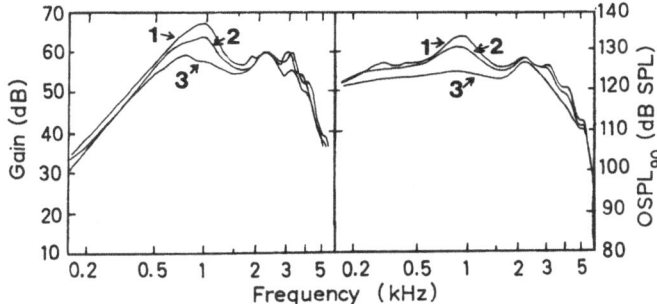

Figure 4.2 Effects of acoustic filters in the earhook of BTE hearing aid. 1, no attenuator; 2, 300 ohm attenuator; 3, 1500 ohm attenuator.

Further variations in acoustic coupling systems are described in the publications cited earlier. More elaborate modifications include the cavity vent earmould (Macrae, 1985), which makes it possible to use a vent with a relatively powerful hearing aid without incurring acoustic feedback. Another type of earmould (Macrae, 1982) creates a notch filter that is useful in cases with good hearing over a narrow range of frequencies (e.g. around 2 kHz). Other special-purpose devices include the 'K-Bass' friction hook (Killion and Wilson, 1985).

(c) Choosing the best hearing-aid-fitting option

Even with an extensive set of performance data, it is impossible to envisage every possible combination of electrical and acoustical variation. It has, therefore, become desirable to use a computerized system in order to make optimal use of the available options. However, in the absence of such a system, certain strategies may be employed to sift through the performance data and make a good choice of fitting option. These would include the following: first, the number of aid models may be reduced by eliminating those that cannot provide the appropriate MPO. Next, the number may be further reduced to those providing appropriate gain within the tolerance of +/− 6–8 dB. It may be appropriate to give most weight to gain from 1 kHz to 2kHz because this frequency range will be least affected by electrical or acoustical modifications. Next, we may consider which low-frequency and/or high-frequency modifications are necessary to achieve the appropriate frequency response. We should remember the general desirability of providing a vent, when feasible, principally for acoustical effect, but also for comfort and health. We should also remember that acoustical modifications will affect the MPO curve as well as the gain (frequency response) curve. Finally, we might look at the gain in the mid-frequency range to decide whether the fitting could be improved by changing the acoustic filter. Such a fitting procedure obviously requires a good knowledge of the effects of various modifications and, in many instances, the combined effects will need to be calculated.

4.4 MEASURING REAL-EAR GAIN
AND FREQUENCY RESPONSE

After a hearing-aid has been fitted on the basis of its coupler-measured performance, it is necessary to verify that the desired performance has been achieved in the ear of the individual client. The three methods commonly used for measuring real-ear gain (REG) are (1) real-ear insertion gain measurements (several systems are commercially available), (2) functional gain and (3) aided threshold testing.

(a) Real-ear insertion gain (probe microphone) measurements

Real-ear insertion gain is the preferred method for measuring REG because (1) it is highly accurate, (2) it can be applied to virtually all cases and (3) it is quick and easy. However, difficulties may be experienced when measuring high-gain aids because acoustic feedback occurs when the probe is inserted beside the earmould. If feedback does occur at the preferred volume setting, the measurements should be made on a lower volume setting (5–10 dB below where feedback first occurs). The real-ear gain for the preferred setting can be calculated by measuring, in a coupler, the difference in gain between the measured and preferred settings.

(b) Unaided minus aided thresholds (functional gain)

Considerable care is required for accurate sound field threshold measurements (see Walker, Dillon and Byrne, 1984 for recommended procedures). When adequate care is taken, functional gain measurements may be comparable in accuracy with insertion gain measurements. However, this method has two significant limitations:

1. Aided thresholds may be invalid for clients having only small hearing losses (about 40 dB HTL or less) because the thresholds will be determined by the internal noise of the hearing aid or by amplified ambient noise. This will result in an under-estimation of the amount of functional gain.
2. Unaided thresholds will not be measurable for the severely hearing-impaired with the equipment usually available.

Because of these limitations this method is only applicable to clients having moderate to severe hearing losses (about 40–80 dB HTL) at all test frequencies. Also, it takes considerably more time than the insertion gain method.

(c) Aided threshold testing

This is a short-cut functional gain method in that the unaided thresholds are not measured but are, in effect, predicted from earphone thresholds. The attractions of this method are that it only takes half the time of the standard functional gain method and it is applicable to the severely hearing-impaired because it avoids the need for unaided sound field thresholds. However, it is inapplicable for small hearing losses (at any frequency) and it is substantially less accurate than either of the other two methods (Dillon and Murray, 1987). This method may have some advantages for the severely hearing-impaired but in general, it is considerably inferior to the insertion gain method.

4.5 EVALUATING AIDED HEARING

After the hearing-aid has been fitted, and after we have verified that the prescribed real-ear performance has been achieved, there remains the question of determining how well the client hears when aided. First, is the hearing aid fitting as effective as possible and hence is there any reason to consider modifying it? Secondly we need to know how well the client functions when wearing the hearing aid in order to advise him appropriately and determine the need for any further rehabilitative measures.

There are three general ways in which aided hearing can be evaluated. First, this may be done in an informal manner by simply asking the client how he is getting on with his hearing aid. The value of this method is undoubted and such follow-up should be universal practice. A more systematic approach may be adopted by administering an appropriately designed and validated questionnaire before and after aid fitting. The third approach involves testing aided hearing. This is used infrequently in clinical hearing-aid fitting, apart from the American hearing-aid evaluation procedure (Carhart, 1946), which is used for selection rather than post-fitting evaluation. Speech-discrimination tests can be used for evaluation but it is difficult to achieve satisfactory reliability and sensitivity within an acceptable amount of testing time (Schwartz, 1982; Studebaker, 1982). It would be valuable to be able to determine whether speech discrimination is as good as possible but unfortunately, there is no way of estimating what this possible score should be. One important, although limited, use of speech-discrimination testing is the evaluation of aided hearing of severely deaf clients who are being considered for cochlear implantation. In this application, speech discrimination with the hearing aid is usually compared with the average score obtained by persons using a cochlear implant.

NAL has recently developed a post-fitting evaluation procedure based on paired comparison judgements of the intelligibility of speech in quiet and the pleasantness of speech in noise (Byrne, 1987b). This procedure is a valuable addition to the use of the NAL selection formula. It does not, however, provide any absolute information on the effectiveness of aided hearing and therefore, additional procedures would be desirable to meet this need.

This chapter has presented an overview of some of the issues involved in the selection and fitting of hearing aids. It is far from comprehensive yet no issue has been examined in depth. Hopefully this material will provide a useful orientation and conceptual framework that the audiologist who is engaged in hearing-aid fitting will follow up with further reading.

REFERENCES

ANSI (1969) American national standard method for calculation of the articulation index. *ANSI S3.5-1969*, Am. Nat. Standards Inst.

Berger, K.W., Hagberg, N.S. and Rane, R.L. (1977) *Prescription of hearing aids*, Herald Pub. Co., Kent, Ohio.

Braida, L., Durlach, N., Lippmann, R., Hicks, B., Rabinowitz, W. and Reed, C. (1979) Hearing aids – a review of past research on linear amplification, amplitude compression and frequency lowering. *ASLHA monograph No. 19.* ASLHA, Rockville, Md.

Byrne, D. (1983) Theoretical prescriptive approaches to selecting the gain and frequency response of a hearing aid. *Monographs in contemporary audiology*, Vol. 4/1.

Byrne, D. (1986a) Effects of bandwidth and stimulus type on most comfortable loudness levels of hearing-impaired listeners. *J. Acoust. Soc. Amer.*, **80**, 484–93.

Byrne, D. (1986b) Effects of frequency response characteristics on speech discrimination and perceived intelligibility and pleasantness of speech for hearing-impaired listeners. *J. Acoust. Soc. Amer.*, **80**, 494–503.

Byrne, D. (1977a) Hearing-aid selection formulae: same or different? *Hear. Instrum.*, **38**, (1), 5–11.

Byrne, D. (1987b) A post hearing-aid-fitting evaluation procedure using speech intelligibility and pleasantness judgments. *NAL Report 112*, National Acoustic Laboratories, Sydney.

Byrne, D. and Cotton, S. (1987) Preferred listening levels of persons with sensorineural hearing losses. *Aust. J. Audiol.*, **9**, 7–14.

Byrne, D. and Cotton, S. (in press) Clinical trial and evaluation of the National Acoustic Laboratories' new hearing-aid selection procedure. *J. Speech Hear. Res.*

Byrne, D. and Dillon, H. (1986) The National Acoustic Laboratories (NAL) new procedure for selecting the gain and frequency response of a hearing-aid. *Ear Hear.*, **7**, 257–65.

Byrne, D. and Murray, N.M. (1985) Relationships of HTLs, MCLs, LDLs and psychoacoustic tuning curves to the optimal frequency response characteristics of hearing aids. *Aust. J. Audiol.*, **7**, 7–16.

Byrne, D. and Murray, N.M. (1986) Predictability of the required frequency response characteristics of a hearing aid from the pure-tone audiogram. *Ear Hear.*, **7**, 63–70.

Byrne, D. and Tonisson, W. (1976) Selecting the gain of hearing aids for persons with sensorineural hearing impairments. *Scand. Audiol.*, **5**, 51–9.

Carhart, R. (1946) Selection of hearing aids. *Arch. Otolaryngol.*, **44**, 1–18.

Christen, R. and Byrne, D. (1980) Variability of MCL measurements: significance for hearing-aid selection. *Aust. J. Audiol.*, **2**, 10–18.

Cox, R. (1979) Acoustic aspects of hearing aid–ear canal coupling systems. Monographs in contemporary audiology (eds D.M. Schwartz and F.H. Bess), Vol 1/3, Maico Hearing Instruments, Minneapolis, Mn.

Cox, R.M. (1983) Using ULCL measures to find frequency/gain and SSPL90. *Hear. Instrum.*, **34**, 17–21, 39.

Crouch, J.D. and Pendry, B.L. (1975) Otometry in clinical hearing-aid dispensing. *Hear. Aid J.*, Sept 12, 42–8; Oct 18, 31–3.

Davis, H. and Silverman, R. (1964) *Hearing and deafness*, Revised edn, Holt, Rinehart and Winston, New York.

Davis, H., Stevens, S.S. and Nichols, R.H. (1947) *Hearing Aids, An Experimental Study of Design Objectives*. Cambridge, Mass. Harvard Univ. Press.

Dillon, H. (1985) Earmoulds and high frequency response modifications. *Hear. Instrum.*, **36**, (12), 8, 11–12.

Dillon, H., Chew, R. and Deans, M. (1984) Loudness discomfort level measurements and their implications for the design and fitting of hearing aids. *Aust. J. Audiol.*, **6**, 73–9.

Dillon, H. and Macrae, J. (1984) Derivation of design specifications for hearing aids. *NAL Report 102*, National Acoustic Laboratories, Sydney.

Dillon, H. and Murray, N. (1987) Accuracy of twelve methods for estimating real-ear gain of hearing aids. *Ear Hear.*, **8**, 2–11.

Haggard, M.P. (1983) New and old conceptions of hearing aids. In *Hearing Science and Hearing Disorders* (eds M.E. Lutman and M.P. Haggard), Academic Press, New York.

Hawkins, D. (1984) Selection of a critical electroacoustic characteristic: SSPL90. *Hear. Instrum.* **35**, 28–32.

Hickson, L., Hamilton, L. and Orange, S.P. (1986) Factors associated with hearing aid use. *Aust. J. Audiol.*, **8**, 42–55.

Hodgson, W. and Wernick, J.S. (1985) Canal aid versus standard custom ITE performance (Part 2). *Hear. Instrum.*, **36**, (4), 26–8, 68.

Killion, M.C. (1982) Transducers, earmoulds and sound quality considerations. In G.A. Studebaker and F.H. Bess (eds) *The Vanderbilt Hearing Aid Report: State of the art–research needs. Monographs in contemporary audiology.* Upper Darby, Pa.

Killion, M.C. and Wilson, D.L. (1985) Response modifying earhooks for special fitting problems. *Audecibel*, **34**, (4), 28–30.

Laurence, R.F., Moore, B.C. and Glasberg, B.R. (1983) A comparison of behind-the-ear linear high-fidelity hearing aids and two-channel compression aids, in the laboratory and in everyday life. *Brit. J. Audiol.*, **17**, 31–48.

Libby, E.R. (ed.) (1980) *Binaural hearing and amplification*, Zenetron, Chicago.

Libby, E.R. (1982) In search of transparent insertion gain hearing aid responses. In G.A. Studebaker and F.H. Bess (eds) *The Vanderbilt Hearing Aid Report: State of the art–research needs. Monographs in contemporary audiology*, Upper Darby, Pa.

Libby, E.R., Johnson, J.H. and Longwell, T.F. (1981) Innovative earmould coupling systems: rationale, design, clinical application. *Zenetron Monograph No. 4*, Zenetron Inc., Chicago.

Lippmann, R.P., Braida, L.D. and Durlach, N.I. (1981) Study of multichannel amplitude compression and linear amplification for persons with sensorineural hearing loss. *J. Acoust. Soc. Amer.*, **69**, 524–34.

Lybarger, S.F. (1944) US Patent application SN 532, 278.

Lybarger, S.F. (1955) *Simplified fitting system for hearing aids*. Radioear Corp. Canonsburg. PA.

Lybarger, S.F. (1978) Selective amplification – a review and evaluation. *J. Amer. Aud. Soc.*, **3**, 258–66.

McCandless, G.A. and Lyregaard, P.E. (1983) Prescription of gain/output (POGO) for hearing aids. *Hear. Instrum.*, **34**, 16–21.

Macrae, J. (1982) Acoustic notch filters for hearing aids. *Aust. J. Audiol.* 4, 71–6.

Macrae, J. (1985) A smaller version of the cavity vent. *Aust. J. Audiol.* 7, 17–21.

Radley, W.G., Bragg, W.L., Dadson, R.S., Hallpike, C.S., McMillan, D., Pocock, L.C. and Littler, T.S. (1947) *Hearing aids and audiometers, report of the committee on electroacoustics*, Her Majesty's Stationery Office, London.

Ross, M. (1978) Hearing-aid evaluation in *Handbook of clinical audiology* (ed. J. Katz), Williams and Wilkins, Baltimore.

Schwartz, D.M. (1982) Hearing aid selection methods: an enigma. In G.A. Studebaker and F.H. Bess (eds) *The Vanderbilt Hearing Aid Report: state of the art – research needs. Monographs in contemporary audiology*, Upper Darby, Pa.

Skinner, M.W. (1988) *Hearing Aid Evaluation*, Prentice Hall, New Jersey.

Skinner, M.W. (1980) Speech intelligibility in noise-induced hearing loss: effects of high-frequency compensation. *J. Acoust. Soc. Amer.*, **67**, 306–17.

Skinner, M.W., Pascoe, D.P., Miller, J.D., and Popelka, G.R. (1982) Measurements to determine the optimal placement of speech energy within the listener's auditory area: a basis for selecting amplification characteristics. In G.A. Studebaker and F.H. Bess (eds) *The Vanderbilt Hearing Aid Report: State of the art–research needs. Monographs in contemporary audiology*, Upper Darby, Pa.

Studebaker, G.A. (1982) Hearing aid selection: an overview. In: G.A. Studebaker and F.H. Bess (eds) *The Vanderbilt Hearing Aid Report: State of the art – research needs. Monographs in contemporary audiology*, Upper Darby, Pa.

Swan, I.R.C., Browning, G.G. and Gatehouse, S. (1987) Optimum side for fitting a monaural hearing aid. 1. Patients' preference. *Brit. J. Audiol.*, **21**, 59–65.

Swan, I.R.C. and Gatehouse, S. (1987) Optimum side for fitting a monaural hearing aid. 2. Measured benefit. *Brit. J. Audiol.*, **21**, 67–71.

Walker, G. and Dillon, H. (1982) Compression in hearing aids: an analysis, a review and some recommendations. *NAL Report 90*. National Acoustic Laboratories, Sydney.

Walker, G., Dillon, H. and Byrne, D. (1984) Sound field audiometry: recommended stimuli and procedures. *Ear Hear.*, **5**, 13–21.

Walker, G., Dillon, H., Byrne, D. and Christen, R. (1984) The use of loudness discomfort levels for selecting the maximum output of hearing aids. *Aust. J. Audiol.*, **6**, 23–32.

Wallenfels, H.G. (1967) *Hearing aids on prescription*, C.C. Thomas, Springfield, Ill.

Watson, L.A. and Tolan, T. (1949) *Hearing tests and hearing instruments*, Williams and Wilkins, Baltimore.

5

ATTITUDE FACTORS AND HEARING-AID ORIENTATION

Denzil Brooks

In Chapter 3 it was noted that the degree of success (or failure) in using a hearing aid was associated with initial attitude to hearing impairment and hearing aids. Individuals with negative perceptions tend to fare less well with amplification than those with a positive outlook. Attitude can be compounded of many interacting factors. In order to clarify the role of these factors, it is desirable to identify them and consider them in isolation, though recognizing that in an individual, the overall effect will be more complex due to interactions. Thus, in counselling, although one seeks to identify, and in some measure to quantify the various factors, the person must be considered as a whole.

For some years, candidates for hearing aids at Withington Hospital, Manchester, have been asked to complete a questionnaire before their first visit to the hospital, that is, before attending the ENT department for medical examination, which precedes the visit for hearing-aid fitting. In this way it is hoped to obtain information about their attitudes before those attitudes have been modified by contact with any professional staff. The current version of the questionnaire has 39 questions seeking information on acceptance of impairment, perception of stigma, motivation, expectation, degree of personal or social withdrawal, role of family and/or friends and strength of personality (Appendix A). Thus a profile on each individual is obtained prior to the provision of the hearing aid. Further information is gathered at the home visit made prior to the issue of the hearing-aid (see Chapter 8) and the degree and nature of the counselling programme is based on this composite picture. The profile may be revised as additional knowledge is gained through reports from volunteer counsellors and at the follow-up visit one month after issue.

Four months after issue an assessment of daily use, performance and satisfaction with the fitted aid is made (Appendix B). These outcome measures can then be correlated against initial attitude.

Similar questionnaire-based data on initial attitude and outcome are obtained for individuals who do not, for administrative and logistic reasons have individualized counselling. These subjects form a control group for assessing the benefits of the counselling programme. Different versions of the questionnaire have also been used on occasion to explore how attitude measures relate to specific descriptors. For example, in an early version the question was asked: 'Do your family and friends get exasperated because of your difficulty in hearing?' The response was positive in almost 100% of individuals. This indicated how frequently hearing loss was a source of mild irritation in social relationships, but did not tell us much about the specific difficulties of the individual. The question was modified, the word 'exasperated' being first changed to 'impatient'. The number of positive responses dropped to 67%. A third version is now employed using the word 'angry'. Around 45% of subjects report that their family and friends are angry as a result of their hearing difficulties. When this question is considered along with another, 'Are your family and friends understanding about your hearing problems?', a group can be identified where relationships appear to be more than normally strained. Hence the limited resources of the counselling staff can be targeted onto those most in need.

Some of the attitude factors will now be reviewed, but again it should be borne in mind that these are only strands in the web of personality that affect the individual's perceptions about hearing impairment and the potential benefits of amplification.

5.1 STIGMA

The dictionary defines stigma as 'A mark of infamy (ill-fame or repute); a disgrace or reproach attached to anyone.' The stigma associated with hearing impairment seems to be of the same historical antiquity as hearing loss itself. As Gilhome-Herbst (1980) observed, probably the most detrimental influence on attitudes towards the deaf came from Aristotle's factually based observation that 'Those born deaf all become speechless. They have a voice but are destitute of speech.' This was misunderstood or misinterpreted as implying that the born-deaf were no better than imbeciles. The 'mark of infamy' in such individuals was the inability to utter normal speech, and this gradually came to be attributed to lack of intelligence. For nearly two thousand years Aristotle has been unjustly blamed for denying the opportunity of education to the deaf.

In medieval times hearing loss was generally regarded, as it is to this day in some cultures, as a direct affliction of the Creator. As such, man could not, and indeed should not, attempt to help the sufferer. Possibly this attitude of passive acceptance has more (but not much more) to commend it than the intolerance of those who viewed the deaf as subhuman.

The stigma of deafness has gradually extended to encompass lesser degrees of hearing loss. There is 'a disgrace or reproach' attached to a diminished ability to communicate in societies in which communication has become the key to social function. Superficially, the hearing impaired are accepted as members of human society, but severe to profound deafness with its associated 'deaf' speech is still frequently, although not intentionally, confused with diminished mental capacity. Hearing impairment of lesser degree is not distinguished by the lay public as anything other than a slightly milder form of the same dysfunction, and thus any hearing loss tends to be regarded as synonymous with a measure of stupidity. Few individuals would admit to accepting the generality of 'deaf, dumb and daft', but behaviour not infrequently belies the denial. The hearing handicapped, as members of the community that has these prevailing attitudes, recognize the stigma attached to hearing impairment, and not wishing to be branded with that mark, seek to deny the existence of the impairment.

When, due to increasing difficulty and family pressure, recognition becomes inevitable, the dominant hope and expectation is that it is a simple matter such as an accumulation of wax. The hope is that 'something can be done' to improve hearing, something that diminishes the difficulties and that does not require the use of a prosthesis. The hearing-aid is perceived as a stigma. A number of studies in the last decade have investigated the possibility that the visual presence of a hearing-aid may elicit negative reactions. Although such studies can be criticized on a number of points the findings suggest that the more obvious the hearing-aid, the more the individual is stigmatized with respect to intelligence, personality, socioeconomic status, achievement and appearance (Danhauer et al., 1985). There does seem, then, to be justification for the desire by the hearing handicapped to have hearing aids that are less and less conspicuous.

In a recent survey of 300 potential hearing-aid candidates, just over a quarter thought that behind-the-ear hearing aids were cosmetically unacceptable, too obvious and conspicuous. For 10%, the degree of concern reached the level of being 'worried' about being seen with an aid. Around 15% expressed the view that the prospect of wearing an aid made them feel older (the average age of the sample was approximately 70 years) or a bit silly.

Use levels four months after issue were obtained for two groups of individuals. One group, the controls, had been supplied with the hearing-aid without follow-up or counselling. The second, experimental group had had not only post-issue counselling, but also a pre-issue domiciliary visit at which worries about stigma were discussed and, hopefully, resolved (Brooks and Johnson, 1981, see also Chapter 6). In the control group, those subjects who had expressed the view that the aid was conspicuous, obvious and cosmetically unacceptable were using the aid 20% less on average than those who found the aid acceptable. In the experimental group, there was no difference in terms of daily use between those who initially thought the aid to be unacceptable and those who had no such feelings. Those subjects who felt that wearing an aid would make them look older were using the aids only just over half as much as the unconcerned subjects in both control and experimental groups.

It seems, therefore, that the counselling currently provided diminishes the stigma directly associated with the aid itself, but is less effective in overcoming the perceptions of the hearing-aid as a token of aging.

What is being done, and what more can be done to minimize the perception of stigma? Miniaturization of hearing aids has undoubtedly made a major contribution to diminishing the stigma, primarily by making the aid less obvious. There may be a second factor associated with the reduction in size. With the older, box-type aids the impression given to the non-hearing impaired was of a crude, inelegant and clumsy device. Hearing aids were a source of thoughtless mirth. The modern behind-the-ear or in-the-ear aid is, to anyone who takes the trouble to consider it, a remarkable example of electro-acoustical development, a high-technology product. This can, of itself, produce a better perception of the aid, and hence a reduction in the stigma associated with it. For a minority of those considering the possibility of obtaining a hearing-aid, the expectation is that the aid they will need is large and obtrusive. The realization that modern hearing aids are truly small and inconspicuous may go a long way towards persuading them to try amplification. For the female patient (and for some of the younger males with trendy, long hairstyles), guidance on concealing the instrument may again be sufficient to overcome the initial reluctance even to try wearing an aid.

For some, a different approach may be justified. This will depend on the assessment of the individual's intelligence, lifestyle and relationships with others. It rejects or reverses the idea of concealment at all cost and suggests that there may be merit in a hearing-aid that is evident, though not obtrusive. The candidate is asked to consider the reaction of the individual seeking to converse with them – the hard-of-hearing person. Perhaps a question has been posed and because their attention was elsewhere, this was not heard at all. A second attempt is made with, probably, a slightly louder voice. This time, the hearing-impaired person is aware of the question, but not sufficiently to make a sensible response. Instead, he responds with some expression such as 'Pardon?'. For the third time, and with growing impatience manifesting itself in tone and quality of voice, the question is posed. Because of the impairment in hearing, only a part of the message is actually heard. A guess is made at the meaning of the enquiry – and the guess may be very considerably wrong. The answer, then, does not relate to the three-times posed question. The questioner, unaware of the difficulty of the hearing-impaired individual assumes that the fault lies at the intellectual level and terminates the interview with a metaphorical, if not a literal, shake of the head or with eyes raised to the heavens as if in supplication! Returning to the hearing-aid candidate, it is suggested that, firstly, the situation would probably not have deteriorated to that level if an aid had been worn and, secondly, that should the situation have been so bad as to require three unsuccessful attempts at obtaining an answer, then the just-visible hearing-aid might have made the speaker realize that the problem lay in defective hearing rather than defective intellect.

For those who perceive the aid as a token of aging, a rather similar line of reasoning may be employed. Failure to hear (i.e. failure to use a hearing-aid effectively) is more likely to be taken as a sign of decreasing intellect than is the presence of a hearing-aid, if the latter enables the individual to remain involved in a wide range of activities. It is the unaided hearing impairment that will lead to age-associated stigma, not the aid.

For a very small minority, the knowledge that rich and famous individuals like former US President Ronald Reagan and former UK Prime Minister Winston Churchill used hearing aids may be a deciding factor in trying amplification.

A major task for the hearing health-care professional must surely be to use every form of publicity to improve attitudes. No opportunity should be missed to correct inaccurate portrayals of the hearing impaired in the media. Likewise, every opportunity should be taken to educate the public and involved professionals. As previously noted, studies in the United Kingdom have indicated that family doctors tend to deter rather than encourage the elderly hearing-impaired to seek for help by means of a hearing-aid, essentially through lack of awareness of the benefits that modern aids, properly supplied, can bring. Education through courses, feedback from successfully rehabilitated patients, or possibly direct mailing may all help to improve the knowledge base and hence, indirectly, the hearing-impaired.

5.2 RECOGNITION AND ACCEPTANCE

It might seem surprising that not everyone coming forward for a hearing aid either recognizes or accepts the reality of hearing impairment. In the pre-issue questionnaire used at Withington hospital, three questions are posed that relate to recognition and acceptance. One question (Appendix A, no. 35) is: 'Do you feel that you are missing out in not hearing some sounds like the song of the blackbird or rain pattering against the window?' Out of 300 consecutive subjects, 273 answered the question and of the latter, 100 gave a negative response. The hearing losses of these individuals were such that it was not likely that they actually heard these quiet sounds. The explanation for their response seems rather to lie in their not being aware that they were not hearing them or that they had forgotten the pleasure that can come from such sounds. Their average amount of daily use assessed four months after the issue was over 30% below that of those giving a positive answer, the difference being highly significant. ($\chi^2 = 20.6$, 3df)

In response to a second question (Appendix A, no. 4). 'In your opinion do people speak as clearly as they did a generation ago?', 30% said that they did not think that this was so. In the group that did not receive counselling, the daily amount of use four months after issue of those who transferred blame to others was down 20% relative to use levels in those who accepted their hearing loss. In the experimental group, the four-month daily use was at the same level in those who initially transferred blame as in those who accepted hearing loss as the reason for their communication difficulties.

Another question that indicates that many potential users, though going forward through the system to the point of delivery of a hearing-aid, have not fully come to terms with their hearing impairment is: 'Do you think your hearing is below normal for your age?' (Appendix A, no. 3). A quarter of the subjects said 'no'. In response to the more searching question, 'Do you think your hearing is absolutely normal?' (Appendix A, no. 24), only 8% gave an affirmative response. Where the response to the latter question was positive, average daily use was down by 20% in the control group subjects, but was not reduced in the experimental group. It seems, therefore, that counselling can help to bring about a realistic acceptance of the hearing impairment.

One approach employed in Manchester commences at the home visit prior to issue of a hearing aid. After preliminary discussion aimed at establishing a friendly relationship with the potential user, it is suggested that a short trial be made with an aid in the home. When the aid has been adjusted to a comfortable listening level, the interview continues with the conversation being, perhaps, about communication within the home. Frequently during the conversation, the individual may be distracted by some sound such as rustling paper, a car passing in the street outside or a bird singing in the garden. It is at such times that realization may slowly dawn that some hearing loss is really present. The clarity of reception when wearing the aid may also bring recognition that acuity is below normal.

Very often, the loudness of the voice diminishes when the aid is switched on, sometimes to such an extent that the spouse, relative or friend present at this home visit remarks on the change. They notice also that the modulation of the voice is better. It is gentler and less aggressive in tone. To the user of the aid it may seem that their voice is louder and different in quality. Explaining the reasons for this helps to bring further awareness of the nature and degree of the hearing impairment and to heighten acceptance.

The recognition of hearing loss is usually most apparent when the aid is removed. The sudden dullness of hearing is commented on. The ease of listening without sitting forward on the edge of the chair and straining to catch each syllable is noted. Scepticism is replaced by a measure of acceptance and even a positive desire to proceed with amplification.

5.3 MOTIVATION

There are two aspects to motivation – motivation to obtain a hearing aid and motivation to use the instrument. The two are so closely interwoven as to be virtually inseparable and can, to all intents and purposes, be treated as one. According to Rupp (1982) strong motivation almost guarantees positive adaptation to a hearing aid. Conversely 'if the patient was forced into appointments with the physician and audiologist by well-intentioned relatives or associates, but maintains a minimal positive attitude, then the likelihood of effective follow-up is markedly reduced.' How frequently is the candidate for a hearing aid self-motivated? Hickson, Hamilton and Orange, (1986) found 30% of their study population of 135 claimed to be self-motivated. Spouse or family were responsible for 24% attending for advice regarding hearing aids. Most of the remainder had gone to their doctor, no doubt with the expectation that 'something could be done' to remove the difficulties and cure the problem. Similar data comes from the Manchester study. Self-motivation is claimed by 24% and a further 23% state that they are reacting to pressure from family or friends. More than half (53%) indicate that they went to their doctor expecting treatment, but not a hearing aid (Appendix A, nos. 1 and 2). Hickson *et al.* did not find any significant relationship between expressed motivation and eventual outcome in terms of hours of daily use, but in the Manchester study, a significant difference was found, though not in the direction anticipated. The 65 subjects who claimed to have set out with the prime intent of obtaining a hearing-aid were using their aids significantly less (p = 0.02) after four months than the rest of the subjects (209) who said either that they had hoped for treatment or were acting as a result of the influence of others. A possible explanation of this unexpected finding may lie in the method of eliciting motivation. When the candidates are seen in their homes (some time after completing the questionnaire but before the issue of the aid), it is evident in a number of cases that even though they claim to have been self-motivated, they are, in fact, reacting to pressure. However, due to pride or stubbornness they are not prepared to admit this. In reality, therefore, they are far from being self-motivated. Experience suggests that perhaps as few as 10% of all persons applying for hearing aids through the NHS are truly acting entirely on their own initiative.

Where the candidate freely admits to reacting to the influence of those who are acting genuinely out of concern for their welfare, the prognosis is usually good. Counselling is more necessary for those who went to their practitioner for advice and in the hope of treatment and who were brusquely told that they would have to have a hearing aid. In such instances the feeling may have been engendered that this is the last resort, and that the prospect of success is poor. Reassurance, and a demonstration of the benefits that can accrue from a well-fitted hearing aid may be all that is necessary in such cases.

The most difficult situation may be where the individual lives in an environment with little auditory stimulation. The motivation for seeking help may be pressure from less well-meaning individuals such as a neighbour who has been driven to distraction by the excessive volume from the TV, or by the relative who visits infrequently, but who complains at having to raise his/her voice to communicate. Ideally, a hearing-aid should be recommended, but there is little personal motivation to wear the instrument in such a situation. Alternative approaches may have to be considered. In the former case, the solution may lie more in the realms of environmental aids – a TV amplifier with headphones or an earpiece. In the latter, both the patient and the relative need help so that a mutual approach can be made to the problem. In an ideal world, the hearing-impaired should be encouraged to use the aid in the widest possible range of situations so that maximum experience in communicating can be gained, but in reality, a compromise usually has to be made.

5.4 EXPECTATION

Most hearing-aid candidates superficially appear to have reasonable expectations as to what the instrument can do to help. Two questions have been asked in the Manchester study to assess expectation (Appendix A, nos. 36 and 37). The first asks, 'How long do you expect it will take you to get used to the hearing-aid?' Three possible answers are available for choice: (a) A day or two. (b) A few weeks. (c) A very long time. No significant difference in amount of daily use four months after the issue was observed in relation to the option chosen (usually either (a) or (b)). Only 15 out of 300 candidates expected to take a very long time to get used to the instrument, but in the event they performed as well as those with 'better' expectations. The second question asks, 'Which of these terms BEST describes how you expect to hear with the aid?' and there are again three options: (a) Quite well after getting used to it. (b) Not very well. (c) Without any difficulty. Only four subjects chose option (b); 226 selected option (a) and 43 opted for (c). No significant difference in use level at four months was observed relative to the option selected.

Undoubtedly, when the aid is supplied a part of the instruction is normally related to adaptation, and realistic targets are discussed at that time. Preconceived expectations do not seem to be so deeply rooted in the majority of those seeking for help with hearing aids that they cannot be brought to a reasonable level. However, there are always exceptions to the general rule. Occasionally one encounters an individual who, regardless of the severity of the impairment, expects that with amplification he/she will hear with the same clarity and facility as a normal hearing person. A careful and patient explanation of the audiogram of that person and the implications of the test results may lead to a more realistic appreciation of the situation. Few persons expect that sight can be restored to the severely vision impaired by the simple provision of spectacles, and analogies such as this may be of assistance in explaining the nature and reality of the problem to certain individuals. In some instances it is the relatives who expect restoration of total hearing function. They anticipate that as soon as the aid is put on, the hearing will be restored to normal and, unless disillusioned, will reproach the hearing-impaired person for not 'listening'. Explanation of the audiogram and its meaning may be helpful in such situations, as may the use of tape recordings of speech made to simulate the effects of different degrees of hearing loss.

5.5 WITHDRAWAL

In response to the question (Appendix A, no. 22) 'When in company do you often get the wrong end of the stick?' around 83% of the potential hearing-aid users admitted that they did. The strength of response indicates that errors and misunderstandings are the common lot of the hearing impaired. In a caring family, or in a company of good and true friends the occasional slip-up may be a source of gentle amusement. Under less auspicious circumstances, the laughter may be at the expense of the hearing-impaired individual. Then that person will feel hurt and diminished.

If the situation occurs repeatedly, the response of the victim may be to withdraw. The first stage may be to withdraw from active participation in the group while retaining as much interest as possible. The hearing-impaired person tries to follow the gist of the conversation, but no longer actively joins in for fear of getting things wrong. In response to the question (Appendix A, no. 32), 'In a group conversation do you keep quiet for fear of saying the wrong thing?' almost four out of five (78%) of those questioned answered in the affirmative. The next stage may be to withdraw subconsciously but not physically. The hearing-impaired individual remains in the group, but abandons all attempts to follow the thrust of the conversation. When asked (Appendix A, no. 31) 'If you are in a situation where several people are chatting, do you give up trying to follow the thread of the conversation?', 72% of hearing-aid candidates said 'yes'. Possibly, to keep a semblance of interest, there may be an occasional nod of the head or, when looked at directly for a response, some non-committal utterance such as 'mm-mm' or 'ah-ha'.

When the strain of even this pretence becomes too great, then physical withdrawal may take place. Efforts are made to avoid getting involved in situations where difficulty is anticipated. Almost two-thirds (64%) of those questioned said that they tried to avoid small talk because of their hearing difficulties (Appendix A, no. 28). Some patients have, in conversation volunteered the information that they resorted to crossing over the road when seeing a neighbour or friend to avoid the difficulty and embarrassment of trying to talk in such circumstances. Others have indicated that before going into the garden to hang out the washing they first checked to see that their neighbour was not in her garden, when failure to converse would be construed as rudeness or ignorance. Such tactics are not always possible. Some situations are unavoidable, for example, family gatherings. While the conversation goes on around the hard-of-hearing individual, they pick up a book or newspaper; they sit back and close their eyes as if dozing or they may even decide to leave the group and retire to another room to watch TV or make a cup of tea. Sadly, the impression created with family or friends is that of disinterest. Not realizing the strain imposed in such circumstances, or the frustra-tion of being unable to keep a toe-hold in the discussion, the other group members feel offended that they have been rejected. So withdrawal leads on to isolation. Around one-third of those questioned admitted that they mixed less, avoided other people and had given up social activities because of their hearing loss. Withdrawal had now become a positive factor. No longer were they merely finding it difficult to keep in company, but they were deliberately shunning the companionship of others. There was an admission by a similar proportion that they tended to stay at home and go out less as a direct result of their hearing impairment. Self-imposed isolation may further lead to ostracism, and bitterness grows.

A few individuals seek to remain in company and avoid the problems stemming from their inability to hear by monopolizing the conversation. A quarter of those questioned admitted to this ploy saying that they tried to control the thread of the conversation. A smaller percentage (10%) admitted that they sought to 'dominate' any discussion (Appendix A, no. 34). This power to dominate requires a strong, even aggressive, personality and though it may appear to be successful, it does not enhance respect or pleasure in one's company.

Undoubtedly, hearing impairment brings much distress through the loss of social contact. Withdrawal is a very real problem that is compounded by additional age-related factors such as diminished mobility, poor health and loss of friends and relatives through death.

On the positive side, those who recognized that withdrawal was taking place tended to make better use of the hearing aids than those who failed to see the signs of impending isolation. Four-month use data indicated significantly higher ($p < 0.01$) daily usage when the questionnaires were answered positively with respect to questions asking (1) if they avoided small talk, (2) if they gave up trying to follow the thread of conversation and (3) if they kept quiet in conversation to avoid saying the wrong thing. Counselling improved use levels in those who answered negatively, but not to the level of those who acknowledged the evidences of withdrawal.

5.6 RELATIONSHIPS WITH FAMILY AND FRIENDS

About three-quarters of those applying for hearing aids live either with their spouse or families. Undoubtedly, these significant others have a substantial influence on the hearing-impaired person. They have probably been the prime movers in getting that person to recognize the existence of a hearing problem – in persuading them to seek advice, and in inducing them to try a hearing aid. Their influence will be substantial in determining what happens after the aid has been supplied. In view of the vital role that families can play in rehabilitation, special considerations will be given to this in Chapter 9.

However, one or two points arising from the questionnaires should be noted. In response to the question 'Are your family and friends impatient with you at times?', the response was positive in 67% of those responding (95% of the whole sample). When the strength of feeling was intensified to 'very impatient' the percentage dropped slightly to 59%, and when the level was raised to 'angry' just 45% replied positively (Appendix A, no. 14). Undoubtedly, hearing loss can produce a great deal of stress in the domestic situation, not only in the hearing-impaired, but also in those near and dear to them. It is interesting to find that the amount of use made of the hearing aid after four months was very significantly related ($p < 0.001$) to the response to these questions. Those responding negatively used the aids considerably less than those responding positively. It may be that among those responding negatively there were families who were more patient and less inclined to become angry over the difficulties encountered. It is at least as likely that the real answer lay in the hearing-impaired individual who failed to recognize the root cause of the impatience in those close to him/her. This view received support from a consideration of self-perception of hearing loss relative to attitude of family and friends. Those who do not perceive their hearing as being below normal for their age tend to report less impatience in their associates than those who accept their hearing as impaired ($\chi^2 = 3.6:1\text{df}$).

Where there is stress in the domestic environment, then counselling may need to be extended not only to the hearing impaired, but also to the other members of the group.

5.7 PERSONALITY

Hearing impairment almost inevitably leads to disability, but the relationship between the two is neither direct nor simple. External circumstances can substantially alter the effect and extent of the handicap. A relatively small hearing loss in a young adult whose work requires extensive communication, may be crippling. It can erode self-confidence, diminish promotion prospects and distort family relationships. A greater degree of hearing impairment in an elderly individual living a self-contained and fulfilled existence may be perceived as creating minimal handicap. However, even where external factors are similar, the degree of disability may be quite different due to personality differences in the individual. Some are able to meet disability head on; to regard it as a problem to be solved, an obstacle to be overcome. At the other extreme, there are those who take hearing impairment as a personal disaster, a major catastrophe, the last straw. Such personality factors are likely to affect outcome in those obtaining hearing aids.

Of those applying for hearing aids in Manchester, approximately 50% stated that they were unable to cope with their hearing difficulty without a lot of embarrassment (Appendix A, no. 12). A similar proportion admitted to feeling upset if others commented about their inability to hear normally (no. 18). These appear to be individuals of more-than-average sensitivity. There is a significant relationship between this tendency to be upset and embarrassed and the trend towards withdrawal from company and keeping quiet for fear of saying the wrong thing ($\chi^2 = 9.8$:1df). The inhibiting effect of hearing impairment is seen also in the responses to the question 'Are you as outgoing and talkative as you were before becoming hard of hearing?' (Appendix A, no. 30). Half of those asked indicated that they were not. Nearly as many (40%) said that they were not as self-confident as they used to be (no. 20).

A higher proportion – almost two-thirds – said that they felt their ability to think quickly had deteriorated since the onset of hearing impairment (no. 21). It is possible but usually not the situation that ability has genuinely deteriorated because of aging. The more likely reason for the apparent deterioration is the insidious effect of encroaching hearing loss. Normal speech contains much that is redundant, even when conveying important information. There is redundancy at the semantic, lexical and phonological levels, but diminished hearing progressively reduces the redundancy. Firstly, the soft fricatives and sibilants may become inaudible, resulting in occasional confusions and mistakes. With increasing deterioration of hearing, the number of clues to the subject matter further declines. The hearing-impaired individual then has to build up the context from isolated fragments – rather like seeing the picture in a jig-saw puzzle when only a fraction of the pieces are present. But building up the picture in this way takes time – and hence the perception that the thought processes are slowing up. Increasing the number of clues improves the speed of response – and the provision of a hearing aid with counselling support is the most effective tool for that purpose.

In a very small number of subjects, the frequent mistakes and constant rebuffs can give rise to an almost total loss of self-esteem. Unaware of the extent and nature of their hearing impairment but very conscious of the fact that they are failing repeatedly to grasp what is said to them, they begin to believe that their mental faculties are failing. Fortunately, in such cases, the provision of a correctly fitted hearing aid with appropriate counselling can work wonders, not only for the hearing, but also for the bruised personality. Indeed, the long-term use data indicate that in those who recognize their loss of confidence, their growing introversion, their embarrassment and difficulty in coping, in such individuals the level of use is significantly higher than in those who either have not reached that stage of withdrawal or who do not recognize the effects of their hearing loss in terms of personal diminishment.

5.8 THE WHOLE PERSON

A somewhat analytic approach has been adopted in looking at attitude factors relevant to hearing impairment and rehabilitation. When seeking to assist an individual, the separate strands can be identified and to some extent quantified, but in designing an approach to that individual's rehabilitation, all the factors must be considered together. Some will wish to know the nature and extent of their hearing loss in order that they can comprehend the effects it has on their ability to communicate. From that base of factual knowledge, a step-by-step model for rehabilitation can be constructed. Others may have little interest in the mechanics of the problem, seeking only for answers to specific difficulties.

Forming a profile based on attitudes and including other data can be helpful in preparing the rehabilitative approach to each person. Accompanying this must be adequate technical knowledge so that the hearing aid is tailored to that individual's need. Auditory rehabilitation can only be fully effective when the two strands of personal insight and technical skill are combined.

REFERENCES

Brooks, D.N. and Johnson, D.I. (1981) Pre-issue assessment and counselling as a component of hearing aid provision. *Brit. J. Audiol.* **15**, 13–19.

Danhauer, J.L., Johnson, C.E. Kasten, R.N. and Brimacombe, J.A. (1985) The hearing-aid effect. *Hear. J.* **38**, (3), 12–14.

Gilhome-Herbst, K. (1980) Psycho-social consequences of disorders of hearing in the elderly in *Medicine in old age; hearing and balance* (ed. R. Hinchliffe), Churchill Livingstone, Edinburgh.

Hickson, L., Hamilton, L. and Orange. S.P. (1986) Factors associated with hearing aid use. *Aust. J. Audiol.*, **8**, 37–41.

Rupp, R. (1982) Predicting hearing aid use in maturing populations: the feasibility scale. *Hear. Aid J.*, **35**, (1), 10–15.

APPENDIX A
Hearing assessment questionnaire

For questions 1 & 2 please circle either (a) or (b)

1. When you first went to your doctor about your hearing, was this
specifically to see about getting a hearing aid? .... (a)
or
in the hope of having treatment other than an aid? .... (b)
2. IF your ideas was specifically to obtain a hearing aid, was this
your own idea, uninfluenced by anyone else? .... (a)
or
as a result of continued pressure from relatives or friends? .... (b)

For questions 3 to 35 please circle either YES (Y) or NO (N)

3. Do you think your hearing is below normal for your age? .... Y/N
4. In your opinion do people speak as clearly as they did
a generation ago? .... Y/N
5. Can you hear children's voices as clearly as you would wish to? .... Y/N
6. Do you feel that if you concentrated harder you would hear more? .... Y/N
7. Do you get upset if you cannot follow the conversation? .... Y/N
8. Does the thought of wearing a hearing aid make you feel older? .... Y/N
9. Do you go out as much as you did before becoming hard of hearing? .... Y/N
10. Does your poor hearing sometimes make you feel inadequate? .... Y/N
11. Are you concerned about being seen wearing a hearing aid? .... Y/N
12. Can you cope with your hearing problem without a lot
of embarrassment? .... Y/N
13. Are you looking forward to getting a hearing aid? .... Y/N
14. Do your family and friends get angry because of your hearing
difficulty? .... Y/N
15. Have other people's comments made you unhappy about
getting an aid? .... Y/N
16. Do you think behind-the-ear aids are tiny and *IN*conspicuous? .... Y/N
17. Do you feel OTHERS associate wearing a hearing aid with stupidity? .... Y/N
18. Do you feel hurt if people comment on your hearing difficulty? .... Y/N
19. Are you constantly ignored because of your hearing difficulty? .... Y/N
20. Are you as self-confident as you were when your hearing was normal? .... Y/N
21. Do you think as quickly as you did before becoming hearing impaired? .... Y/N
22. When in company do you often get the wrong end of the stick? .... Y/N
23. Do you get into regular arguments about the loudness of the TV? .... Y/N
24. Do you think your hearing is absolutely normal? .... Y/N
25. Do your family or spouse frequently tell you to listen harder? .... Y/N

26. Do you think your family and friends find it a strain talking to you? .... Y/N
27. Do you mix less with others (not family) because of your hearing loss? ..... Y/N
28. Do you try to avoid small talk because of your difficulty in hearing? .... Y/N
29. Do you dread meeting new people since becoming hearing impaired? .... Y/N
30. Are you as outgoing and talkative as you were before becoming
     hearing impaired? .... Y/N
31. If you are in a situation where several people are chatting, do you
     give up trying to follow the thread of the conversation? .... Y/N
32. In a group conversation do you keep quiet for fear of saying
     the wrong thing? .... Y/N
33. Are your family and friends understanding about your hearing
     problems? .... Y/N
34. Do you try to dominate conversation so you don't have to listen? .... Y/N
35. Do you feel you're missing out in not hearing some sounds,
     like the song of the blackbird or rain pattering against the windows? .... Y/N

For questions 36 to 39 please circle either (a) or (b) or (c)

36. How long do you expect it will take you to get used to the aid?
        A day or two .... (a)
        A few weeks .... (b)
        A very long time .... (c)
37. Which of these terms BEST describes how you expect to hear
     with the aid?
        Quite well after getting used to it .... (a)
        Not very well .... (b)
        Without any difficulty .... (c)
38. Which of these terms BEST describes your hearing loss?
        Not a serious problem at all .... (a)
        A grievous burden .... (b)
        A difficulty that can be overcome with help and determination .... (c)
39. How would you rate yourself in terms of hearing?
        Hearing-impaired .... (a)
        Hard of hearing .... (b)
        Deaf .... (c)

THANK YOU FOR YOUR HELP

IT WILL HELP US TO HELP YOU

APPENDIX B
Four-month hearing-aid review

NAME: .... AGE: ....

Do you live: (a) With your spouse   (b) With family or relatives   (c) Alone   (d) Other

---

1. Do you use your aid ....
   - (i) Every day
   - (ii) Most days
   - (iii) Some days
   - (iv) Only occasionally
   - (v) Not at all

---

2. When you wear the aid, do you use it ....
   - (ii) All day long
   - (ii) Most of the day
   - (iii) About half the day
   - (iv) Less than half the day
   - (v) Only short periods

---

3. How many hours a day do you think you use it on an **average day**
   - (i) Less than 2
   - (ii) Between 2 and 4
   - (iii) Between 4 and 8
   - (iv) More than 8

---

4. Have your family, friends and close associates been helpful to you in getting used to the aid?
   - (i) YES
   - (ii) NO
   - (iii) There is no-one to help me.

---

5. Are you getting more enjoyment out of life since you obtained the hearing aid?
   - (i) YES
   - (ii) NO

---

6. In the following situations, how do you rate the hearing aid? Please circle the appropriate word.

   (a) In person to person conversation: Very Good/Good/Average/Poor/Useless
   (b) In a group of family or friends at home: Very Good/Good/Average/Poor/Useless
   (c) Listening to music: Very Good/Good/Average/Poor/Useless
   (d) Listening to TV (or radio) news: Very Good/Good/Average/Poor/Useless
   (e) With a group of people in noisy
       conditions (i.e. club, bus, pub, etc.):   Very Good/Good/Average/Poor/Useless

---

7. Please indicate – by putting a circle around them – which of the following words or expressions describe your feelings NOW about the hearing aid and its use: ....

   DIFFICULT TO INSERT: CONSPICUOUS: HELPFUL: TIRESOME: MAKES ME LESS TENSE:

   BOOSTS MY CONFIDENCE: MAKES ME FEEL STUPID: EASY TO USE: NOT VERY HELPFUL:

   NOISY: DIFFICULT TO MANIPULATE: BENEFICIAL IN COMPANY: UNCOMFORTABLE:

   INVALUABLE: UNNECESSARY: INDISPENSIBLE: RFGRET NOT OBTAINING ONE SOONER:

---

8. Please try to assess your satisfaction with the hearing aid on the ten-point scale below. Circling 1 means that you are totally **dis**satisfied. Circling number 10 means that you are completely satisfied. Try to assess how satisfied you are:

   Totally
   Dissatisfied   1   2   3   4   5   6   7   8   9   10   Completely Satisfied

---

Please write on the other side of this page any comments you have about any aspect of the hearing aid, or of the service you have received. Such comments, whether good or bad, help us to improve the service we provide.

Thank you for your help.

JN 687

6

HEARING-AID FITTING – PRE-FITTING CONSIDERATIONS

Denzil Brooks

In the previous chapter consideration was given to some of the factors contributing to the attitude of the potential hearing-aid user. Each individual hearing-aid candidate may manifest each of these to a different degree, a reality implicit in the use of the term 'individual'. Nevertheless, to a certain extent, specific attitudes and behaviours tend to cluster together and form common patterns or types of subject. Goldstein and Stephens (1981) suggest that there are four basic types of subjects who come forward for hearing aids.

The Type I subject is positive, looking forward to the aid as a helpful step towards restoration of communication and keen to commence the process of rehabilitation. Interest and involvement can be taken for granted. There is minimal need for attitude modification.

The Type II individual is essentially positive, but not as straightforwardly so as the Type I. Expectation may have been prejudiced by contact with an unsuccessful hearing-aid candidate or by uninformed opinion about the difficulties of using an instrument. Worries about stigma, possibly based on misconceptions about the size and visibility of the aid may be present, especially if in employment; even more so if there is any element of job insecurity. There may be submerged fears about the effects of regular use of a hearing-aid on residual hearing, or that such use may make the ears 'lazy'. In this group, Goldstein and Stephens also include those with positive attitude but difficult audiometric configurations. The latter may include unusually small hearing losses, losses in the high frequency only, and unilateral losses as well as the more bizarre patterns seen only rarely. For such configurations of hearing loss, the potential benefits of amplification need to be considered alongside the undoubted disadvantages of hearing-aid use. In such situations, it is wise to indicate beforehand that obtaining the maximum benefit from amplification can sometimes be an extended procedure involving a number of trials.

Type III subjects, though seeking help for their communication difficulties, are essentially negative towards the hearing-aid. As seen in the consideration of attitude, there may be a failure to accept the hearing loss as real, transferring the blame for all difficulties to others or to circumstances. There may be deep-seated resentment at having to wear something that is perceived as being a hallmark of old age (and encroaching senility), or at being persuaded against their will to accept any help for the difficulties they experience. There may even be resentment at having the even tenor of life disturbed, even though that life was becoming ever more restricted.

Fortunately, Type IV subjects are rare, at least at the clinical level. These are individuals who reject the whole concept of help, be that a hearing aid or any other rehabilitative measure. Such individuals only arrive at the point of delivery of service after strenuous efforts by family, relatives or other carers, but unless there is some degree of flexibility, the whole effort is doomed to failure.

Goldstein and Stephens (1981) suggest that about two-thirds to three-quarters of subjects fitted with aids may be categorized as having an essentially positive attitude – Type I. The majority of the remainder are seen as fitting the description of Type II.

In a later paper (Stephens, 1982), the distribution of attitude types in a population of new applicants for hearing aids was described. It was slightly less optimistic than the original assessment, but still suggests an essentially positive attitude in those seeking for help through amplification. Just under 5% were categorized as Types III or IV, the majority of these being in Type III. The bulk of the candidates were distributed almost evenly between attitude Types I and II.

In the rehabilitation scheme developed in South Manchester, a questionnaire is sent to all hearing-aid candidates before their first attendance at the hospital clinic. One question asks if the individual is looking forward to getting a hearing-aid, and 76% indicate that they are. When asked how well they expect to perform with the instrument, 83% expect to do 'quite well'. By contrast, only 1.5% expect not to hear very well with the aid and 6% expect to take a very long time to get used to the aid. Kapteyn (1977) has shown that those who do take a long time in adapting to a hearing aid tend to be poor users and to benefit less from the aid than those who adapt rapidly. Thus a broad measure of agreement can be seen between the Manchester data and Stephens's London data with the majority of potential candidates for hearing aids being basically positive in attitude.

However, underlying the basic positive attitude are some concerns and worries. Of the potential aid users in Manchester, 24% were *not* looking forward to getting a hearing-aid, although perceiving the need for some help with their communication difficulties, and 20% were concerned at being seen wearing a hearing aid, of whom half indicated that the thought of being seen wearing an aid worried them. When asked the question 'Does the thought of wearing a hearing aid make you feel older?', 16% responded positively.

Thus, although basically positive in their attitude towards the need for remediation, there are substantial numbers of candidates with very real concerns and worries about the use of amplification. These concerns and worries should be allayed before the aid is provided, otherwise the process of rehabilitation will be delayed and the prospect of ultimate success diminished. There is good reason to suggest that rehabilitation should commence before the aid is provided, and should be concerned with ensuring that attitude, motivation and expectation are optimized before proceeding to the actual fitting of the amplification system. The system in operation in South Manchester will be described in Chapter 8, with some indication also of measured benefit.

6.1 THE FITTING PROCESS

The provision of a hearing aid has two major aspects – technical and personal.

(a) Technical aspects of the fitting

The technical process commences with the examination of the ears by a suitably qualified medical specialist. This is desirable as there are many conditions in the adult that might require some form of remediation other than, or in addition to the provision of a hearing aid. Wax in the ear canal is a common problem, especially so in the more elderly and in those in institutional care. In the study by Martin and Peckford (1978), over 27% of residents in homes for the elderly were found to have wax in one or both ears. Hart (1980), in a review of 1152 residents in both private and social services homes for the elderly, reported that when examined by an otologist, 33.4% had wax occluding the external meatus. Milne (1976) reported wax as a significant factor in 49% of men and 38% of women in a random sample of 489 persons over the age of 62 years. The high incidence of wax is relevant, not only in terms of the possible hearing loss it might create in addition to the basic organic deficit, but also because it may conceal other, possibly serious conditions such as attic perforation or discharge. Furthermore, the presence of wax will militate against making a good earmould, which is vital to success with any hearing aid. If wax is not removed, it may be responsible for early onset of acoustic feedback with all the consequences implicit therein.

In addition to the incidence of wax there are other less-common conditions of which the hearing-aid provider should be aware. Active disease of the middle ear is fortunately rare – under 1% in the Hart (1980) study. Obviously it is unwise to proceed with a hearing-aid fitting in such circumstances, except where medical clearance has been given. Perforations may be present in as many as 2–7% (Hart, 1980; Milne, 1976) and although normally not creating any obstacle to fitting an aid, medical clearance for proceeding with the fitting of an earmould is advisable.

Medical examination is also necessary to ensure that the hearing problem is not secondary to some more fundamental disorder or symptomatic of some condition for which treatment might be appropriate instead of or in addition to the provision of amplification. All potential hearing-aid users should first be encouraged to obtain a qualified medical opinion. Perhaps a cautionary note may be added. The medical opinion should be confined to medical aspects of the hearing loss. Regrettably, too often, the opinion is also expressed that a hearing aid will be of little or no assistance, an unjustified opinion based on inadequate knowledge of the benefits of amplification. Such an opinion should be disregarded.

The technical process of hearing-aid fitting will then proceed to an evaluation of the hearing loss and, in all probability, the recommendation of a hearing aid. In Chapter 4 Denis Byrne described the procedures that lead up to the 'prescription' of the aid. Having decided on the configuration appropriate to the individual in terms of the hearing aid(s) and earmould(s), an impression or pair of impressions will be necessary. There are several texts outlining the procedures vital to the production of a high quality earmould. (Berger, 1984; HAAG, 1984; Fifield, Earnshaw and Smither, 1980).

Undoubtedly a poor earmould can destroy all the effort put in to achieve the best technical hearing-aid fitting. The impressioning needs to be precise, the instructions to the processing laboratory equally precise, and the materials and production techniques employed by the laboratory of the highest quality.

(b) The personal aspects of hearing-aid fitting

Preliminaries

The potential hearing-aid user, though basically positive in outlook, is likely to be apprehensive. The majority of adults seeking for a medical opinion about their communication difficulties hope that some cure can be effected by the doctor (Brooks, 1972). Frequently, they are shocked to hear that their hearing is defective and that the condition is irreversible and progressive. Too often their question: 'But I don't need a hearing aid, do I?' is answered with some remark such as 'Not yet – your hearing is not very bad.' Even when the problem is not deferred, the shock of being told: 'There is nothing we can do to cure you. You'll have to have a hearing-aid' can be traumatic. Hearing aids are for 'old' people. Wearing an aid is an admission to oneself and others that one is old – with all that is implied in that admission. Ideally, the news should be broken gently and with a more upbeat emphasis. The doctor or specialist who is responsible for telling the hearing-impaired person that medicine and surgery cannot overcome the hearing loss should present the hearing aid as a logical method of assistance on a par with spectacles for vision defects. The stark statement, 'You are deaf and will have to have a hearing aid' can be like a blow in the face – and the person fitting the aid may be the one who has to heal the wounded personality.

Even if some time has elapsed between the announcement by the medical practitioner of the need for an aid, and the actual fitting visit, the subject is likely to be worried. 'Do I really have to have an aid? Will it show? Do I have to wear it outside or in company?' Recognizing these underlying fears and worries is vital to a successful first meeting between the dispenser of the aid and the subject. The patient should be greeted with a cheerful voice, a genuine smile and a warm handshake. Eye contact should be made and held for a few moments. The person should be courteously ushered into the room and offered help if necessary.

The room should not be clinical. Ideally it should be as like a home as possible. Carpets, curtains to the windows and pictures on the wall all add to the homeliness and hence help to produce a relaxed subject. In fostering the same non-clinical atmosphere, the fitter should preferably not wear a white coat, which tends to give a pseudo-medical appearance and to increase rather than relieve tension. Instead of a desk and office-type chairs, it is preferable to have a table and easy chairs, though these should not be too low in view of the difficulties many elderly persons have in getting up and down from very soft, low armchairs. The lighting should be good and arranged so that the face of the instructor/ audiologist is well illuminated to assist speechreading. It should not need to be said that the room should be quiet, situated away from sources of noise such as an air-conditioning plant or lift machinery! Some external indicator that a patient is being interviewed is also advisable in order that other staff or patients do not knock and enter, thus breaking the train of events and disturbing concentration.

For the majority of potential hearing-aid users, be they elderly, middle-aged or young, a close relative or friend should be encouraged to accompany the potential user. Unless there are indications to the contrary, it is desirable for that person to join in the session, particularly if the person is the spouse or a relative living with the hearing-impaired individual. In such circumstances, the hearing problems are usually joint problems. One person may be unable to hear clearly; the other has difficulty in getting messages across. Both are handicapped in communication and both can contribute to the rehabilitation process. Explanations about the hearing aid and potential benefits are valuable to both. Realistic expectations can then be explored and established. Tactics to improve communication can be discussed in addition to the use of the aid.

Having ushered the parties into the room, some introductory remarks unrelated to the hearing-aid fitting are often helpful in breaking the ice. The weather may be a fair opening gambit, but other remarks may be related to the subject's means of transportation, or general health. From this point, the conversation can be led gently into some enquiries about aspects of communication. Information about the medical and audiological aspects of the hearing should be to hand, but the essentials should have been committed to memory. If the professional fitting the hearing aid is constantly having to check up on basic information, the confidence of the potential user will be diminished. If the professional has not only briefed him/herself on the technical aspects of the fitting, but has also some more personal knowledge of the candidate's feelings and perceptions, a better rapport is likely to be achieved. Ideally therefore, information should also be available on the subject's attitude, motivation, expectation, personality, etc. This can, to some extent, be acquired beforehand from questionnaire-based investigations, and the questions at interview can be used to further explore that individual's needs and hopes.

The ability to actively listen is vital in a counsellor – and the word is used advisedly because the individual fitting the hearing aid must needs be a counsellor also. 'Listening' in this context includes not merely perceiving the sounds of the words, but also the nuances that underly the statements or questions. In its broadest sense it will include not only the acoustical aspects of listening, but also the physical attitude of the patient, the tensions in posture as well as in expression and vocalization. It will include the responses, spoken or silent, of the accompanying 'significant other'.

With active listening there must needs be empathy, a non-judgemental understanding of the individual's feelings. It may seem ludicrous that the old lady of 90, confined to a wheelchair and resident in a local authority home, is vain about the prospect of wearing a hearing-aid that can be seen, but the feelings are real, deeply felt and worthy of respect.

The counsellor may try to rationalize the attitude, but the approach must be with understanding and not merely authoritative. It may be counterproductive to state that other people of the same age wear aids without such concerns, or that aids are much better now than they used to be. It is better to explore the reasons for the worries and fears, to accept their reality and possibly to suggest that embarrassment can come in different guises. The embarrassment in wearing the aid might conceivably be less than that brought about by constant repetition of 'pardon', or worse, the blank look of incomprehension or the irrelevant answer following a dimly perceived question.

In the younger candidate, there may be fears about using the aid at work. A little good-natured joking can be accepted by all except the most sensitive individuals, but if the humour is tinged with malice, the situation is very different. Only the candidate can anticipate with any reliability the reaction of colleagues, but undoubtedly the more experienced they are in handling the instrument and in coping with sound, the better the prognosis is likely to be. A further concern may relate to security of employment. 'Will I be able to cope with my work with the aid?' The answer to this question requires some knowledge of the nature of the work, and the counsellor can and should discuss this, explaining in what situations the aid will be most helpful and where benefit may be limited, perhaps due to background noise.

Other fears that may emerge even before the aid is considered relate to the use of the instrument. Will it make the ears lazy? Will regular use cause a deterioration in the hearing? Once again these worries should not be treated as trivial or silly. Depending on one's judgement of the potential user, an answer may be given in rational or even scientific terms. Usually reassurance backed up by a logical explanation is adequate. The relaxation brought about by easier, aided listening may be contrasted with the tensions involved in straining to hear unaided. Parallels may be drawn between the skill of effective listening and other skills where practice improves performance and neglect results in deterioration. For the more scientifically orientated, the concept of disuse atrophy and evidence regarding the safety of amplification may be considered.

Concerns such as those indicated should be dealt with before proceeding to a consideration of the aid itself, otherwise they will remain as inhibitory factors, diminishing the value and benefit of the hearing aid and hence reducing the potential for rehabilitation. Sanders (1975) puts the situation succinctly in his statement: 'Even the most advanced technology is completely useless if through ignorance, negative attitudes, or unrealistic expectations, the hearing aid is improperly used, or, as not infrequently happens, is not worn at all.'

Proceeding then to the fitting process, it should not need to be stated that all necessary preparations for the fitting should have been made before ushering in the candidate. The aid(s) and earmould(s), the explanatory information and any accompanying papers should all be to hand. Relevant tools and accessories should be within easy reach – screwdrivers for adjusting controls, scissors, a hand or wall mirror, a dummy ear with earmould for demonstration purposes, a supply of batteries, etc. The individual can then be introduced to the aid.

It is unnecessary at this stage, for the majority of hearing-impaired persons, to explain the nature and degree of their hearing loss. This is best considered either before the fitting, perhaps at the medical interview, or at some later stage. At the fitting visit, time is inevitably limited, not primarily by constraints on the hospital or clinic staff (although such constraints may be very real) but by the concentration span of the hearing-impaired individual. A young adult may be able to absorb a great deal of information during a fitting visit, but bearing in mind that the great majority of those seeking hearing aids are elderly, a shorter attention and retention span must be recognized and taken into account. There is a certain amount of information to be imparted at the introductory visit that is essential. An understanding of hearing loss, even the hearing loss of the specific individual is not generally an essential part of that information. Time should therefore be concentrated on aspects of the hearing aid and its use that are most relevant during the first days or weeks of possession, such as the basic controls and inserting the earmould correctly. Time should be concentrated on appropriate patterns of adaptation and wise choice of situations for use. Other, more sophisticated aspects of use, and the interesting but not fundamentally essential aspects of hearing correction can be deferred to further visits, and it is assumed that such visits will be arranged. Supplying a hearing aid in a single session, without structured follow-up, is a practice to be deplored.

Basic instruction

A considerable amount of information has to be imparted to the potential hearing-aid user. A booklet should be supplied at the time of issue so that the new user can have a source book of information to which he/she can refer later about any points in doubt. Even with this back-up, it is desirable that the maximum amount be heard and retained at the initial fitting. There is wisdom therefore in using amplification during the actual period of instruction about the instrument. It is not practicable to employ the aid to be supplied as a means of communication during the fitting and to use it at the same time for demonstration purposes. There is considerable merit in using, for demonstration purposes, an aid of identical type to the one being supplied as the 'listening aid'.

Behind-the-ear aids are, with the exception of the USA and Canada, still the most commonly supplied type of instrument. Hence the ensuing discussion will be centred around postaural aids. In-the-ear and in-the-canal aids will require some modification to the method of issue and instruction.

After explaining what is about to happen to the subject, the earmould can be placed in the ear, the aid placed behind the ear and the appropriate length of the tubing estimated and connected. The controls on the aid should already have been adjusted to the proposed settings, based on the fitting protocol adopted. The earmould can then be inserted, and the aid snugly placed behind the ear. With the volume control set to minimum, the aid is switched on. The gain is then adjusted while talking to the subject. A comment that the speaker's voice sounds hollow, or that there is an echo effect suggests that some slight reduction in gain is required. Once a comfortable level has been achieved, the aid can usually be temporarily 'forgotten' and effort concentrated on the instructional aspects of aid provision.

The second aid can now be used to demonstrate the position of the essential user controls – the switch and gain control. All aids supplied by the National Health Service, and many commercially available aids have a three-position switch marked O–T–M. At the first instructional stage, especially with elderly adults, it is probably advisable to suggest that the 'T' setting be disregarded. The switch can then be viewed as a simple on–off control. There is a real danger that if too much information is imparted at the initial interview, the less-important aspects crowd out the really vital points. Explanation of the function of the T setting and when and how to employ this type of input is best left to a follow-up visit. Volume-control rotation for increasing and decreasing gain can be demonstrated both visually and physically. The subject can get the feel of the controls without, for the moment, disturbing the adjustment of the aid being worn.

Programming use Advice on when and how to use the aid can and should be given at this time. A carefully structured approach to using the instrument is essential in view of the fact that most potential users have a poor recollection of the nature and extent of environmental noise. A study in the UK (Brooks, 1979) revealed that the average period of time from first noticeable indication of hearing loss to point of delivery of service for those applying for NHS aids was 16 years. Even if the period is considerably less than this, it is likely that the new aid user will have forgotten quite how 'unquiet' is the world to which he/she is returning. Unless forewarned they may well be taken aback by the sounds that the normal-hearing person takes for granted and hears only at the subconscious level. Depending on age and adaptability, the new user should be strongly advised to use the instrument in the home only for a period of a week or two to a month or two. At home, the environment is normally reasonably quiet and reasonably controllable. Outside, one can be assailed by sudden, uncontrollable noises – the overflight of a noisy jet, the rasp of a motorcycle exhaust or the barking of a dog. Such noises are best avoided until skill has been developed in quickly and efficiently adjusting the gain control.

The best time and place to commence using the instrument is normally at home, in the evening, when listening to a single source of sound. A practicable suggestion is to put it on when settling down to viewing the TV. At this point, a problem may well arise – getting the earmould into the ear. For this reason, if for no other, it is helpful to have a relative, preferably the spouse, daughter or son, or a close friend at the fitting session. They can then be shown how to tell if the earmould is in correctly, and how to insert it if need be. Ideally, the new hearing-aid user should try and insert the earmould, but frequently the necessary degree of skill is lacking. We suggest that two or three attempts be made, but if unsuccessful, then help should be sought from the spouse or other informed person. Continuing to struggle with a recalcitrant earmould will probably result in mounting frustration and irritation, and a sore ear. Better to seek help on that occasion, and try again the next evening. It may take several days or even weeks before the skill is acquired to efficiently and swiftly insert the mould, but with patience and help that skill will come.

Once the earmould has been inserted, the aid can be switched on and adjusted for volume. For the elderly, this can be a difficult operation, not only because of the small size of the volume control, which can be hard to adjust with stiff, insensitive fingers, but also with respect to getting the level of amplification at the optimum level. New users tend to underestimate the degree of amplification they require, setting the level more in relation to background noise than to speech. It is suggested that, where possible, the sound level of the TV be set by the non-hearing-impaired individual to a normal listening level instead of at the level that probably has been customary for the hearing-impaired person. If the new user lives alone, it may be difficult for them to know what is 'normal'. The help of a friend can be valuable in such a situation, in setting the volume level of the TV and, perhaps, drawing attention to that position of the volume control. Alternatively, a softly ticking clock may be used to set the gain before settling down to using the aid with the TV.

For the first few evenings, the new user should be encouraged to experiment with the gain control. This is to get some 'feel' for the range of movement, the sensitivity and the degree of adjustment needed for different levels of input. The aid might then be worn for an hour or two, depending on the feelings of the user. Some may well find that after a time, the ear feels peculiar. The earmould is noticeable as a foreign body. The ear feels warm. Others may find the experience of hearing so many things tiring. They may wish for a little peace and quiet. Such feelings can be anticipated and profitably discussed. It is understandable that, at first, the sound and feeling of the aid/earmould will be strange, but the way to get used to this strangeness is by practice. So the new user should be encouraged to repeat the experience the following evening – and the next evening – and the next. They should be encouraged to increase the time of use gradually, though still only within the home. They should also be discouraged from missing out use on the odd day. It is too easy for the 'odd day' then to become a regular event. Learning to use an aid may be likened to learning to play the piano. Regular practice is essential. If the student misses out odd days, the tutor knows because performance deteriorates. So with the aid, practice makes perfect. Soon, both the feeling and the amplified sound becomes acceptable. Indeed, hopefully, they become the norm.

Once the controls have been mastered, which may take a few days, then some further experience-gathering is suggested. Persons supplied through the Withington Hospital Clinic are given a 'sound list'. This itemizes a number of sounds that can be heard in most homes, and the new user is advised to seek out these sounds and identify them, sounds such as the striking of a match; water running into the sink; the ticking of the clock; the click of a cupboard door; the sound of a spoon stirring in a cup; footsteps on a hard floor; the flush of the toilet. Seeking out the sounds in this way helps in building up a knowledge of environmental sounds. The characteristics of those sounds can then be lodged in the memory and called forth when the sound is heard next. This reduces the distracting effect of background sounds at other times, such as when in conversation.

With a younger individual, the process may be accelerated somewhat, but the basic advice remains the same. Use the aid only in the home at first. Gain experience with handling the controls and with identifying environmental noise before launching out into wider and more extensive use.

While explaining the tactics for the first month or so, a view of the longer-term objective should also be given. The limited daily use is only a short-term measure. For most candidates the long view is for full-time use. This often requires explanation, as many potential users feel that their needs are restricted to just one or two specific situations. They only want the aid for going to the club, for visiting the family or for when friends call to see them. Such unrealistic ideas have to be dispelled – gently, but firmly. A hearing-aid cannot be used effectively under such circumstances, and the reasons for this have to be explained. Allowing the individual to go away with such illusions is dishonest and can only lead to disappointment. It is vital to explain carefully that listening is a highly developed skill that can be maintained only by constant practice. The sifting of the meaningful from the meaningless cannot be performed by the hearing aid. A simple illustration often helps, and one frequently employed in the Manchester area concerns those persons who live close to the railway. When first moving into the house, the regular passing of the trains was disturbing. Conversation stopped. Sleep was disturbed. But within a few days, a process of adaptation took place. Soon the trains were no longer noticed. Only when a visitor drew attention to the noise were the residents aware of the passage of the trains. The sounds were still heard as loudly as before, but they were no longer listened to. In other words, to adapt to environmental noise requires regular experience of those sounds. Occasional exposure will not generate the listening skill essential to easy conversation in the presence of background noise.

Hence, the long-term objective put before most potential aid users is that of regular use. The merit of wearing the aid when in the house alone is described. Only in this way will the occasional caller at the door be heard. And only in this way will the hiss of the gas fire, the hum of the fridge and the ticking of the clock fade into the background, allowing more relevant sounds to enter the forefront of consciousness.

The earmould   Having covered the basic controls of the aid and outlined a programme of use for the first few weeks, attention may then be turned to the earmould. This can be a source of difficulty for many new users, especially the elderly. The earmould is complex in shape, the ear canal is also complex in shape, and inserting the mould into the canal can be taxing on skill and patience. As already noted, the assistance of spouse or relative can be invaluable, but it should not be regarded as a substitute for learning to insert the mould oneself. A particularly useful role of the relative is to ensure that the mould, when inserted by the user, is correctly positioned. The majority of earmoulds used with postaural hearing aids have an upward projecting tip that slips into the helix/anti-helix groove. This provides anchorage to the earmould/aid combination. Many first-time users fail to position this tip behind the helix, placing it on the surface of the skin instead. This may seem a trivial point, but in fact may be the make-or-break for the aid. When so placed, the mould is liable to slip out, and this is particularly so if the individual wears spectacles. As the side arm slides over the ear the tubing is pushed, and the aid falls to the floor. Leaving aside the possibility of damage to the aid, the reaction of the user is to become irritated at the trouble the aid is causing. Another problem with incorrect insertion is that the earmould will be positioned incorrectly in the ear canal. It will be at a slant, and as such may well create pressure points in the canal, and also on the skin where the helix tip lies outside the fold of the auricle. A further likely outcome of an ill-fitting or poorly inserted earmould is acoustic feedback. There will be a tendency for sound to leak around the mould giving rise to howling, a potential cause of embarrassment and a source of distortion in the performance of the aid. Correct insertion is vital to long-term comfort and efficiency.

Where difficulties persist, a different approach to earmould insertion may be necessary. The increasing gap technique outlined by Corcoran (1984) is especially helpful in such situations. In this approach, the usual method is reversed. Instead of starting by having the aid/mould on the table and proceeding from that point to pick it up in a specific manner and lift it to the ear canal, the teaching begins with the mould in the ear and the aid snugly behind the pinna. The new user is encouraged to feel the mould, then to grasp the tubing close to its point of emergence from the mould, but not to remove it. Instead, they are shown how to ease the back of the mould out from close contact with the concha, but then to slip it back again. In this way contact with the concha is maintained. Once confidence in that manoeuvre has been developed, the next stage is to ease the mould a little further out, but not to the point where physical contact between the tip of the mould and the skin of the ear is lost. Again, the mould is re-inserted, and the step repeated until confidence is assured. The next step may be to actually break contact, but not to move away from the immediate vicinity of the pinna. Thus slowly, and in a progressive manner, always working from an established base of confidence, the earmould can be removed, brought to the front, and placed on the table.

The technique may take 10 to 15 minutes for an elderly individual lacking in dexterity and confidence, but that is a small time to contribute if the end result is a competent and satisfied user.

At the initial visit it is wise to give some information about what to do if things go wrong. The probability of breakdown for the hearing aid is very low, but there are other difficulties that can arise during the first few weeks, and these should be covered at this time, and reinforced at a later stage.

Wax in the earmould is a common problem, not necessarily in such quantities as to completely block the sound passage, but sufficient to worry some individuals who are meticulous about cleanliness and hygiene. They should be shown how to remove the wax with something like a cocktail stick – pointed, but not too sharp. Likewise they can be shown how to detach the earmould from the aid so that it can be washed in warm water, and a caution should be given that water is not to be allowed to enter the aid.

When and how to change a battery should obviously be explained at this time, and especially with the elderly, care should be taken that the correct method of inserting the battery is understood. If the aid is a high-power model, it may also be necessary to explain that zinc–air batteries may be unsuitable, although this piece of information might well be left until the follow-up, provided this is not too long after the issue.

New users should be cautioned against using hair sprays, lacquers, etc. near the aid, as these can stick up the controls and damage the casings. Even where aids are provided at no direct cost to the patient, a sense of responsibility should be encouraged. Hearing aids are expensive and should be treated with care and consideration.

Follow-up A number of considerations discussed in the preceding passage suggest that some review of the new hearing-aid user is essential. When that review should be is dependent on the assessment made of their likely progress. A young or relatively young individual may make excellent progress over the first few weeks. A review at one month after issue might be adequate. An elderly person living alone with little help from anyone might be best reviewed after a week or ten days. If the review is deferred until a month after supply, frustration with the earmould, volume control or switch may have so built up that no amount of additional help can undo the damage.

The review session is normally best conducted at the clinic where facilities exist for modifications that might be deemed necessary, but for the elderly client as noted above, a domiciliary visit may be preferable. If the purpose of the visit is essentially to assist with the initial difficulties experienced with an aid, then the use of a trained voluntary counsellor may be sufficient. The use of such counsellors will be discussed in Chapter 8.

As suggested above, a period of from one month to six weeks after initial issue is a reasonable interval for a review. It is valuable at the beginning of the session to ask the new user how they have fared with the aid; what their feelings have been; and whether they have had any problems. Indeed, with some first-time users, the suggestion may be made at the initial fitting that a note be made of any difficulties encountered with the aid, or any puzzling features. These can then be brought to the review session. From either the verbal or written comments, it might become apparent that some modification is needed to the aid characteristics. For example, individuals with somewhat reduced dynamic range may initially require a substantial amount of compression for comfort. After a period of experience in listening with the aid, tolerance increases and the compression can be reduced somewhat. Similar changes may take place with regard to high-frequency emphasis, more being tolerated as the ear/brain becomes accustomed to a less-deficient, high-frequency content than was experienced before amplification. Careful listening by the audiologist may reveal other areas where counselling, either to the hearing impaired or to the family, might improve enjoyment and communication.

Hopefully, in the first few weeks, the new user will have learnt to insert the earmould, to regulate the volume efficiently and to differentiate between background noises in the home and the sounds that have relevance and meaning. Having checked that this is so, then a programme of more extended use can be discussed. Use should include groups of people if this has not already been tried. Use outside should be considered, but under carefully controlled conditions at first – in the garden, at church, in quiet streets are suitable introductions to external use. Use in very noisy conditions such as on busy roads or in public houses, bars or noisy restaurants should be deferred until much more experience has been gained.

At this session, the use of the T setting may be explored. Many theatres and churches have now installed loop systems for the benefit of hearing-impaired patrons or parishioners. The merits and demerits can be discussed and the system tested (provided the clinic has a functioning loop system). The various ways of using a hearing-aid with the public telephone system can also be considered. The position of the microphone should be demonstrated so that the telephone receiver can be placed in the most efficient position for acoustical transfer.

In the protocol operating in the author's hospital, it is at this time that consideration is given to the possibility of speechreading as an adjunct to amplification. As already indicated, the philosophy of the audiology department in the hospital is that the primary approach to minimizing the disability brought about by hearing impairment is the provision (with appropriate counselling) of a hearing-aid that has been individually tailored to the requirements of the client. If, after this reasonable period of trial, it appears that further assistance is needed, and if the hearing-impaired individual is willing and able to attend classes in speech-reading, then referral is made to the instructor.

If, on the other hand, it appears that that need might be more appropriately met by provision of suitable environmental aids, then these will be discussed and tried.

Fitting an aid is a process that irrespective of age cannot be rushed if one conscientiously seeks to help the candidate to an effective level of rehabilitation. The professionals involved must have an appreciation of the attitudes, expectations and perceptions of the client and take these into account in structuring the rehabilitation. They must be adaptable, pacing the information to the capacity of the listener.

REFERENCES

Berger, K.W. (1984) *The hearing-aid. Its operation and development*, 3rd edn, National Hearing Aid Soc., Livonia, Mich.

Brooks, D.N. (1972) The use and disuse of Medresco hearing aids. *Sound*, **6**, 80–5.

Brooks, D.N. (1979) Counselling and its effect on hearing aid use. *Scand. Audiol.*, **8**, 101–7.

Corcoran, A. (1984) Teaching earmould fitting. In *The earmould. Current practice and technology*, Hearing Aid Audiology Group, British Society of Audiology, Reading, Berks.

Fifield, D.B., Earnshaw, R. and Smither, M. (1980) A new ear impression technique to prevent acoustic feedback with high powered hearing aids. *Volta Review*, **82**, 33–9.

Goldstein, D.P. and Stephens, S.D.G. (1981) Audiological rehabilitation: Management model I. *Audiology* **20**, 432–52.

HAAG (1984) *The earmould. Current practice and technology*. Hearing-Aid Audiology Group, British Society of Audiology. Reading, Berks.

Hart, F.G. (1980) *The hearing of residents in homes for the elderly – South Glamorgan*. University Hospital South Wales.

Kapteyn, T.S. (1977) Satisfaction with fitted hearing aids. I. Analysis of technical information. *Scand. Audiol.*, **6**, 147–56.

Martin, D.N. and Peckford, R.W. (1978) Hearing impairment in homes for the elderly. *Social Work Service*, **17**, 52–62.

Milne, J.S. (1976) Hearing loss related to some signs and symptoms in old people. *Brit. J. Audiol.* **10**, 65–73.

Sanders, D. (1975) Hearing-aid orientation and counseling. In *Amplification for the hearing impaired* (ed. M.C. Pollack, Grune and Stratton, New York, pp. 323–72.

Stephens, S.D.G. (1982) Audiological Rehabilitation – extending the model. Memorandum of the Royal National Throat, Nose and Ear Hospital, London.

7

BINAURAL AIDS

Denzil Brooks

A complete chapter is being devoted to binaural aids to emphasize the importance of this form of assistance to the bilaterally hearing-impaired. It is relevant and instructive as an introduction, to consider the professional and public attitude towards alleviation of a different form of sensory handicap such as vision impairment. From the time of the invention and development of lenses to correct vision, it has been the accepted practice to compensate both eyes as effectively as possible. The wearing of a monocle has never been adopted as a routine method of treatment, being seen rather as an indication of eccentricity. At no time has the concept of having lenses for both eyes had to be justified on the grounds of cost/benefit relative to one lens only.

Partly for historical reasons, the approach to compensating hearing loss has been a much less-straightforward process. Ear trumpets were usually used for one ear only to leave one hand free for other activities such as writing. The development of the electrical amplifier was the most important step in providing help for the hearing-impaired, but early aids were large, cumbersome and ugly. No-one would choose to wear two such bulky devices. Thus the concept of single-ear assistance became firmly rooted in the minds of the public and the professionals involved, and consequently, has been accepted as the norm by health administrators. When aids were reduced to the size that could be worn at or in the ear, the philosophy remained essentially monaural. Even now, two or three decades later, the prevailing attitude of many health-care providers is still that one aid is sufficient.

Yet, as Bentzen (1980) stated 'When we fit a monaural hearing-aid on an individual with a bilateral hearing loss, we are trading one handicap for another.' The pioneering work of Bentzen in Denmark has gradually changed attitudes, and the benefits of binaural assistance are now being appreciated by a growing proportion of the hearing-impaired.

The potential benefits of having two ears are many, but can these benefits be realized by hearing-impaired persons wearing two hearing aids? Specific aspects of binaural hearing will be considered and information on aided benefit reviewed.

7.1 ASPECTS OF BINAURAL HEARING

(a) Binaural summation of energy

At hearing threshold the effect of using two ears rather than one produces an increase in sensitivity of about 2.5 dB (Hirsh, 1948; Tempest, Bryan and Marsh, 1968). Normal listening is usually at supra-threshold levels and the summation effect rises to 6–10 dB in the mid-level range (Reynolds and Stevens, 1960). For a person with normal hearing, binaural summation of energy may appear to be of minimal significance, but for the hearing impaired these small gains confer a number of benefits in terms of hearing-aid use. Primarily, to achieve the desired level of comfortable listening, the gain controls on the two aids can be set at lower levels than for a single aid in the same situation. This diminishes the probability of acoustic feedback, which is not only a potential source of embarrassment to the user, but also a significant factor in reducing the effectiveness of a hearing aid. As harmonic distortion is related to output and hence gain level, lower gain reduces the amount of distortion in the output, especially if the aid(s) are being used towards the upper end of the gain-control span. With lower gain, output is less likely to reach loudness discomfort level, thus increasing comfort in use and diminishing the (admittedly unlikely) possibility of further damage to hearing from high-output levels.

(b) Binaural summation of information

Having two inputs should double the probability of receiving information. Evidence to support this hypothesis comes from studies on filtered speech. Bocca (1955) presented speech to one ear at a level such that only about 30% was discriminable. To the other ear, he presented the same speech material after passing through a 500 Hz low-pass filter, and at an intensity level such that around 30% was again discriminable. When the stimuli were presented binaurally the discrimination score improved substantially, demonstrating the summation of information with binaural inputs. Since Bocca's initial investigations, many researchers have developed tests for assessing central auditory dysfunction based on integration of binaurally presented signals (for a review of these see Korsan-Bengtsen, 1973). Further support for binaural integration of information came from Groen and Hellema (1960) in their studies on binaural speech audiometry. They observed that the speech performance versus intensity ogive was steeper for the binaural condition than for either ear independently, as predicted by probability theory.

Are these benefits realized for the hearing-impaired user of binaural hearing aids? Ross (1980) reviewed 19 studies in which speech-discrimination scores obtained binaurally and monaurally were compared. He concluded that clinical research had demonstrated the superiority of the binaural condition, although the extent of benefit is difficult to quantify, depending very considerably on the exact details of the test protocol.

Franklin (1975), using split-band amplification demonstrated significant improvements in consonant recognition scores when the two bands were presented binaurally (i.e. one band to each ear) as compared to presenting both bands simultaneously to the same ear.

Support of a somewhat subjective nature comes from performance ratings of monaural versus binaural listening in different situations. Brooks (1984) obtained assessments on a five-point scale ranging from 'very good' through 'good', 'average' and 'poor' to 'useless' from 150 experienced binaural and 296 monaural-aid users. Similar situational ratings were also sought from 125 persons with hearing self-judged to be within normal limits. For listening situations where there was a single sound source without competition from noise, the ratings of the binaural users were not significantly different from those of the normal-hearing individuals. The monaural user ratings were notably poorer. Where there was a small amount of competing noise, the binaural rating lay below that for normal-hearing listeners, but above that for the monaural-aid users.

(c) Improved localization

Normal-hearing individuals are able to localize sounds in the horizontal plane to within approximately one degree. This high degree of accuracy is achieved by using interaural time and phase difference cues from low to mid-range frequencies and interaural intensity differences from higher frequencies. In a monaural fitting the likelihood is that only one ear will be effectively receiving acoustic information and that no significant interaural cues are available for localizing the source of sound. Binaural amplification should restore the potential for interaural cueing.

Markides (1977), after a most detailed and thorough investigation of binaural benefit stated 'There was a remarkable improvement in localization ability with two hearing aids as opposed to one.' Byrne and

Dermody (1974) likewise found that localization with binaural aids was far superior to localization with one aid, though somewhat less accurate than localization ability of normal-hearing individuals. Westermann and Topholm (1985) suggest that with in-the-ear hearing aids, localizing skill approaches normal levels, the ability improving with experience.

(d) Improved intelligibility of signal in noise

In 1950, Koenig noted a reduction in the masking effect of noise on a signal when switching from monaural to binaural listening, and used the term 'squelch' to describe this effect. The degree of benefit experienced depends on the aspect relationship of the sound and noise sources. In the monaural condition, the most unfavourable situation will be where the noise is on the axis of the better ear and the signal on the axis of the poorer ear. Not only is the signal at the side of the poorer ear, but to reach the better ear it has to overcome the 'head shadow'. This monaural disadvantage can be distressing, indeed almost catastrophic in some situations, such as at a dinner party where one's host sits on the side of the impaired ear. It is possible, to some degree, to overcome the problem by turning the head through almost 180°, but this is an impracticable approach in situations such as that described above. In the opposite situation, there may be some monaural advantage (and monaural listeners frequently use this effect, for example, lying in bed on the better ear to eliminate the noise of snoring from one's spouse).

The magnitude of the squelch and head-shadow effect has been investigated by many researchers with different results dependent on the experimental conditions. Markides (1977) assessed the binaural advantage attributable to squelch as between 1.5 and 2.5 dB. For head shadow the effect was greater at 6 to 7 dB. Byrne and Dermody (1974) found the binaural squelch to add about 7% to speech-discrimination scores, and the head-shadow effect contributed 11%. Valente (1982) reviewed a number of studies on squelch and head shadow and suggested that the binaural advantage was of the order of 3 dB for the near-ear condition (equivalent to the signal being on the side of the aided ear) and up to 16 dB for the far-ear condition (equivalent to the signal being on the side of the unaided ear). This may represent an improvement in discrimination of from 10 to 50%, depending on the nature of the speech signal and the competing noise.

(e) Quality of sound

Even though in some studies there has been little evidence of measurable improvement in performance (possibly due to a poor choice of test material and listening conditions) there is no doubt that many hearing-impaired persons prefer the use of two aids rather than one. Killion (1982) suggests that a very important reason is that with two aids, the quality of sound is better. He cites some experimental work on sound-quality assessments of 16 amplification systems. At one extreme there was a very high-fidelity amplifier/speaker system; at the other extreme a $5 pocket radio. When one channel of the binaural listening system was switched off, the subjective quality ratings fell dramatically. In the monaural condition, even the high-fi systems were rated as poorer than all the systems heard binaurally, except for the $5 radio, which was driven into severe overload. In the study reported above (Brooks, 1984), binaural-aid users rated listening to music on a par with normal listeners. Monaural-aid users gave lower ratings.

(f) Enhanced frequency discrimination

Average binaural frequency discrimination is considerably better than in monaural listening (Versteegh, 1954). In that speech perception is dependent to a substantial degree on recognition of frequency changes, this advantage should significantly assist the individual with binaural inputs.

(g) Increased speed of response

Groen and Hellema (1960) stated that when performing speech audiometry, there was a very marked difference in response time between the monaural and binaural conditions. In the rather difficult test situation of listening for isolated words close to threshold, each acoustic clue perceived has to be weighed up and related to linguistic knowledge. Probabilities have to be judged before making a response. The studies of the above authors indicated that judgements were quicker and more accurate in the binaural than in the monaural condition. Causey and Bender (1980) noted that binaural-aid users were significantly faster in their responses in a test of localizing ability than were monaural users.

(h) Ease of listening

Over 30 years ago, Bergman (1957) noted that binaural listening was adjudged as easier by hearing-impaired persons fitted binaurally. In a follow-up study of 204 persons supplied with binaural postaural aids in the Manchester region, Brooks and Bulmer (1981) listed 18 possible descriptors and requested users to circle those regarded as most apposite to their experience. Of the 155 who said they were using the binaural aids regularly, 36 (23%) circled 'relaxing'. Even in the irregular and non-user category, four of the 49 subjects indicated this as a feature of binaural aids. In the same study, 111 (72%) of the regular users indicated that binaural aids were superior to one aid; 68 (44%) indicated that localization was improved, and 64 (41%) that using two aids boosted their confidence. In a replication of this study Briskey (1982) reported 22% finding binaural aids 'relaxing' and 36% 'confidence boosting'.

However, for the author, the most convincing demonstration of the benefits in terms of ease of listening came from a professional colleague. This audiologist had been hearing-impaired for the largest part of his adult life. His audiogram indicated a bilateral loss of around 60 dB in the low frequencies falling to 75 dB at the higher speech frequencies. For over 20 years an aid had been worn in the left ear with a considerable measure of success. However, at professional meetings he would never ask a question from the floor, partly because he was unsure as to whether someone else had already asked that question, and partly because he would often be unable to hear the reply, a situation that could be particularly embarrassing if that reply included a question to him. Adapting to binaural aids was a process that took a number of weeks, as the right ear seemed at first to contribute little information, only noise. Once full integration was achieved, communication improved dramatically, especially in group situations. He became a lively contributor at professional meetings, seemingly no longer inhibited from asking questions. He stated that his general standard of health had improved, a fact that he attributed to the very strong sense of relaxation derived from use of the binaural system. In company he no longer had to watch faces with the same intensity to see who was speaking. With the two aids, his directional ability was excellent, and localization of the speaker almost instantaneous. Since that time, some ten or a dozen years ago, similar reports have been made by other binaural users. There can be little doubt that ease of use is a very significant benefit deriving from the use of binaural aids.

(i) Dominant ear benefits

Kimura (1967) suggested that although both ears are connected with each cerebral hemisphere, the right ear has a more efficient connection with the speech area in the contralateral temporal lobe. The left hemisphere normally is dominant in the processing of verbal information and therefore there should be a right-ear advantage for speech material.

Thus fitting a hearing-aid to the left ear when hearing loss is symmetrical might be to the disadvantage of the user.

Noonan and Axelrod (1981) found that ear preference was more strongly influenced by minor environment and instrumental factors than by 'eardness'. For example, telephone listening was strongly influenced when there was an expectation of having to take down a message. The phone was then held in the left hand to leave the right hand free for writing. Surwillo (1981) similarly found a left-ear preference for telephone use in those who made heavy use of the telephone and suggested that these findings cast doubt on the supposed advantage of right-ear listening. Alhuwaizi (1983) tested two groups of patients with symmetrical hearing loss to whom hearing aids had been issued. The groups were closely matched on an individual basis with the major difference being the ear fitted. For one group the aids had been fitted to the left ear; for the other group to the right ear. Using speech in noise, use data and subjective responses judged by questionnaire, no significant difference was found between the two groups. Even if there are subtle differences not revealed by the rather simplistic speech tests employed in these studies, binaural fitting is more likely to ensure that any dominant ear effect is preserved than is monaural fitting.

7.2 BINAURAL CANDIDACY

With so many potential advantages why is not every candidate for amplification recommended to use, and supplied with two hearing aids? One basic reason has been indicated above. The prevailing attitude of those responsible for providing hearing aids is that one aid has been conventional in the past and that, by tradition and practice, one hearing-aid is sufficient. This attitude has received support from some publications by eminent audiologists who have reported studies showing no advantage from binaural amplification under specific test conditions. It is no surprise therefore to find the US Bureau of Consumer Protection (1978) stating in its Final Report to the Federal Trade Commission:

Audiologists are less enthusiastic principally because of the dearth of clinical evidence for binaural superiority. The advantages cited for binaural amplification include improved localization ability, better speech discrimination ability, greater ease of listening and better sound quality. These advantages are essentially subjective and therefore often cannot be demonstrated with existing clinical techniques

The thrust of this, and of the policy of health-care administrators tends to be that if some advantage cannot be proven by current test practices, but is only reported by the majority of subjects tested, then that advantage cannot be accepted. However, a new dimension has been added to the situation as a result of a law suit in the United States. A hearing-impaired individual was struck by a moving vehicle from the side on which there was no hearing aid, his audiologist having recommended only one instrument for him. He argued (apparently successfully) that, had he been issued with binaural aids, the accident could have been avoided. Further suits are being brought against audiologists who recommended only one hearing aid on the basis that quality of life would have been significantly better had two instruments been recommended (and worn).

Assuming that the attitude of the service providers who advocate only monaural instrument provision can be rectified, is the implication that every candidate for amplification should be fitted binaurally? No. There are good and valid reasons as to why binaural aids are not suitable for every individual seeking help with their hearing deficiency. These reasons become more explicit when the diversity of characteristics of the individuals who make up the hearing-impaired population are considered. Several factors then become apparent that either preclude the use or limit the applicability of binaural aids. These can be classified under three broad headings of technical, physical and attitudinal problems.

7.3 TECHNICAL CONTRA-INDICATIONS TO BINAURAL FITTING

(a) Asymmetry

Obviously asymmetry can occur with an infinite range of possibilities, not all unsuited to binaural aids. If one ear is close to normal there is clearly no need for amplification on that side. Conversely, if one ear has a total loss of function it cannot be aided. A CROS configuration may be beneficial to the individual with this impairment, but two aids (or two microphones, one on each side of the head) would not provide true binaural hearing. Between these extremes there are two primary elements contributing to asymmetry, degree of loss and audiometric shape or slope. Additionally, there may be differences in speech-discrimination capacity, in tonal perception (diplacusis), and possibly in other more subtle aspects of auditory perception.

A number of authors have suggested that a difference between the average thresholds on the two ears of 15 dB or more should be taken as contra-indicating binaural hearing aids (Pollack, 1975; Briskey, 1980; Davis and Haggard, 1982). Others have suggested that benefits may accrue from binaural use where greater degrees of asymmetry exist (Bentzen, 1980; Byrne, 1980; Markides, 1980; Mercola and Wenke-Mercola, 1985). The evidence cited in these studies suggests that even with quite marked asymmetry some benefits may accrue from the use of binaural aids, but that the probability of benefit is greater as the two ears approach complete symmetry. The decision as to benefit with degrees of assymmetry greater than 15 dB becomes a cost/benefit decision that will depend for an answer on the resources available.

Where the asymmetry is in shape rather than by degree, Markides (1980) found that subjects with a relatively flat hearing loss on one ear and a steeply falling audiometric pattern on the other derived little benefit from binaural aids. However, the range of aids used to compensate for the hearing loss was limited. It is possible, indeed probable, that with amplification tailored closely to the requirements of each ear the benefit might have been greater. Contrasting with the findings of Markides, Byrne and Dermody (1974) reported advantages in fitting binaural aids to persons who had better low-frequency hearing on one ear combined with better high-frequency hearing on the other. By fitting both ears, a wider frequency range of effective hearing could be provided than was possible with a single-ear fitting.

(b) Diplacusis

Markides (1977) reported that subjects with pitch differences between the ears exceeding 10–15% in the speech frequency range, derived no benefit from binaural amplification. Fortunately this degree of diplacusis is rare. Jones and Pracy (1971) suggest that diplacusis is only significant in individuals with sensorineural loss with recruitment. The majority of the subjects tested by Markides had sensorineural hearing loss, although there were a few subjects with conductive loss that appeared to have diplacusis. Usually, but not always, the loss was assymmetrical.

(c) Retro-cochlear and central impairment

There is general agreement that amplification of any kind is of less benefit when the hearing deficit lies central to the cochlea. The problem in such subjects lies in the processing of the incoming signal, not in the reduction of intensity, and consequently amplification, either monaural or binaural, is less likely to be of benefit.

7.4 PHYSICAL LIMITATIONS TO BINAURAL FITTING

(a) Organic limitations

The use of binaural aids may be made more difficult by a number of physical conditions such as hemiplegia, frozen shoulder, arthritis, loss of digits or upper limbs and chronic discharge of one or both ears. However, it should not be assumed automatically that such conditions preclude the use of two aids. A blind, one-armed lady in her 80s was successfully fitted with two aids at the author's hospital. At first there was considerable difficulty experienced in inserting the earmould into the ear on the side of the missing arm. With help and determination, a highly successful outcome was achieved. Each case must be treated on its own merits.

(b) Age associated limitations

Hearing impairment is strongly associated with advanced age, and with increasing years come many problems. Finger-end sensitivity diminishes through deterioration or loss of touch receptors. For the person who wears only one hearing aid, the approach may be to fix the volume control of the aid at a comfortable level or to rely on the carer to adjust the gain to a comfortable level, either on the basis of the numbers on the gain control, or by carefully monitoring the response to the live voice. Such approaches tend to be less practicable for binaural aids and the general recommendation in such cases, with regret, has to be for a single hearing-aid.

7.5 ATTITUDINAL PROBLEMS OF BINAURAL FITTING

(a) Poor motivation

Among the elderly in particular, there are those who, though they have the fine-motor control to handle delicate controls on the hearing aid, yet lack the motivation to use binaural aids. If they are satisfied that their limited needs are being met by a single aid, then their wishes should be respected. The potential benefits of binaural aids should be explained to them, but the final decision remains theirs.

(b) Aberrant attitude

Many persons, indeed probably the majority of those with hearing impairment, will recoil in horror if the suggestion is made that they should use two hearing aids. 'I'm not that bad' is the usual response. Binaural aids are perceived as necessary only for those with the most severe degrees of hearing loss. With this knowledge in mind, there is much to be said for a softly-softly approach to the idea of binaural fitting.

If the individual has a suitable audiometric configuration and does not appear likely to have significant difficulty in manipulating the controls of the aid, then a comparison may be drawn between their hearing disorder and the commoner types of visual impairment. Where short or long sight occurs it is usually of roughly the same magnitude in both eyes. The optician or optometrist will then, in the vast majority of cases, prescribe a pair of spectacles. The suggestion that a monocle might be adequate would be rejected as ridiculous. Monocles are for the eccentric. Moving on from this standpoint the potential binaural user may view the prospect with more favour, recognizing the appropriateness of assisting both ears to achieve balanced listening.

Although many persons with symmetrical hearing loss will accept the force of the argument for two aids, not all will concede to that argument and proceed to the (seemingly) logical conclusion of accepting two aids. Some, though themselves convinced of the logic of the proposition, will reject the idea of wearing two aids because, they believe, other persons will be unaware of the reasons for their having a binaural system. They opine that colleagues or friends will assume that their hearing problem must be severe for them to have to wear two instruments. Other suitable candidates are reluctant to try two because 'I've never seen anyone else with two'. They fear that they will be regarded as freaks. Some potential binaural aid users initially reject the second aid on the basis that they feel unable to cope with two lots of controls.

In such instances it is worth reviewing the potential benefits of binaural amplification, not so much to try and persuade them to change their mind there and then, but to plant a seed in the mind. The hope is that in time, when the benefits of the first aid have been realized, it will mature so that the concept of wearing two aids may be reconsidered. It is better that the trial with two instruments be delayed in this way than that too much pressure be applied too soon. In such circumstances the reaction may be to discard even the one aid. A structured programme for reviewing monaurally aided patients is recommended in order that those whose reluctance to try two has disappeared can be reviewed and provided with the second instrument. The second aid may be provided on a trial basis: if no benefit is achieved after a reasonable period it can be returned without penalty.

7.6 BINAURAL AIDS FOR TINNITUS

Although the majority of hearing aids are supplied to help compensate for diminished acuity in hearing, there are increasing numbers being supplied to assist individuals afflicted with tinnitus. In that the majority of those with this distressing complaint also have some degree of hearing loss, a well-fitted hearing aid may bring considerable relief from the head noises. Where the hearing loss (and the tinnitus) is binaural, supplying a single hearing aid may bring considerable benefit on the aided side, but frequently the subjects indicate that the tinnitus has now 'switched' to the unaided ear. In such cases binaural fitting should be considered.

The treatment of tinnitus is considered at greater length in Chapter 13.

7.7 BINAURAL FITTING PROCEDURES

A question to be considered with regard to binaural-aid fitting is, should the two aids be provided together as soon as amplification is accepted, or should there be an interval between the provision of the first and the second aid? Experience with unilateral fittings shows that many individuals, especially those who are more elderly and who have limited dexterity, take many days to learn how to insert the earmould and manipulate the controls of the aid. It would seem likely that for such persons, the difficulties of manipulating two aids and, in particular, the difficulty of achieving balance between the two units, would suggest staggering the provision of the two aids. Once the basic hand skills have been mastered for the first aid, their acquisition for the second will usually be only a matter of days. Having found how to achieve the optimal gain setting for one aid, balancing the second to provide a central sound image is fairly straightforward. If too long an interval is allowed between the issue of the first and second aids, difficulty may arise in adaptation. If the delay amounts to several months, then the central processing may well have adapted to unilateral input and the use of a second aid will require a further period for adaptation to binaural inputs. Bentzen (1980) stated that both methods (simultaneous issue of both aids and staggered issue) were employed in their programme at Aarhus, Denmark. One prescribing doctor fitted the second aid after a period of three to four months; others commenced amplification with two aids. A follow-up extending over several years indicated that the second method resulted in more rapid acceptance and higher long-term success. However, the report does not indicate whether eventual success depended on the age and adaptability of the subjects. Our experience in Manchester, also over several years, is that a small interval of a month or so does not diminish eventual success. On the contrary, as noted above, it is easier for many elderly persons to adapt to a second aid once the skills necessary for effective use of a post-aural aid have been acquired.

A second consideration has to do with the attitude of the potential binaural user. As noted above, if there is some reluctance to accept two aids, for whatever reason, it is unwise to try and pressure that individual on the basis of professional expertise, however enthusiastic one may be about the potential benefits. Too much pressure exerted too soon can deter a patient from trying. A softly-softly approach is therefore adopted for such individuals.

Where the hearing loss, though symmetrical, is relatively small the use of skeletal, open earmoulds can be helpful, not only by improving the acoustics of the aid/mould combination, but also by reducing the visibility of the earmoulds.

At the one-month, post-issue, follow-up visit the merits of two aids may be mentioned, but if the response is still cool, then further discussion of the topic is abandoned. If the review at four-months post-issue indicates that the person is using the aid with satisfaction and for substantial periods of time, then once more a tentative suggestion regarding binaural use may be made. Not infrequently, having found that public reaction to the hearing-aid is less extreme than had been feared; having also found that the aid is a very considerable help in a wide range of circumstances, but that sometimes a little more help would be welcome, there may be a willingness to give binaural aids a trial.

If there is still reluctance at the four-months post-issue visit, a further attempt to convince of the merits of binauralism may be made at the 12-month review. Those who still resist the idea are informed that should they at any time change their minds and decide to give two aids a trial, the clinic will always be willing to arrange that trial and give full support. Enthusiasm in the audiologist, based on experience, is un-doubtedly a vital factor in encouraging the wider use of binaural hearing aids and, in consequence, easier, better listening for the hearing impaired.

REFERENCES

Alhuwaizi, F.H. (1983) Cerebral dominance and hearing aid fitting. Unpublished MSc. thesis, University of Salford.
Bentzen, (1980) Binaural hearing-aid applications – Denmark. In *Binaural hearing and amplification* (ed. E.R. Libby), Zenetron Inc., Chicago, Vol. II, pp. 133–57.
Bergman, M. (1957) Binaural hearing. *Arch. Otolaryngol.*, **66**, 572–8.
Bocca, E. (1955) Binaural hearing: another approach. *Laryngoscope*, **65**, 1164–71.

Briskey, R.J. (1980) Selecting and fitting a hearing-aid: binaurally. In *Binaural hearing and amplification* (ed. E.R. Libby), Zenetron Inc., Chicago, Vol. II, pp. 187–204.

Briskey, R.J. (1982) A consumer evaluation of binaural hearing aids. *Beltone Colloquy*, **6**, 1–5.

Brooks, D.N. (1984) Binaural benefit: when and how much. *Scand. Audiol.* 237–41.

Brooks, D.N. and Bulmer, D. (1981) Survey of binaural hearing-aid users. *Ear Hear.*, **2**, 220–4.

Byrne, D. (1980) Binaural hearing aid fitting: research findings and clinical application. In *Binaural hearing and amplification* (ed. E.R. Libby), Zenetron Inc., Chicago, Vol. II, pp. 23–73.

Byrne, D. and Dermody, P. (1974) Binaural hearing aids – findings of a three-year study. Paper presented to ASHA Conference, Las Vegas.

Byrne, D. and Dermody, P. (1974) An incidental advantage of binaural hearing aid fittings – the 'cross-over' effect. *Brit. J. Audiol.*, **8**, 109–12.

Causey, G.D. and Bender, D.R. (1980) Clinical studies in binaural amplification. In *Binaural hearing and amplification* (ed. E.R. Libby), Zenetron Inc., Chicago, Vol. II, pp. 75–96.

Davis, A.C. and Haggard, M.P. (1982) Some implications of audiological measures in the population for binaural aiding strategies. *Scand. Audiol.*, suppl. 15, 167–179.

Franklin, B. (1975) The effect of combining low- and high-frequency passbands on consonant recognition in the hearing impaired. *J. Speech Hear. Res.*, **18**, 719–27.

Groen, J.J. and Hellema, A.C.M. (1960) Binaural speech audiometry. *Acta. Otolaryngol.* **52**, 397–414.

Hirsh, I.J. (1948) Binaural summation and interaural inhibition as a function of the level of masking noise. *Amer. J. Psychol.* **61**, 205–13.

Jones, R.O. and Pracy, R. (1971) An investigation of pitch discrimination in the normal and abnormal hearing adult. *J. Laryngol. Otol.*, **85**, 795–802.

Killion, M.C. (1982) Transducers, earmolds and sound quality considerations. In *The Vanderbilt Hearing Aid Report* (eds G.A. Studebaker and F.H. Bess). *State of The Art Research Needs. Monographs in Contemporary Audiology*, Upper Darby, Pa., pp. 104–11.

Kimura, D. (1967) Functional asymmetry of the brain in dichotic listening. *Cortex* **3**, 163–78.

Koenig, W. (1950) Subjective effects in binaural hearing. *J. Acoust. Soc. Amer.* **22**, 61–62.

Korsan-Bengtsen, M. (1973) Distorted speech audiometry. *Acta Otolaryngol.*, suppl. 310.

Markides, A. (1977) *Binaural hearing aids*, Academic Press, London.

Markides, A. (1980) Binaural hearing aids: results of a four-year experiment. In *Binaural hearing and amplification* (ed. E.R. Libby), Zenetron Inc., Chicago, Vol. II, pp. 97–110.

Mercola, P. and Wenke-Mercola, C. (1985) A new test for determining binaural candidacy. *Hear. J.*, **38** (3), 19–26, 31.

Noonan, M. and Axelrod, S. (1981) Eardness (ear choice in monaural tasks): its measurement and relationship to other lateral preferences. *J. Aud. Res.* **21**, 263–77.

Pollack, M.C. (1975) Special applications of amplification. In *Amplification for the hearing impaired* (ed. M.C. Pollack), Grune and Stratton, New York, chap. 7.

Reynolds, G.S. and Stevens, S.S. (1960) Binaural summation of loudness. *J. Acoust. Soc. Amer.*, **32**, 1337–44.

Ross, M. (1980) Binaural versus monaural amplification for hearing-impaired individuals. In *Binaural hearing and amplification* (ed. E.R. Libby), Zenetron Inc., Chicago, Vol. II, pp. 1–21.

Surwillo, W.W. (1981) Ear asymmetry in telephone-listening behaviour. *Cortex*, **17**, 625–32.

Tempest, W., Bryan, M.E. and Marsh, J.A. (1968) Binaural advantage at the absolute threshold of hearing. *Int. Audiol.*, **7**, 294–301.

Valente, M. (1982) Binaural amplification. *Audiology – A Journal for Continuing Education*, **7**, 79–93.

Versteegh, R.M. (1954) Frequency modulation and the human ear. Thesis (Utrecht). Cited by Groen and Hellema. Op. cit.

Westermann, S. and Topholm, J. (1985) Comparing BTE's and ITE's for localizing speech. *Hear. Instrum.*, **36**, 20–4, 36.

8

COUNSELLING FOR THE FIRST-TIME USER

Denzil Brooks

In the early 1970s a number of studies were undertaken in Manchester to try and determine how well first-time users coped with, and how much use they made of the hearing aids supplied to them free of direct cost through the UK National Health Service. The findings were not encouraging. One in five said they were dissatisfied with the aid. A quarter were having problems with the aid or earmould such that they were getting only minimal benefit. As many as one-third were either not using the aids at all, or using them only infrequently. In those that were using their aids, average daily use was very low – only an hour or two, and that primarily for watching TV. A number of factors were seen as contributing to this low level of satisfaction and use. One was the Medresco aid, which had all the disadvantages of a body aid – unsightly appearance, clothes rub and a fragile cord that tended to become entangled in clothing and was difficult to conceal. A second factor was the inflexibility of the amplification characteristic. There was virtually no possibility of tailoring the frequency response to the differing require-ments indicated by the wide range of audiogram patterns. A third factor was that many persons possessing NHS aids had very poor understand-ing of even the essential aspects of hearing-aid use. A year after receiving the aid, many were unable to correctly insert their individual earmould, to replace the battery or to cope with noise (external or due to clothes rub). This lack of basic knowledge was largely due to the inadequate initial instruction. The time allocated to provide a hard-of-hearing individual with a hearing aid was sufficient only to impart the most fundamental information. There was no time to get to grips with the problems and worries of the individual. Hearing impairment was given a very low priority by Health Service administrators, so the service was underresourced and understaffed, and the technical staff that were responsible for instructing new hearing-aid users were undertrained and undermotivated.

Another factor underlying the poor use of many hearing-aid candidates was a poor attitude to the whole procedure. They were frequently acting under pressure from well-meaning (or exasperated) relatives or friends and had not truly come to terms with the hearing loss. They were worried about getting a hearing aid and worried about visiting hospital. These subconscious fears diminished the prospects of successful rehabilitation.

A substantial move towards reducing the first two causes of poor take-up and use was made in 1975 when a range of postaural hearing aids was introduced. Not only were the aids more acceptable cosmetically, but they were also more versatile in terms of performance. Substantial variation in frequency response was attainable either in the aids themselves or through modifications to the earmould 'plumbing'.

However, increasing knowledge and understanding of and overcoming poor attitudes to hearing loss and hearing aids cannot be dealt with by technical improvements alone. This is the role of the counsellor.

Counselling is usually seen as commencing when the hearing aid is supplied. The Manchester study demonstrated that many candidates had anxieties and fears that lurked at the back of their minds prior to and during the issue procedures, thus reducing the attention given to the audiologist imparting the essential information about adapting to amplification. *Prima facie*, there would seem then, to be justification for initiating counselling before the aid is issued. Better to have worries and concerns faced up to and dispelled before rather than after the technicalities of amplification are discussed.

With these considerations in mind, a rehabilitation programme was developed to provide a service tailored to the requirements of each and every hearing-aid candidate. Regardless of age or circumstance, each person is visited in their home a few days prior to the fitting of a carefully selected hearing aid. Thereafter, counselling is provided as need is perceived until optimum results have been achieved. It is accepted that such a scheme may not be the ideal; that it may not be unique; that it may leave much undone. However, it is the system of hearing-aid supply with which the author is most closely associated and it will be described as one possible approach to hearing rehabilitation, an approach that is economic and practicable in terms of time and staff, and that produces higher levels of use, satisfaction, reduction in handicap and performance than where such therapy is absent.

8.1 THE SOUTH MANCHESTER
AUDITORY REHABILITATION SCHEME

On receipt of a request for an NHS hearing aid at Withington Hospital, an appointment for an ear, nose and throat (ENT) consultation is sent to the candidate, along with a questionnaire (Chapter 5, Appendix A) for completion and return to the clinic when attending. This questionnaire can be seen as a first step in the counselling process; the acquisition of knowledge about underlying feelings and perceptions of the subjects, including some indication of relationships with significant others.

At the hospital visit, apart from the otological examination, pure-tone audiometry is performed from which the hearing-aid gain/frequency response prescription is derived. This indicates which aid is most appropriate, and also any modifications required to the aid and coupling system. Appropriate instructions are sent to the earmould manufacturing laboratory for such requirements as venting, open-mould construction or the use of a Killion horn.

On receipt of the earmould, a personal (not officialese) letter is sent to the candidate. It is designed to help in relieving anxiety about the impersonal nature of modern hospitals and medicine, and to commence the building of a bridge between the patient and the professional staff.

The letter sets out two appointments. The second of these is for the hospital visit at which the aid will be supplied. The first is for a home visit by the author and the hearing therapist, and it is stressed that this is part of the normal routine. This was found to be important because previously, some individuals had expressed concern at having a home visit for something that seemed to be quite straightforward – the supply of a hearing aid. They feared that the reason for a home visit was some untoward finding at the ENT examination of such gravity that it could not be discussed at the clinic. The clear statement that the procedure is routine allays this fear. Also in the letter a request is made that, if possible, the spouse, or a relative or friend be present during the visit. This again is a planned part of the counselling programme. Hearing loss almost invariably involves the 'significant others'. It is advisable, therefore, to draw them into the rehabilitation exercise. The greater their understanding about the problems of their partner, relative or friend, the more they will be able to offer assistance based not just on goodwill, but on a foundation of knowledge. An additional facet of this request for another person to be present is that, for some individuals, this may be the first time they have admitted their disability to another person (excluding the doctor). It can be seen as a small step along the road to acceptance.

(a) The home visit

The home visits are planned to take into account age, working times and any other known, relevant factors in order to minimize any possible inconvenience to the potential user. They are arranged at hourly intervals and as the district served by the hospital is fairly compact, this timing allows for an average of 45 minutes for discussion in the home.

The purposes of the home visit are detailed as follows, with some indication of the rehabilitation/counselling that may be commenced at that time.

To allay anxieties and establish a rapport between the patient and the professionals

Apprehension, anxiety, worry, even fear are almost inevitable components of the feelings of those about to attend hospital in the role of receivers of service. For the elderly, the stress and fear may be associated with a number of negative experiences. Possibly as young persons, many years ago, they attended hospital. Conditions then were often spartan, and there may be memories of fear and pain. Friends and relatives have probably entered hospital within the last few years – and not returned. Bereavement is a common, but sad reality in the elderly, and it is frequently associated with hospitals. Further anxieties may be associated with worries about not hearing their name called at reception, or not hearing the doctor and making wrong or silly responses to only partially heard questions. These factors can unite to generate a vicious cycle of worry, uncertainty and stress. The home visit has, as one of its functions, the breaking of this cycle, the allaying of anxieties, the assurance of understanding and the reduction of stress. It creates a personal relationship between the patient and the therapist/professional. It diminishes the perception of the hospital as a monolithic, impersonal institution, and helps to eliminate the feeling that one is just another 'case' thereby enhancing the sense of personal worth.

To obtain a more comprehensive appreciation of the communication problems

A limited grasp of the problems the individual is experiencing can be obtained during an interview in the hospital, but the attitude of medical staff, the atmosphere and the surroundings often inhibit the patient. The doctor wants the medical data and appears not to be interested in the day-to-day problems that distress the hearing-impaired person. It is taken for granted, perhaps even made crystal clear, that time is precious. So the answers to questions inevitably tend to be specific and short rather than the long, rambling and complicated truth as it affects the handicapped person.

By contrast, at the home interview the patient is on his/her own territory, and there is no stress or pressure on time. The interviewers allow, indeed encourage, the hearing-impaired to unburden their worries and anxieties in their own way and in their own time. This should not be taken as implying that there is no structure or direction to the interview. Certain fundamental facts need to be established, but this can often be achieved by careful listening, by observation and by gentle and subtle probing, with the same exactitude as by direct questioning – and with far less stress on the subject. Seeing the home, its location, environment, proximity to other dwellings, layout, and even furnishings, can provide insight into the specific difficulties experienced by the individual. Modification to some of these factors may be advisable and practicable. Some may require intervention by other arms of the statutory services with whom close links are maintained. But the difficulties can often only be identified, and approaches to their remediation instituted, as a result of the knowledge gained by the home visit.

To further assess attitude and commence modification, where necessary

Prior to the home visit some indication of attitude towards hearing impairment and hearing aids has been obtained from the questionnaire. The picture can be rounded out by information obtained at the home visit. Not infrequently, the attitude pattern observed by the counsellor(s) talking with the candidate in the home differs significantly from that indicated by the same person in their responses to the questions. For example, the candidate may indicate that there are few problems in communication at home, and few socially, these latter being essentially the result of some people's habit of muttering instead of articulating clearly. The home visit, and particularly the reactions of the spouse, may demonstrate that there are very long-standing and deep-seated communication problems. The partner may have almost given up attempts at small talk; may have taken on some roles formerly those of the hearing-impaired person; may indicate that the reason for few social problems is that social activity has been drastically curtailed since the onset of hearing impairment and may state that the reason there are not many arguments about such matters as the loudness of the TV is that they, the non-hearing-impaired have given up arguing due to the futility of trying to get their partner to hear.

Again, in response to the questionnaire it may be evident that the candidate is worried about the thought of wearing a hearing aid. They fear it will be very obvious, and that wearing it will brand them as 'old', 'senile' or 'decrepit'. Very often these fears are allayed when the aid is seen, and when indications are given as to how to wear it inconspicuously. Some individuals receive further reassurance when they are persuaded that wearing a hearing aid effectively will help them to appear more, rather than less, alert. With better hearing ability their responses will be both quicker and more appropriate. Admittedly, such revision of attitude might take place at the issue of the aid, but it is better to clear these issues out of the way before that time. The mind can then be concentrated on the essentials necessary to a good understanding of aid usage.

Other fears about the use of a hearing-aid may surface spontaneously at the home visit, or may be raised by the interviewers. There is a common belief in many of the elderly, and in some of the younger subjects also, that using a hearing-aid will either 'make the ear lazy' or cause further deterioration of the hearing. Hence the concept arises that an aid should be used only sparingly; only when absolutely necessary. At other times it is thought better to keep the hearing 'exercised' by straining to listen. It is vital that such myths and misconceptions should be dispelled by more informed consideration. For some, reassurance may be all that is necessary; for others, hard scientific data may be more convincing, but for anyone who nurses these false notions, it is important that they are cleared out of the way before the aid is supplied. Otherwise they will remain in the background undetected and unrecognized, but inhibiting full and pleasurable use of the aid.

To determine the extent to which withdrawal has taken place and take appropriate action

One of the most distressing aspects of hearing impairment is that it tends to produce isolation. Beethoven expressed this in moving terms in his Heiligenstadt Testament where he said:

For me there can be no relaxation in human society, no refined conversations, no mutual confidences. I must live quite alone and may creep into society only as often as sheer necessity demands; I must live like an outcast. If I appear in company I am overcome by a burning anxiety.

In the early stages of hearing impairment, the withdrawal may be more subconcious than physical. Even a small degree of hearing loss can make it difficult to follow a swiftly moving conversation in a group. Not infrequently, the hearing-impaired individual will try to keep up with the ebb and flow of the discussion, but after a time, this becomes both tiring and frustrating. Superficially it seems easier to sit back and merely pretend to be following, perhaps giving an occasional nod or ambiguous murmur to give the impression of involvement. Usually the only persons deceived by such tactics are the hearing-impaired persons themselves! Others may well interpret the vacant expression as indicating lack of interest, and the nods and murmurs as a ploy to try and disguise this disinterest. Failure to respond at appropriate times may be construed as rudeness. After a time, the hearing impaired find the effort of appearing interested too great. They may then opt out by picking up a newspaper or book. Sometimes they may even withdraw physically, going into another room, thus confirming the view of the others that they have no interest in the conversation. Other social activities begin to diminish. Visits to the theatre or cinema become infrequent or stop. The reason for this may be rationalized as being due to rising costs or transport difficulties; to deterioration in acting skills, especially voice projection. The spouse may tell a different story. The visits were marred by the hearing-impaired individual constantly asking their partner what was said, which spoiled the enjoyment of both, and drew forth adverse comments from those seated nearby. And so withdrawal increased.

Where this is happening, or has happened, a first step towards rehabilitation is to bring about recognition both of the situation and the underlying reasons for its development. This is necessary in both the hearing-impaired and in those closely associated with them so that the misunderstandings can be cleared up, and the reasons for the apparent disinterest and rudeness revealed. Explaining the nature and degree of the hearing loss with the help of the audiogram can be instructive and illuminating in many instances. Discussing the reasons for withdrawal with significant others can heighten understanding and improve relationships. Then the process of re-entering company can be considered and realistic goals can be set.

To explore the relationships with significant others

To some extent, this area has already been touched on and a more detailed consideration will be made in the next chapter, but the role of spouse, family and friends can hardly be exaggerated. A supportive partner or relative can greatly enhance the prospects for rehabilitation and conversely, an unsympathetic, unfeeling, or ignorant (of the effects of hearing impairment) person can almost totally destroy the benefits of the aid, and the work of the professionals involved in the rehabilitation. Often the attitude of the significant other lacks sympathy because it lacks understanding. Hearing loss can be very misleading. The poor high-frequency hearing associated with the majority of hearing impairments explains why the impaired individual sometimes hears the door knocker, but misses the telephone bell; why they hear some men's voices, but do far less well with their grandchildren's piping voices; and why background noises may cause more trouble to them than to their hearing partner. An appreciation of the nature and effects of the individual's hearing impairment can often improve relationships and enhance the prospects for successful rehabilitation.

To prepare the potential user for exposure to environmental noise

Absolute silence is rare. It might be experienced on a windless night in the open countryside, but even here, there may well be the rumble of distant traffic, the sound of an aircraft passing overhead or the cry of an animal. We are immersed in noise; the chatter of conversation; the noises of the home such as the heating system, the clock, or the washing machine; street noise; or the working environment. These sounds are processed by the ears, but, because they have no communicative value, are perceived only as background. We are aware that they are there, but only barely so. They do not rise to the level of conscious attention. From this background our brain selects those sounds which are important and meaningful. This sophisticated process of selection by relevance is maintained at a very high level of efficiency by constant use, 24 hours a day, every day of the year.

When hearing begins to deteriorate, it is the quiet sounds that disappear first. The tick of the clock fades away. The birds cease to sing. The rain no longer patters against the windowpanes and the strength of the wind is apparent only by its effect on the trees. Due to the lack of practice, the skill of differentiating sounds with meaning from environmental noise diminishes, and a false perception of what is normal develops. If no thought has been given to, and no preparation made for, a return to the living, noisy world, the shock can be such as to totally discourage the new user. Unless warned, the sound of turning a page of the newspaper or flushing the toilet can be traumatic. The hearing aid can be blamed for producing a ticking noise or a steady hissing when these are actually sounds made by the clock or the gas fire. The naive user may well discard the aid because it does not immediately sort out the sounds required – voices, the phone bell, the radio – from the background. The home visit provides an opportunity to reacquaint the candidate with the sounds within their own home. Assurance is given that the ability to listen selectively will be largely regained provided the task of re-educating the hearing is approached correctly and patiently. The professional can help by providing a programme for growth of listening skill, but the main effort has to be put in by the hearing-aid user. Based on the home visit, objectives can be set dependent on the motivation, circumstances and personality of the individual.

Advice is usually given to use the aid only within the house for around a month (although this period may be reduced for younger candidates) until handling the controls has become automatic and environmental noise can be disregarded. Initially, it is also suggested that the aid be used only in one-to-one situations. To help the new user to become familiarized with different sounds of the house, a 'sound list' is supplied at issue. This itemizes a couple of dozen common domestic sounds and it is suggested that the new user deliberately creates or listens out for these sounds. Once identified, the pattern is then mentally stored for future reference. The sounds are soon accepted as part of the background and no longer interfere with listening to more meaningful stimuli. As experience grows, the input can be widened to include small groups of family or friends. The aid might then be tried in the garden where a new range of sounds will be noted – birdsong, wind in the trees, traffic noise or children playing close by. Steadily experience is built up, the range of use situations increased, the number of sources of sound listened to at one time is enlarged. With increasing skill comes increasing confidence and over a period of time that may be months rather than weeks, amplification is accepted with the same nonchalance that characterizes the regular wearer of spectacles.

To assess potential needs for environmental aids (assistive listening devices)

Although the hearing aid is the amplifying device that has the widest possible range of applications, there are circumstances in which an alternative may be superior. There is little doubt that for many elderly persons the communication situation engaged in most extensively is television. For the hearing-impaired individual living alone the simple answer to the difficulty of hearing the TV would seem to be to turn up the volume, but this may be a short-lived solution if the home is a flat or a semi-detached house with thin partition walls. The neighbours may not wish to listen to the same programmes. For the hard-of-hearing person living with spouse or family, turning up the volume may lead to friction, arguments and angry words. Around 50% of patients admit to frequent arguments about TV volume. The hearing aid is an effective solution to this difficulty for the majority, but for some, a dedicated TV listening device may be a more appropriate solution. Need can best be determined at the home visit where all appropriate factors can be assessed.

   The telephone is another potential cause for concern both for those living alone and for those living with the family. It is not uncommon when exploring this area, to hear of situations where the son or daughter tried to telephone the parent but to no avail. Fearing that there had been an accident or sudden illness, a hurried trip had been made only to find the hard-of-hearing individual watching TV with the volume at such a level that the ringing of the telephone had gone unnoticed. Occasionally, a solution can be suggested immediately, such as moving the phone into the room from the hall, or obtaining a plug-in phone with sockets in one or two rooms. Alternatively, a phone with a louder or differently pitched bell, or an extension bell may be suggested.

Where the difficulty is in hearing the message rather than the ringing tone, the usual approach is to wait and see if the aid provides a satisfactory solution. An amplified telephone or one with an induction coil built into the handset may ultimately prove to be a better method of resolving the problem, but as these can be quite expensive, a decision is postponed until some skill has been acquired in using the aid. A working display of telephone-listening devices and television adapters is maintained at the hospital and if the initial visit to the home indicates a possible need for such a device, a trial can be made, but this normally takes place at the follow-up visit one month after issue. By this time there will be some indication as to whether the aid alone will be adequate or whether additional help is needed.

Another common cause of difficulty may be hearing callers at the home. The noise of the TV, vacuum cleaner or washing machine may blot out the sound of the knocker or bell, especially if the bell is in the entry hall and the hearing-impaired person is in the kitchen at the rear of the house. Seeing the layout of the home enables the professional to make suggestions that are both practicable and within the scope of the individual or a member of the family. Moving the bell, adding an extension or changing to a low-pitched buzzer may be simple and cheap solutions should the aid not prove satisfactory. For the severely hearing-impaired, and occasionally the less impaired with a normal-hearing family or spouse, a flashing-light door-alerting system may be necessary and steps can be taken to provide this.

To identify any special factors that may need attention

The home visit enables the counsellor(s) to see if there are any particular features about the individual's situation or environment that need special attention. Many families or elderly persons have a pet. Indeed, for some, this may be more effective than any doorbell in making them aware of callers, but what may be a boon when hearing-impaired, may be almost disastrous when wearing an aid. The sharp bark of a terrier can be painful to the unaccustomed aid wearer. It is wise to warn of such possibilities.

Living in a home located close to a railway, a busy main road or on the flight path of an airport raises unusual problems. The noise levels indoors will probably be acceptable, but the candidate should be prepared for the extra noise of the trains or planes. Extra care is advised when first using the aid outside the house.

If the patient is bedfast or wears a spinal collar, or if the favourite chair has high sides, a rearward facing microphone is liable to give rise to acoustic feedback. In such circumstances an aid with top microphone is provided. If, perhaps due to stiff arthritic fingers, or lack of adaptability, the capacity to adjust the volume control of the aid accurately does not exist, and if there is no-one else who can help, then the volume control may be taped up at a suitable gain setting. This can be a successful strategy, just as that employed with deaf young children who cannot adjust their own volume control.

To determine if additional assistance is required

Where there is a co-operative and helpful spouse or relative, the initial difficulties of using a hearing aid can be mitigated. Help can be given in inserting the earmould. Encouragement to use the aid as advised can also be forthcoming. But where the person is elderly and lives alone, the seemingly simple tasks of inserting the earmould and adjusting the volume control can present almost insuperable difficulties. When the home visit indicates that this is likely, arrangements may be made for help to be given by a volunteer counsellor who is usually a successful hearing-aid user (Brooks and Johnson, 1981). The first visit usually takes place by prior arrangement within 10 days or so of the issue of the aid. The timing is felt to be important. Enough time has to be given to allow for a reasonable attempt to be made by the new user to handle the instrument, but not so long that frustration and despair set in. Further visits may be made as need is perceived, and after each visit a report is forwarded to the clinic staff so that progress can be monitored and any necessary action taken. If at any time the volunteer counsellor feels that additional help is required from the professional staff, this is arranged. Using voluntary semi-skilled help in this way ensures that scarce and expensive professional time is used most effectively.

To obtain a complete picture of the subject's attitudes and needs
and to prepare an individual programme to help in meeting those needs

In combination with the completed questionnaire, the home interview enables the clinic staff to form a reasonable assessment of the candidate's attitudes to hearing loss and the prospect of using a hearing aid. To some extent the counselling commences with the initial letter to the patient. It continues in the home by reducing worries and fears, by seeking to correct aberrant attitudes, by advising those in close contact with the hearing impaired and by setting out realistic expectations about progress with amplification. The value of the home visit has been commented on by many potential users. It has also been commented on by the technical staff who fit the aids. They have spontaneously volunteered the information that patients visited in their homes prior to the issue of the aid at the clinic are more receptive and relaxed than those who, for various reasons, are not visited.

Immediately after the home visit, and based on the information obtained, a target is set for each new user in terms of the amount of daily use to be made of the aid. This may range from 'full-time use' through 'regular substantial use' and 'regular limited use' to 'occasional use only' or 'nil use' depending on many factors. For an active, relatively young person with a moderate degree of hearing loss, the target might well be for full-time use. For an elderly person living alone, with only a mild degree of hearing loss, whose desire is to converse more easily with her son or daughter on their occasional visits, a realistic target may be for occasional use only. Progress towards the target is reviewed at the one-month follow-up and on receipt of the four-month questionnaire on use, performance and satisfaction. If the level of use appears to be below that expected, an effort will be made to try and determine the reason for the reduced level of use and then to take whatever action is necessary to progress towards the target.

(b) The hearing-aid issue

Four days after the home visit, issue of the hearing aid takes place. Prior to this the salient information about each subject will be discussed with the technician delegated to carry out the issue. Particular attention can then be paid to any needs or idiosyncrasies of the patient. The fitting procedures were discussed in Chapter 6 and will not be repeated here.

One month after issue, a follow-up appointment is sent to the new users and 98% keep this appointment. Usually the 2% who do not have valid reasons for their inability to attend. As with the home visit and issue session, it is suggested that the spouse, or other close associate accompanies the hearing-impaired individual at the review.

(c) One-month post-issue counselling

Recall that the advice given to the patient before and at issue is to use the aid initially only within the confines of the home so that experience can be gained in manipulating the controls and becoming familiar with environmental noise. For younger adults, a few days may suffice for gathering this experience, but for the elderly, a period of a month is usually advocated. At the follow-up session progress is reviewed. Usually, some improvement in attitude and self-image can be seen that can be fostered and used as a springboard for further development. For the majority, more extended use can be recommended, initially perhaps in the garden, when visiting family or friends, or at church. Thereafter, progress can be steadily made to more complex listening situations. To help in familiarizing the patient to new sounds a second 'sound list' may be issued at this time, this containing outdoor noises such as the wind in the trees, a barking dog, a bicycle bell and so on. As with the first sound list, identifying sources of noise assists in future recognition. It also has the merit of involving the individual in a positive way with their own progress in rehabilitation.

Caution is advised in using the aid in situations where there is either a high level of noise or the likelihood of sudden noises – noisy bars or busy streets. Using the hearing aid in such circumstances should only be contemplated when the user feels totally in control of the instrument, able to instantly and accurately adjust the gain to the appropriate level.

A minority may still be having difficulty in handling the earmould and the aid. For those who have not mastered the art of correctly putting in the individual earpiece, the 'increasing gap' technique (Corcoran, 1984) may be tried. Alternatively, or additionally, where the major problem lies in manipulating the aid/earmould, arrangements may be made for a volunteer counsellor to visit and give help.

At the review, information is sought about the performance of the aid. Is the tonal quality satisfactory? Do voices sound clear and natural? Are loud noises painful, or merely noisy? On the rare occasion when the answers suggest the need for a change, adjustments will be made and subjective tests undertaken. If necessary, a different model of aid may be tried, perhaps with more sophisticated circuitry.

At this time explanation is given, where relevant, on how to use the aid with the telephone. As several different approaches to this situation are possible, the audiologist will probably discuss the options with the aid user to decide which is the most appropriate. For those where the aid has been fitted to the poorer ear, and the better ear is not too impaired, it may be preferred to continue using the telephone directly on the better ear. For some, direct acoustical input from the telephone handset to the hearing-aid microphone may be satisfactory, but advice is often required so that the 'speaker' of the telephone is appropriately placed adjacent to the microphone port of the hearing-aid. Without such guidance, many persons press the handset to the earpiece of the hearing-aid – not surprisingly with very little benefit. For others the 'T' setting may be more suitable, dependent on the type of telephone being used. Models designed to be used with hearing aids on the 'T' setting are available (at extra cost), and a trial of such an instrument can be arranged for a potential user. Alternatively, a clip-on acoustic to inductive coupler can be employed, this having the advantage of being usable on any telephone.

Frequently in the discussion, comments are made that indicate that relationships with spouse, family or friends have improved. Communication has been easier, with consequent reduction in tension and strain. Arguments over television volume have diminished. Where appropriate, suggestions may be made regarding renewal of some social activities abandoned through encroaching hearing loss. Information may be offered as to which theatres and churches have loop systems – and how to benefit from such installations.

Free classes in speechreading are available and at follow-up, aid users are asked if they would like to attend. More than three-quarters express themselves as fully satisfied with the help they receive from the aids. The others are invited to attend the next series of classes.

For a few persons, group therapy may be recommended. The group size is usually under 10, small enough to be intimate, but large enough to ensure a spread of abilities and personalities. The short course consists of four sessions each lasting around two hours, partly didactic, partly informal and including a tea/coffee break. Relatives and friends are encouraged to come. If, at the earlier interviews, binaural aids have been suggested, the question is again raised at this time. Some persons will not wish to pursue the possibility, preferring to continue with a single instrument. A number will express a measure of interest, but indicate that they would like to have a little longer to think about wearing two aids. A substantial proportion will express readiness to try using a second aid now that they have discovered the benefits of one and appropriate action is taken.

(d) Four-month review

Four months after the issue of the hearing aid a questionnaire is sent to every patient seeking to evaluate the effectiveness of the aid. Amount of daily use, performance and satisfaction ratings are sought, as are the individual's opinion of the aid. Comments and criticism are encouraged, because this type of feedback is valuable in indicating where improvements in service are required.

Almost 70% of those supplied with aids indicate a satisfaction rating of 8 to 10 on the scale where 10 is equated with complete satisfaction. Only 10% give scores of 4 or less, a score of 1 indicating total dissatisfaction with the aid. These patients, and any indicating very low performance scores are offered further counselling. Unfortunately at least half of these poorly satisfied and poorly performing individuals are very elderly and living alone or with an equally elderly spouse. Even with a great deal of personal help the outcome tends to remain poor. As Alberti (1977) stated 'a geriatric hearing-aid program is highly cost result/ineffective and effort would be much better directed at a younger still active age group'. The hope is that with better awareness, better public and professional attitudes and, in consequence, earlier referral, candidates for hearing aids in the future will be younger, more adept and alert, and more able to cope with amplification.

Where review indicates that progress towards the predetermined target has been less than expected, further reviews are made and additional help offered. Always, the hearing-aid user is assured that a listening ear and the professional skills of the clinical staff are available, even after the passage of months or years.

8.2 THE ECONOMICS OF COUNSELLING

A number of studies have been made into the benefits of counselling and aural rehabilitation with the elderly. Stephens (1977) cites a number of studies that indicate very positive benefits in terms of hearing-aid use as a result of fairly extensive programmes of aural rehabilitation. Alberti (1977) showed that attending an aural rehabilitation programme reduced the drop-out rate among those provided with hearing aids, but as noted above, the benefit/cost ratio diminished with advanced age. Hardick (1977) suggested that in the less elderly, only a quarter require more than basic hearing-aid orientation, but with increasing age, a higher percentage need more extensive counselling. Brooks (1979; 1985) found marked improvement in the use of hearing aids, handling skills and satisfaction, accompanied by significant reduction of handicap, where counselling is provided.

There seems little doubt that hearing-aid benefit and use improve as a result of aural rehabilitation, but this form of assistance is relatively expensive in terms of trained staff. Can criteria be determined for assessing cost/benefit? Ward, Tudor, Gowers and Morgan (1978), demonstrated that even a small amount of time devoted primarily to handling skills could result in a significant improvement in use time for many elderly persons. Their studies indicated that one hour of counselling over and above the basic instruction should be sufficient for three-quarters of the adult population currently applying for hearing aids in the UK. For the remainder more extensive support is required. The same authors further suggested that providing such a rehabilitation service gave definite cost benefits to the NHS in terms of reduced wastage of resources (hearing aids). The benefit to society as a whole of improving communication function in the elderly and reducing stress in family relationships cannot be costed out, but is surely substantial. There can be no doubt that a little aural rehabilitation can improve the quality of life for many persons, not just the hearing impaired, but also those who live with, care for, or are in regular contact with them.

REFERENCES

Alberti, P.W. (1977) Hearing aids and aural rehabilitation in a geriatric population. *J. Otolaryngol.*, suppl. 4.

Brooks, D.N. (1979) Counselling and its effect on hearing aid use. *Scand. Audiol.*, **8**, 101–7.

Brooks, D.N. (1985) Factors relating to the underuse of postaural hearing aids. *Brit. J. Audiol.*, **19**, 211–17.

Brooks, D.N. and Johnson, D.I. (1981) Pre-issue assessment and counselling as a component of hearing-aid provision. *Brit. J. Audiol.* **15**, 13–19.

Corcoran, A. (1984) Teaching earmould fitting (with particular reference to post-auricular aids). In *The Earmould. Current Practice and technology.* Pub. HAAG Brit. Soc. Audiol., Reading.

Hardick, E.J. (1977) Aural rehabilitation for the aged can be successful. *J. Acad. Rehab. Audiol.*, **10**, 51–66.

Stephens, S.D.G. (1977) Hearing aid use by adults: a survey of surveys. *Clin. Otolaryngol.*, **2**, 385–402.

Ward, P.R., Tudor, C.A., Gowers, J.I. and Morgan, D.C. (1978) Evaluation of follow-up services for elderly people prescribed hearing aids. Report of a pilot study. *Brit. J. Audiol.*, **12**, 127–34.

9

THE ROLE OF THE FAMILY AND ASSOCIATES

Karen Pedley

Definition of terms

Hearing impairment is not just a problem for the person with the hearing loss – it affects all those in close proximity. It is for this reason that hearing loss is referred to as a 'dual handicap'. Our lives are a succession of exchanges from a brief acknowledgement to the postman or shop assistant, to involved discussions with family members or work colleagues. In all instances the communication necessarily involves at least one other person and it must flow both ways if the interaction is to be sustained. Therefore, if one party cannot hear, both parties are affected. Although many elderly hearing-impaired people live alone, approximately two-thirds of patients seen for aural rehabilitation live in a family unit with at least one other person. In most cases this is a spouse but it may be a son or daughter, parent, brother or sister. It is these individuals, who are in regular close contact with the hearing-impaired person, that the psychologists term the 'significant others'. By definition, significant others can be friends living in the same house or even a neighbour who spends a significant amount of time in their company. I shall use the term 'family' in its broadest sense to mean all those living together in the same home.

The notion of 'dual handicap', however, is more far-reaching than merely conversation. Part One of this chapter will highlight the many and varied ways in which the relationships between the hearing-impaired person and the family can be affected by the hearing loss.

At present, the protocol concerning the extent of involvement of significant others in rehabilitation is rather *ad hoc*; it is rarely a deliberate component of the hearing-aid fitting. If they happen to accompany the patient, significant others may be invited to 'sit in' but may not be deliberately involved or personally counselled and certainly not all clinics specifically ask them to attend.

In Part Two of this chapter, it is hoped to persuade the sceptical reader of the benefits to both parties of involving the significant others from the early stages. Practical suggestions will be made on points to include when counselling family members (or other significant others) and the ways in which their assistance can be employed to accelerate acceptance of the hearing aid by the hearing-impaired person.

It is probably true to say that, compared with other aspects of audiology, the area of aural rehabilitation has received relatively little attention in the audiological/ENT literature and the reports on the effect on family life constitute only a very small proportion of this. Despite the potential influence of the family on the outcome of a hearing-aid fitting, this area has only recently begun to attract more interest. For this reason, the observations and suggestions put forward are necessarily based more on experience and anecdote and less on empirical evidence.

9.1 THE EFFECT OF HEARING IMPAIRMENT ON FAMILY RELATIONSHIPS

(a) The early stages

Even in the early years of hearing impairment, before the patient recognizes or acknowledges the hearing loss, the significant other can affect the attitude of the hearing-impaired person in a way that may have far-reaching consequences. Both parties may battle through social situations in a charade of normality, admitting neither to themselves nor to each other that something is wrong. A spouse may encourage the hearing-impaired person to hide the hearing loss because of its associations with the elderly, senility and stupidity. Over the years, the hearing loss may begin to affect other aspects of their lives, in particular their social life may be diminished and friends lost. Some spouses will carry the burden of all the subsequent changes rather than 'allow' the hearing-impaired person to bring the hearing loss into the open. Eventually though, a crisis point is reached and either the hearing-impaired person goes to their family doctor on their own initiative, or more usually, they are 'persuaded' by members of their family. Unfortunately, by this time the attitudes of non-acceptance and fear of stigma that the significant other has encouraged or complied with, may be so ingrained that the hearing-impaired person may refuse to take action or makes excuses not to do so. Now, instead of working towards the same goal of concealing the hearing loss they are opposing factions and the family relationships are at risk. The same is true when the hearing-impaired person chooses to acknowledge the hearing loss while the significant other does not. Warfield (1957) observed that her marriage began to deteriorate when she began admitting openly to her disability. Previously, her husband had assisted her efforts to hide and deny it.

(b) Family life

The extent and the way in which family life is affected depends on the patient's age, the speed of onset of the hearing loss, the degree of handicap, the family lifestyle, the ability to adapt to change and the strength of previous relationships. An acquired hearing loss in a young person when it is unexpected and uncommon can be a tragedy, whereas the same hearing loss in an elderly person when it is an expected part of growing old may be considered to be just a nuisance, or there may be a resigned acceptance by those living with them. The impact of a sudden hearing loss is totally different from the consequences of the same hearing loss acquired over many years when the family have, often quite unwittingly, compensated for it. The demands made on the family extend over a continuum from slightly raised voices, occasional repetition and sometimes drawing attention to the doorbell for a mild hearing loss through to always having to attract the person's attention and the necessary implementation of environmental aids for a profound hearing loss.

There is little evidence that close family relationships protect the family against the disruption that accompanies hearing loss. In fact a family with disparate ties may be drawn together by their efforts to overcome the disability.

The relaxed atmosphere in family life depends on the interactions between its members, the most important mode being verbal communication, which allows the exchange of news, ideas, gossip, experiences and humour. Even a mild hearing impairment or one affecting only high frequencies, can turn an everyday conversation into a source of great irritation, impatience, anxiety, fatigue and frustration for both the hearing-impaired person and the family members. Wood and Kyle (1983) found that 93% of people they interviewed with a mild/moderate hearing loss first became aware of a hearing problem during conversation. They felt left out if they could not follow the conversation, sometimes suspicious that they might be the subject of it. They may feel distressed, humiliated and embarrassed if their impaired hearing has led to misunderstandings. A frequent comment is 'But you never told me about so and so', to which the usual reply is 'You weren't listening properly'. Some comments may be trivial, requiring no action or information from the recipient but under normal circumstances would be acknowledged. The common reply, usually because they feel rather silly repeating such a mundane remark, is 'Oh, it doesn't matter' – a reply that causes much resentment. There can be constant repetition and raised voices that all too quickly take on an overtone of irritability. It is easy to see how the significant other can quickly tire of the effort required and begins to exclude the hard-of-hearing person from the conversation because it is the easier option. Of patients completing a questionnaire developed in the Manchester Study, 67% said family and friends became 'impatient' with them. Indeed, 45% stated that they became 'angry'. Over 50% of those interviewed by Beattie (1980) felt that they were missing out often or sometimes on family conversations. Of patients in the Wood and Kyle (1983) study, 36% considered that they were not always included in conversation at home. The significant other, then, feels guilty for not making more effort to include them in family discussions or not explaining what is going on. They may also feel upset because the hearing-impaired person is 'living in a world of their own'. In some families, the conversation may be reduced to the bare essentials, silence being preferable to the frustration of trying to communicate. The absence of everyday comments that make us feel part of the world, maintain rapport with one another and show that we acknowledge one another's presence certainly diminishes the quality of life and leads to *both* parties feeling isolated. In some cases, the isolation has been so great that the patient has resorted to generating 'noise' of their own such as drumming on a table. One wife found her husband's humming so annoying that she spent most of the day in a separate room.

The loudness of the television is one of the commonest complaints from families. It is a frequent source of arguments and one of the commonest trigger factors for referral. Of the Manchester respondents, 50% reported frequent arguments over the volume of the TV. Significant others may suffer in silence or find an excuse for watching a spare set in an adjacent room. This increases the isolation and communication barrier and leads to loneliness and anger for the hearing-impaired person and guilt and resentment for the normal-hearing person. The need to 'fill in the plot' of the programme is also a frequent source of annoyance.

Another source of irritation is the amount of noise unwittingly generated by the hearing-impaired individual around the house. The clatter of pots and pans and the excessive noise of cutlery on the plate when they are eating are common examples.

(c) Social life

In social situations outside the home, there may be other effects on the significant other. Hearing impairment is poorly understood by the majority of people, who can be confused when the hearing-impaired person sometimes hears them correctly and sometimes mishears them. It is a more difficult handicap to understand than an obvious problem such as blindness, a stroke or loss of a limb, which attract almost instant sympathy. Many significant others admit to embarrassment when their spouse gets the wrong end of the stick, interrupts conversations that they didn't realize were taking place, laughs inappropriately or talks too loudly because they are unable to monitor their own voice. One wife described feeling 'mortified' when her husband mistakenly replied 'very nice' to a neighbour's news of bereavement!

In their confusion and irritation, people may talk to the hearing-impaired person through the significant other, causing embarrassment to both parties. The stigma of impaired hearing makes it too difficult for many significant others to openly explain the problem to their friends. Instead they find themselves paraphrasing sentences during a lull in the conversation, making sure their spouse keeps abreast of changing subjects and more frequently, stepping in to answer the questions for them. Other significant others have admitted to attempting to cover up for the hearing-impaired person and even walking away from the situation altogether. With these additional responsibilities for the significant other, and the strain for both parties it is not surprising that there is a gradual reduction in social encounters. In the Manchester study, one-third of respondents said that they stay at home more or go out less since becoming hearing-impaired and about two-thirds said that they now avoid small talk. Comments made by hearing-impaired respondents to Orlans and Meadow Orlans' (1985) questionnaire are typical: 'I tend to enjoy being by myself because its easier' (woman, aged 21); 'As for social activities, I'd rather stay at home' (woman, aged 29). Of those completing Wood and Kyle's (1983) questionnaire, 74% perceived a decline in social life. The authors argue that this leads to the family necessarily spending more time together, which then exacerbates any existing tension.

Some significant others admit to worrying about the hearing-impaired spouse when they are at work and unable to rely on them in social situations. One wife in the Harris, Lamont and Thomas (1986) study was constantly worried lest her husband should fail to hear the factory warning sounds.

Leisure activities may have to be tailored to suit the needs of the hearing-impaired person. There is less risk of misunderstandings in one's own home with familiar faces than when meeting new people in a crowded room. Of those who completed the Manchester questionnaire, 40% said they 'hate', 'avoid' or 'dread' meeting new people and nearly half said that they are not as outgoing or talkative as they used to be.

Parties, clubs and talks may be avoided altogether and concerts, cinema and theatre replaced by ballet, museums, spectator sports and exhibitions. The family may have to watch a captioned or sub-titled foreign film rather than a film in English that is not thus aided. Of the 27 families interviewed by Harris *et al.* (1986), seven had curtailed visits to the theatre and/or cinema and two of the normal-hearing wives had ceased going to evening classes because they disliked going alone. Conflicts of interest are inevitable and resentment may be felt when the normal-hearing significant other has made sacrifices. One wife insisted that her husband accompanied her to church even though he was unable to follow the sermon. One husband became angry with his wife because she disliked dining out – she would make excuses rather than explain the increased difficulty of hearing and speechreading with background music, low-lighting conditions and people talking with their heads down in between mouthfuls of food. When the differences become too great, couples can resort to leading almost separate lives.

(d) Role change

Over a period of time, if the hearing loss remains unaided, subtle role changes begin to take place at home in which the hearing-impaired adult may gradually relinquish some of his/her usual responsibilities. One father noticed that his children had begun to seek help with their homework from their mother because of the difficulties in making him understand what was required. A mother was upset because her teenage daughter now talked about her boyfriends and social outings with her father as she herself missed the subtleties of the conversation. This can lead to feelings of inferiority and redundancy on the part of the hearing-impaired person – meanwhile the significant other has all the additional responsibilities to carry and many feel overburdened. Problems can arise if the family member is obliged to take on roles for which he/she is not suited. It is possibly true to say that the role change is relatively easier for most hearing-impaired people as for them there is an obvious and acute cause – they are adapting to the 'sick' or 'patient' role.

The reversal of roles is perhaps particularly noticeable when the husband is hearing-impaired and has to become dependent on his wife, the wife may find herself negotiating with the bank manager or insurance agent because the husband is afraid of appearing stupid. One mother had to take on the sole responsibility for all her children's parents' evenings because her husband was afraid of appearing a fool in front of the teachers. The comments from the respondents in Beattie's study (1980) are typical: 'My wife has tended to do that sort of thing, anything important for some time now.' 'My wife takes the initiative for me. She goes to the doctor with me. . . .' The significant others may find that they are answering all the phone calls and calls to the door and relaying messages later. Some resent the extra work involved, particularly if there is an uneven distribution of duties. Stress, conflict, tension and resentment in the family can also result when reason dictates that a particular responsibility should be relinquished yet the hearing-impaired person refuses to let go and imposes his/her own solution. A paradox exists that can make these decisions difficult – the hearing-impaired person may want to hand over the reins but still wishes to be accepted as a valued member of the family.

It goes without saying that the reduced opportunities for leadership for one accustomed to the more dominant role of head of the household can have shattering effects on the husband's self-confidence and self-esteem. The burden on the wife of all the new responsibilities is less-often appreciated.

For some individuals the hearing loss can result in stagnation at one level of employment, the loss of promotion prospects or even the loss of a job and the subsequent change of status or circumstances can add even more pressure to the already burdened family who perhaps feel resentful or may fear for the future.

(e) Marriage

Certainly a hearing loss puts a marriage to the test. One young woman with a moderate hearing loss explained that she felt it difficult to feel close to her husband as the whispered intimacies had become impossible. Those studies that have investigated this aspect of hearing loss, however, suggest that most marriages survive despite the extra effort and sensitivity required by the hearing spouse, for which the hearing-impaired partner is usually very grateful. It would seem that the deeper level of understanding brings them closer. For example, 'He has saved me from a great deal of embarrassment and I love him for it.' 'I do not know how I could relax without him' (Orlans and Meadow-Orlans, 1985). In Beattie's (1980) study, 32% of the 50 married respondents felt that their marriage had been affected to a greater or lesser degree, and the majority of these were men. Beattie suggests that this is due to men being more affected by role change than women. Only one person indicated that their marriage had been affected 'a lot'. This relatively undramatic effect on marriage is supported by Thomas and Gilhome-Herbst (1980) who found no evidence that a hearing-aid group had a higher level of marital rows, divorce or separation than a control group. However the hearing-impaired group were significantly more likely to have rows over one of them not showing enough affection for the other partner.

(f) Effects on children

A hearing impairment can potentially destroy the natural bond between a parent and child. Children easily become frustrated at having to repeat everything. In Beattie's (1980) study, five respondents pointed out that whereas the spouse was understanding, their children could be very impatient. Daughters were mentioned as relatives most likely to show impatience although they are perhaps more likely to spend time with and have more responsibility for the deafened adult. Some children comment that they miss the conversation at meal times and the exchange of comments during TV programmes, which they are forced to watch in near silence.

Children will admit to feeling embarrassed about bringing friends around to their house because the TV is so loud, or because their mum or dad misunderstand, or worse, appear to ignore comments made by their friends. In nearly half of the 27 families of severely hearing-impaired individuals interviewed by Harris et al. (1986) children said that their friends were embarrassed or uneasy in the presence of their hearing-impaired parent. In the Breed, van den Horst and Mous (1981) study some children were reluctant even to go shopping with the hearing-impaired parent or they would go on ahead or lag behind when walking together. In Beattie's (1980) study some respondents tended to avoid taking problems to the hard-of-hearing parent. Several older children in Harris's study recalled having 'played up' the hearing-impaired parent by refusing to speak clearly or making impertinent comments in a deliberately soft voice. The interviewers noted that, while some children had ceased to behave in this way as they grew up, in other cases the unco-operative attitude had persisted. Children are often accused of mumbling, this made worse by an excited child eager to relate the events of the day and the fact that children's voices are difficult to hear with the more common high-frequency hearing loss. One parent in the above study assumed that her children were plotting against her when she could not hear their conversation and had frequently punished them only to find out later that she had mis-understood the situation. Fortunately, some children show remarkable perception and understanding and will help hearing-impaired members of the family with the plot of a TV programme, will answer the phone and take messages and politely will explain the hearing-impaired person's difficulties to other people.

The problems of adjusting to hearing impairment cannot be underestimated. Unfortunately, the drain on the hearing-impaired person's emotional resources may be so great that the effects on the rest of the family and the adjustments that they have made sometimes do go unnoticed. This is one of the areas in which joint counselling can be valuable.

9.2 THE ROLE OF SIGNIFICANT OTHERS IN THE REHABILITATION OF THE HEARING-IMPAIRED

Involvement of the family in rehabilitation is more often an after-thought than part of a deliberate effort to assist the hearing-impaired person to return to as normal a life as possible. This is partly due to a historical emphasis on the hearing aid itself and the concentration of professional attention on the practical aspects of the hearing-aid fitting. Wood and Kyle (1983) found that 96% of hearing-aid owners in their study stated that they had received no information regarding adjustment within the family from either the ENT consultant or the audiology clinic and 98% said that no information was received on communication strategies from the audiology service.

As an alternative to the family's presence at the hearing-aid issue, Berest (1977) suggests that family involvement can be achieved through the use of two complementary letters – one to the hearing-impaired person, the other to the family or friends. The latter outlines what should be expected from the hearing aid, initial problems that will be encountered and lists some of the hearing tactics that can be employed by the family. A letter obviously does not permit feedback from the significant other or personal individual counselling, nor can the relationships or attitudes be examined, but it provides information and support – someone has taken an interest in them and the suggestions that have been put forward should benefit both parties. In the absence of adequate resources to allow the significant other(s) to attend the clinic, it is a good second-best alternative. It is certainly better than no guidance at all.

Experience at a local clinic has shown that around 40% of significant others will respond to a simple invitation included on the appointment card such as 'it would be helpful if a relative or friend could accompany you'. Where pre-issue visiting of the patient and family is a component of the service as at Withington hospital, approximately 90% of patients are accompanied.

Generally speaking, there are four reasons for involving the significant others in rehabilitation:

First, to help them gain some insight into the problems experienced by the hearing-impaired person and to dispel any misconceptions about the deafness or the hearing-aid.

Second, to make sure both parties realize that the process of overcoming the hearing loss will require them to work together.

Third, to assist with the practical aspects of the hearing aid.

Fourth, to provide moral support to the patient in the intimidating environment of the hospital and to enable emotional support to be given to the significant other.

The last point perhaps raises the issue as to *who* should counsel the family. The information counselling is certainly within the scope of the audiology technician but in some cases the support, especially where marital disharmony is a strong factor, may be more appropriately offered by the hearing therapist.

(a) Preliminary observations

It is always worth taking a few moments to observe the patient and significant other together in the waiting room, as this can provide valuable clues as to their rapport and attitude. Is the significant other reading the posters and leaflets in the vicinity? Are they interested in what is happening to the other patients or are they sitting separately or reading a book, with the car keys at the ready? When the patient is called in, does the significant other follow automatically, eagerly wait to be invited in or require some persuasion. It is usually a sign of disharmony if the patient requests that the spouse waits outside. When they enter the consulting room it is interesting to note whether the spouse chooses to sit close to the patient indicating an interest and a willingness to be involved. If they choose to sit some distance from the patient, this can suggest that they feel the hearing aid is nothing to do with them and that they do not wish to make it so.

It is important to choose the approach to the significant other carefully – those who have not really given the hearing loss much thought will feel overawed if they suddenly find themselves deeply involved with the hearing aid, and all future co-operation may be lost. It is better in these circumstances to make significant others aware of the ways in which they are already implicated and encourage general rather than specific support. At the other extreme, some significant others will be very interested in the device and readily volunteer their assistance. It is important to take careful note of the hearing-impaired person's reaction to this as some initially are not too keen to allow their spouse to become close to a problem that they see as being highly personal.

The fact that both patient and spouse will have been told by the time of the issue appointment that there is no medical or surgical cure for the hearing loss, does not prevent some people from clinging to the idea that a miracle cure may somehow be found. The promise of restored hearing may prevent acceptance of the hearing loss, even after the aid has been fitted. Until *both* patient *and* significant other accept the aid as the only form of treatment, there will be only half-hearted commitment to hearing-aid use.

(b) Use of self-assessment questionnaires

The recent proliferation of hearing-handicap assessment scales suggests that audiologists are becoming increasingly aware of the need to supplement audiological data with information about the individual's attitude, motivation and the social and emotional effects of their hearing problem. McCarthy and Alpiner (1983) not only feel that family counselling is an essential aspect of hearing-aid fitting, but in addition they have developed a self-assessment questionnaire designed to provide information concerning the family's assessment of the problems to enable the audiologist to make the most appropriate use of the time. In their study of 60 families, a parallel form of the scale was completed by the hearing-impaired person. Where the patient was asked 'Do you tend to avoid people because of your hearing loss?', the family member received the same question in third-person format. Correlation coefficients were computed for the psychological, social and vocational sub-sections of the scale by comparing the responses of the hearing-impaired subject with the response of their family member. Overall, a low level of agreement was found in all three items. It is suggested that this is due to differences in the perception of feelings and behaviours – one party may have failed to accept the hearing loss or may not have recognized a particular problem. The authors suggest that the areas of discrepancy would indicate areas in need of family counselling. However, it is important not to overburden the significant other with too much knowledge at the beginning – rather it should be built up in a series of layers as is done with the patient's skills.

(c) Counselling

Support

The audiologist may be the first person the significant other has felt able to talk to about the deafness. Indeed many are visibly relieved that someone else understands *their* difficulties and worries. It may be sufficient just to be a listening ear on the first visit. The fact that this takes place in the presence of the hearing-impaired person is a key factor in the rehabilitation. In the Wood and Kyle (1983) study, 86% of mild/ moderately hearing-impaired subjects agreed that deafness places a strain on hearing members of their families. Beattie (1980) reports that about one-third of respondents felt that members of their families experienced stress when communicating with them. However, there was little recognition that their families might benefit from help. Only one of the 33 who admitted to family stress felt that their family might appreciate advice or help on how to cope with the problems. Overall, this suggests only a shallow understanding by the patients of the difficulties imposed on the significant other as a result of the handicap. Some of the statements from the significant other can come as quite a shock to the hearing-impaired person. For one husband, it was the first time he had realized that his wife had needed to shout to him virtually all the time. A blind lady heard for the first time that her husband had found the level of the talking book uncomfortably loud but did not complain because of the additional handicap. A young wife confessed to making frequent phone calls to her family because her husband did not talk to her anymore – in fact, this was because he was afraid of making her angry with all the constant repetition, so refrained from initiating conversation in the first place. A few misunderstandings aired in the presence of an informed and neutral listener clears the air, strengthens relationships and provides a better base for beginning rehabilitation. It may be more helpful in certain situations to see the significant other separately – some feel unable to voice their anger, frustration and fears for the future in the hearing-impaired person's presence.

While the stigma of hearing loss is strong, the audiologist may be the only individual with whom the significant other feels able to discuss the hearing loss.

Information

Few people understand the problems of hearing loss, even when living in close proximity to a deafened person. The hearing-impaired themselves are only too aware of this as shown by Wood and Kyle's (1983) survey where 86% felt that other people did not understand their problems. Of the 236 people interviewed by Thomas and Gilhome-Herbst (1980), 42% felt that their hearing problem was not understood by those nearest to them.

The amount of information given at each stage will depend upon the significant other's attitude, current awareness, memory and overall intellectual ability. It is a good starting point to explain the extent of the hearing loss, e.g. a normal voice sounds like a whisper, the clock or the closing of curtains cannot be heard. If the hearing loss is mainly high-frequency, it is worth explaining that the high-pitched sounds like the telephone bell are inaudible yet the rumble of traffic outside can be heard normally. The notion that 'he only hears when he wants to' can be dispelled by explaining that only the soft sounds in speech may be missing, for example, 's', 'th', 'sh', 'f', so that some words can be heard quite well, while others may have no beginning or ending.

Significant others are often puzzled if the patient cannot hear a normal voice yet cringes if someone shouts – an explanation of intolerance of loud sounds as a side effect of deafness can help.

The expectations of the significant other from the hearing aid must be realistic from the start. Those who believe that the hearing aid will do for the deafness what glasses do for poor eyesight must realize that the device is an *aid* to hearing and will not return the hearing to normal.

The difference between the instant results with glasses and the more gradual adaptation to false teeth can be a helpful analogy. Above all, it should be emphasized that one *learns* to use the hearing aid over several weeks.

The sudden awareness of background sounds is usually apparent when the aid is inserted in the clinic. This can be used as a lead to emphasize the need for patience in the first few days when the inexperienced hearing-aid user may overreact to the banging of a door or the clatter of cutlery until the tolerance for sudden loud sounds has been re-established.

An understanding of the fear that can accompany hearing loss can be valuable. Fear of not hearing someone in the street, friends in a pub or the neighbour over the garden fence can lead to all kinds of evasive and odd behaviour that may bewilder the significant other.

If tinnitus is present, it may encourage empathy if a similar sound can be demonstrated using an audiometer. The hard-of-hearing person may have had difficulty even convincing the significant other of its existence.

Practical guidance

The extent to which help is received will depend on the way the assistance is offered. Those significant others whose primary aim is to restore harmony to family relationships fare much better than those who constantly seek credit for their efforts and want everyone to know how much they are doing.

Many small but significant difficulties can be overcome with a few simple hearing tactics. The significant other should be encouraged to attract the attention of the hearing-impaired person before speaking by using their name and pausing momentarily before continuing. Questions can be reworded so that the important information comes at the end of the sentence when the person is most attentive, for example, 'John . . . we'll go shopping on Friday'. It should be pointed out that shouting as a way of overcoming the hearing difficulties will no longer be effective as the hearing aid will distort loud sounds. Another common misconception is that one must speak very deliberately and the family members should be encouraged to speak without exaggerated lip movements as this makes lipreading more difficult. The significant others should be encouraged to reduce the distance between themselves and the hearing-impaired person whenever possible as an alternative strategy. Family members should also be encouraged not to shout from another room, to try to remember to face the hearing-impaired person when speaking and to avoid covering the mouth. It can be pointed out that a person with a pen or cigarette in their mouth is more difficult to lipread. Many significant others will not be aware of the effectiveness of doing something as simple as closing a door to reduce background noise during conversation from, for example, the noise of the washing machine or children's voices in an adjacent room.

One of the initial problems when the hearing aid is first worn is the competing nature of background noises that distract the hearing-aid user's attention from the important sound. If the hearing loss has developed gradually over many years, some sounds in the home may have been forgotten. The hearing spouse can assist in identifying the unfamiliar noises that have, in some cases, caused the patient considerable alarm. This is particularly important if the patient is also blind. Once identified, the noises become familiar sounds that can then be ignored.

Our ability to correctly localize sounds depends on the symmetry of our hearing. A first-time hearing-aid user will usually only be issued with one aid and this makes localization difficult. The significant other can help the patient by using simple exercises to practise identifying the direction of sounds.

In conversation outside the home, the hearing partner can help to maintain the flow of conversation. Some spouses repeat occasional statements, rephrasing, or paraphrasing parts of sentences at a convenient lull in the conversation. This can be done quite subtly with practice, if a good rapport exists between the patient and significant other. One man with a slight hearing loss interviewed by Vognsen (1976) says 'In social life my wife is always a relay station. If she notices that I cannot follow the conversation, she will interrupt with questions about the central topic in such a way that I am able to catch on.' Significant others can also gently indicate when the voice becomes too loud and can help by sitting on the aided side in group conversation. It can be difficult to provide assistance when the hearing-impaired person and their spouse are involved in different conversations, yet many spouses describe how they can 'keep one eye on them' for blank or frustrated expressions. The significant other can help to break down the social barrier of stigma by being relaxed and matter of fact when explaining their spouse's hearing difficulties. If the spouse is embarrassed, the rest of the company will be embarrassed also. The significant other should discourage people from using them as an intermediary. Ashley (1985) explains how she achieves this by avoiding eye contact with the person speaking to her husband so that they are forced to speak directly to him.

As a result of the often dramatic improvement in ease of communication, many significant others are too keen to see the hearing aid in full use too soon. They can *encourage* the hearing-impaired person towards regular use but should understand thoroughly the need to begin with short spells, as long periods using a hearing aid can be very tiring for the inexperienced user. The complaint 'Why aren't you wearing your hearing aid?' is the result of a failure to grasp this important point and many patients, to avoid this sort of nagging, will resort to wearing the hearing aid switched off. The spouse or significant other should encourage the hard-of-hearing person to involve themselves in family conversation and ensure that the hearing-impaired person is consulted on family decisions, particularly if there has been significant withdrawal. Of the 236 hearing-aid owners in the Thomas and Gilhome-Herbst (1980) study, 27% reported that they were still left out of discussions and decision-making at home. (However it should be noted that 33% of the sample admitted that they wore their aid 'rarely' or 'not at all'.) Whilst encouraging increasing involvement, it is equally important that the significant other learns to recognize when the partner has had enough. Even with the hearing aid, conversation can be tiring, especially in the learning stages with the new aid. This is particularly true when only one ear has been aided. The patient often communicates so much better that they are assumed to hear normally. However, a person listening with one good ear certainly has to concentrate harder than if they were listening with two. The significant other should appreciate that concentration leads to tiredness, which reduces the attention span and impairs lipreading, which therefore means that more effort is required to listen. Thus it is a vicious circle.

Family members can remove some of the stress of hearing loss by making sure they are aware of what is going on. For example, pointing out the comings and goings of people in the house, remarking on decisions that have been made and avoiding the use of phrases such as 'forget it, it wasn't important'.

Television viewing can be aided with the minimum of effort from the significant others. The family should be instructed to set the TV to a level that is comfortable for them and to *leave it* at that level for the evening. This may present problems if someone else in the house has diminished hearing as it may then be too loud for the patient. This issue will be discussed in more detail later. When watching TV together, the spouse should make a point, where possible, of sitting on the aided side so that the person does not have to turn away from the set to reply to comments made. As many patients know, the added effort of repeatedly picking up the threads of the story afterwards can greatly reduce the pleasure.

The most common reason for non-use of a hearing aid is the inability to insert the earmould (Brooks, 1985). The spouse's help can be invaluable in assisting with the unfamiliar aid and ensuring that the helix portion is correctly positioned. It should be stressed, however, that the patient must not (except in particular circumstances) rely on the significant other to insert the aid for them and independence is to be encouraged. With elderly patients whose short-term memory may be deteriorating, it can also be useful if both are able to change the batteries.

A patient with a severe hearing loss should be encouraged to make maximum use of visual clues and must learn to integrate this with the information available from the hearing aid. In connected discourse tracking, the hearing partner reads from a text (e.g. a newspaper) phrase by phrase, each phrase being repeated by the hearing-aid user. The length of phrase is gradually increased as skill improves. This not only gives the hearing-aid user valuable practice at listening in a non-stressful environment, but it also gives the significant other some appreciation of the extent of the handicap.

As the person's skills with the hearing aid increase, the significant others should be encouraged to relinquish some of their former responsibilities such as allowing the hearing-impaired persons to answer questions for themselves. By assuming some of their former roles, the hearing-impaired persons will regain their confidence and begin to feel a more worthwhile member of the family group instead of a burden. This must be done gradually – a person struggling to come to grips with a new hearing-aid will be overwhelmed if he/she is told 'Now that you can hear again I can hand all the negotiating back to you'. Some relatives may be too eager to encourage dependency because it makes their life easier.

Beattie (1980) suggests that some patients use the hearing loss for 'secondary gain', i.e. as justification for dependency or laziness that is enjoyed or as an excuse for failure or ill-success – a crutch on which to lean. It is these cases where independence should perhaps be most encouraged. The degree of dependency will be determined by the individual's ability to accept this role and stress may result due to a paradox that exists – the attitude of the public at large is to expect dependence from a handicapped person whilst the audiology clinic may encourage independence. Ideally, the significant other should encourage independence, but the hearing-impaired person may have to accept a degree of dependency if family life is not to be too greatly disrupted.

Above all, the significant other should be encouraged to offer support, empathy, patience and comfort.

(d) Special cases

The cases where the significant others are themselves hearing-impaired can give rise to particular problems. The way in which it can affect the progress with the new aid depends on whether the significant other is aided or unaided.

An unaided significant other will probably require the TV to be turned up and may talk too loudly, being unable to monitor their own voice properly. Both can result in loudness discomfort for the hearing-aid wearer and more often than not, this leads to underuse of the hearing aid.

It can be difficult to convince the significant other of their own defective hearing as they commonly use the other person as a reference and assume that since they hear better, they must hear normally. As the hearing-impaired spouse has previously had everything loud, this further disguises their own impairment. By far the best way to encourage the hard-of-hearing spouse to take action is to let him/her try a hearing aid for a few minutes on a temporary tip. More often than not they are surprised at just how much they are missing!

The aided significant other can be a valuable source of encouragement and assistance. However, almost invariably, they have forgotten how difficult it was in the first few weeks with their own aid and expect too much progress too soon. It should be emphasized that progress depends on the individual, and the type, extent and duration of a hearing loss, which may be quite different to their own. The 'You don't need to show him that, I'll do it for him' attitude is not uncommon and must be discouraged.

(e) Cost-effectiveness and implementation into current services

In the UK, the failure to recognize the importance of including the significant other as an integral part of aural rehabilitation has led to almost complete neglect of this valuable source of assistance. It has been found at our clinic that less voluntary visitor support has been needed since significant others were invited to be involved in the pre-issue home visit and hearing-aid issue. It can be predicted that in the long term, less domiciliary visits will be requested for minor problems such as dead batteries and blocked earmoulds. A review of 170 patients returning four-month follow-up questionnaires showed that those who were accompanied by a family member or friend were significantly less likely to need subsequent follow-up appointments than those who came alone. It has been observed that accompanied patients require less reiteration of basic instruction at follow-up. Thus overall, less follow-up support can be envisaged, giving the technicians and audiologists more time to spend with difficult patients and family members.

The question has been raised as to whether the responsibility of providing support for the family in aural rehabilitation is that of the audiology clinic at all or whether it is more of a community responsibility. However, several studies have shown that only an insignificant minority of those with acquired deafness contact local organizations, voluntary bodies and charities. Social workers for the deaf certainly would be an appropriate and able source of assistance but they 'are few in number and are already hard put to cater for the prelingually hearing-impaired' (Harris *et al.*, 1986). The report of the Advisory Committee on Services for the Hearing-Impaired (DHSS, 1975) suggests that this can be overcome if social workers for the deaf act in an advisory capacity to other social services staff who have to deal with families of hearing-impaired people.

Beattie (1980) suggests that the need for objective advice and support can be met (in the UK) by the hearing therapist attending the health centre at regular intervals. Referral would be made for social-work help or voluntary visiting, etc. where necessary.

There is also the view that the need for family support can be met by the existing prelingually deaf community and the network of organizations that exists to help them. However, as Wood and Kyle (1983) point out, the fact that the family and social life of the patient is orientated towards hearing people and indeed, because they themselves have been part of the hearing world for most of their lives, this approach would not be realistic nor would it be acceptable to the majority of the hard of hearing. There is also no practical gain to be had in establishing a 'partially hearing club' since it is more relevant to understand the problems and learn communication tactics with one's own family than with other hearing-impaired people, whose situation and difficulties may be quite different.

REFERENCES

Ashley, P. (1985) Deafness and the family. In *Adjustment to adult hearing loss* (H. Orlans ed.) Taylor and Francis, London.

Beattie, J.A. (1980) Social aspects of acquired hearing loss in adults, unpublished PhD thesis, University of Bradford.

Berest, S. (1977) Family involvement in aural rehabilitation. *Hear. Instrum.*, **28**, (10), 22–49.

Breed, P.C.M., van den Horst, A.P.J.M. and Mous, T.J.M. (1981) Psycho-social problems in suddenly deafened adolescents and adults. First International Conference of the Hard of Hearing, Hamburg. Deutscher Schwerhorigenbund eV, Hamburg, 313–30.

Brooks, D.N. (1985) Factors relating to the underuse of postaural hearing aids *Brit. J. Audiol.*, **19**, 211–17.

Department of Health and Social Security, ACSHIP (1975) *Report of a Subcommittee Appointed to Consider the Rehabilitation of the Adult Hearing Impaired.* Advising Committee on Services for Hearing-Impaired People, London.

Harris, M., Lamont, M. and Thomas, A. (1986) Hearing loss and family life, *Community Care*, February, pp. 22–4.

McCarthy, P.A. and Alpiner, J.G. (1983) An assessment scale of hearing handicap for use in family counselling. *J. Acad. Rehab. Aud.*, **16**, 256–70.

Orlans, H. and Meadow-Orlans, K.P. (1985) Responses to hearing loss: effects on social life, leisure and work. *Shhh*, **6**, (1), 4–7.

Thomas, A.J. and Gilhome-Herbst, K.R. (1980) Social and psychological implications of acquired deafness for adults of employment age. *Brit. J. Audiol.*, **14**, 76–85.

Vognsen, S. (1976) (ed.) *Hearing tactics*, The State Hearing Institute, Frederiksberg, Denmark.

Warfield, F. (1957) *Keep listening*, The Viking Press, New York.

Wood, P.L. and Kyle, J.G. (1983) Hospital referral and family adjustment in acquired deafness. *Brit. J. Audiol.*, **17**, 175–81.

10

THE DIFFICULT PATIENT

Valerie Cleaver

Within the average population attending for rehabilitation, there will usually be a number of patients who will be categorized, for one reason or another, as 'difficult'. It is fairer to these people to recognize from the start that what makes them acquire this epithet is not usually any deliberate contrariness on their part, but rather that circumstances exist that limit the benefit they can gain from routine rehabilitation procedures. They might thus more appropriately be termed 'atypical' patients, particularly since the difficulties involved are often essentially, a reflection of the audiologist's inability to recognize the real problem and the subsequent failure to deal with it. Of course, no two people have exactly the same problems, and ideally all rehabilitation should be tailored to the individual patient's needs, but in reality a range of normal procedures is adopted to which the majority of patients respond well. It is an exciting challenge to the audiologist to recognize that the patient has special needs, so that time is not wasted on standard procedures when an alternative approach to that patient's rehabilitation problems is required.

This chapter considers the main difficulties that can be encountered during the course of rehabilitation, and suggests possible solutions. The majority of problems arise because hearing-aid use is either unacceptable or insufficient to compensate completely for the hearing-impairment. The patient is likely to remain handicapped unless further measures are taken. The distinction is made here between psychosocial, physical, medical, acoustic and auditory problems, but this categorization is purely descriptive of the main source of the difficulty, and not necessarily indicative of the nature of the solution. The methods employed to resolve these problems are also considered to fall into distinct groups – those where the remedy is essentially practical, those orientated around the provision of information or education and those where a support–counselling role is involved.

10.1 PSYCHO-SOCIAL PROBLEMS

(a) Acceptance of the hearing loss

The problems experienced by some people in coming to terms with hearing loss are discussed in Chapter 6. Patients attending for rehabilitation may still need personal counselling to help them complete the necessary emotional adjustment, especially those coerced into attendance by desperate families. Most hearing-impaired people naturally compensate for a high-frequency hearing loss by subconsciously using visual cues, but the resultant erratic ability to hear tends to be blamed by the patient on the speaker, and by the speaker on the patient's lack of interest. An audiovisual presentation of speech material, where the visual channel can be removed for comparison, is usually a very effective demonstration of how much the patient is missing when using the auditory channel alone, as well as showing the patient and others the importance of visual cues. Usually, the significant others will also benefit from immediate counselling and advice on coping with the practical difficulties and frustrations they are encountering. On the other hand, it is preferable that relatives and friends should not be over-protective to the extent that they deprive the patient of the motivation to come to terms with his problem and help himself.

(b) Acceptance of the need for rehabilitation

A patient may recognize and accept a hearing loss but still not wish to do anything about it. This probably reflects the patient's perceptions of how he/she is coping with the hearing impairment and how much rehabilitation would help. For example, it is typical of many elderly people that they admit to a hearing problem but do not consider that they should do anything about it. This may relate to some generally reduced expectancy-of-life quality, or perhaps to a greater preoccupation with the other practical and medical problems attached to the aging process.

More rarely, a younger person experiencing a life crisis, such as an employment problem or a domestic trauma, may feel that all his/her available attention is required to cope with this, leaving none left to apply to the solution of a coincidental hearing problem. The audiologist needs to ensure that these other problems are not being exacerbated by the hearing loss without the patient realizing it. A communication problem can be interacting with a work or marital problem or with a psychological disorder, or with treatment the patient is receiving for such problems, in ways that he/she or those helping have not perceived.

In either case, it may be necessary for the patient's own benefit to direct him/her more positively towards the acceptance of some form of rehabilitation. If appropriate, the audiologist should liaise with the other parties involved in the patient's overall treatment.

A patient may also need directive counselling towards rehabilitation if the hearing loss, although not seen by him/her as a major problem, is causing difficulties to others, so that there is a risk of losing the concern and support of close friends and relatives. This is often the case with elderly patients, who can seem unaware either of the frustration and annoyance they are causing to others or that this can lead to estrangement from those that love or care for them. One of the most demanding counselling roles of the audiologist is to convey empathy to both patient and significant other when they have opposite views regarding the need for rehabilitation. Each needs understanding, support and guidance, but these have to be carefully apportioned so that the audiologist does not lose credibility with either person. Where there is clearly family friction, the author's generally preferred approach is to see the patient alone in the first instance, to establish a degree of empathy and rapport. When this has been achieved, the patient and partner can be seen together to discuss the partner's view of the patient's problems as well as the partner's own experiences and frustrations. It is usually possible in this way to convey sympathy and support to the partner without damaging the relationship already established with the patient.

The goal of the audiologist, whether by individual counselling or group therapy, using open discussion or role-play techniques, is to promote in each person concerned an accurate empathy with the problems of the others. It is this empathy, described so well in his autobiography by the deafened Member of Parliament Jack Ashley (1973), that will help to achieve the constructive behaviour change that is necessary for successful rehabilitation.

(c) Acceptance of hearing-aid use

The most frequently offered form of rehabilitation is the hearing aid. The desire to conceal hearing aids remains quite strong in most users, probably less for simple cosmetic reasons than to avoid encountering the negative attitude towards hearing-aid use, and by inference towards hearing loss, that many patients expect to find in others. In most cases, personal counselling will enable the patient or partner/parent to develop a more positive attitude towards hearing-aid use. Lay counselling by other successful hearing-aid users can be very helpful (see Chapter 8) providing that those involved have some basic counselling skills. However, it is equally important for the audiologist to explore with patients the possible alternatives to hearing-aid use, such as environmental aids or communication training, that may help them cope with their particular problems. These alternative forms of help are sometimes initially more acceptable to the patient and should ideally be available within the context of the audiology department so that the patient sees them as an integral part of the overall rehabilitation process.

(d) Access to rehabilitation

There are occasions when a patient is restricted from taking advantage of rehabilitation due to transport difficulties or to inability to take time away from work or domestic duties. Rehabilitation is more likely to be successful if the audiologist can arrange matters to minimize these problems, by operating a flexible schedule, by carrying out domiciliary visits where appropriate and by being aware of relevant local facilities or agencies from which financial or other help can be sought.

In the case of very elderly or otherwise handicapped patients, suitable transport may theoretically be available to them, but the stress of travelling and of being in an unfamiliar environment can be counterproductive to rehabilitation. This is particularly so where there are problems with continence or strict timing requirements for medication or diet, and in such instances, domiciliary provision of rehabilitation should be available. Visits to a patient's home or place of work may also be appropriate where the audiologist wishes to enlist the help of other people in the patient's environment, such as relatives or neighbours, care staff or colleagues, who are unable or unwilling to accompany the patient to see the audiologist.

Finally, access to suitable rehabilitation can be a problem for minority racial groups where the patient concerned does not have a good command of the audiologist's language. It is extremely difficult to provide anything other than the most basic rehabilitation through the interpreting of a friend or member of the family. In clinics serving large communities where a significant proportion of the population use another language, there is a strong argument for employing staff of the appropriate nationality. Alternatively, suitably bilingual volunteers from the communities concerned could be trained to act as lay counsellors and to assist in dialogue between the patient and audiologist.

(e) Fears associated with hearing-aid use

Most fears concerning hearing-aid use relate to beliefs that the hearing will be made worse or 'lazy' to anticipated difficulties coping with an aid, or to the personal or financial problems that are envisaged after loss or breakage of an aid. In most cases these fears are based on misunderstandings, and should be helped by suitable education and counselling. However, the important thing is that patients should be given the opportunity to express any fears that are inhibiting them from hearing-aid use, and that they should not be made to appear foolish in the process, even if their fears seem irrational to the audiologist.

10.2 PHYSICAL PROBLEMS WITH HEARING-AID USE

Successful hearing-aid use ideally requires that patients should be able to fit, operate and care for the hearing-aid by themselves and that the presence of the aid does not materially interfere with the conduct of their lives. Unfortunately, many hearing-aid fittings are at best a compromise between this ideal and what can be achieved in the face of a variety of physical problems. The audiologist must not underestimate the importance of these problems to the patient. The greater their quantity or severity, the greater will need to be the patient's motivation to persist in hearing-aid use despite them, and the audiologist has a responsibility to try and overcome or minimize them.

(a) Hearing aid use and care

Difficulties with hearing-aid fitting are the most commonly reported problems with aid use amongst the older population (Ward, Gowers and Morgan, 1979; Brooks, 1985). Unfortunately, this is often the result of insufficient time and attention given to making or modifying the earmould for optimum insertion and to instructing the patient appropriately. Skeletonized earmoulds or moulds with added 'handles' help overcome dexterity problems, and the importance of correct instruction methods is discussed in Chapter 7. However, despite careful choice of earmould and painstaking instruction, there are certain patients who remain unable to fit the hearing aid themselves, in which case suitable advice and training may have to be given to other people in the patient's life. The patient must, of course, be consulted first and be in full agreement before such a step is taken.

If a patient has sufficient comprehension and mobility to be able to fit a hearing aid, he/she will normally be able to operate it satisfactorily, although considerable practice may be required to enable suitably fine adjustments of the controls to be made. It is better for a patient to learn to operate the aid when it is in place rather than develop the habit of switching it on and setting the volume before insertion, as this latter procedure tends to deny the patient the opportunity to make

subsequent adjustments to the aid according to his/her listening requirements.

For the same reason it is highly desirable that a patient, whose aid is
fitted by someone else, should still be able to operate the aid without
assistance. Patients with poor dexterity can be encouraged to practise
manipulating the aid while holding it in their hands, first looking at it
and then with eyes closed, so that they can subsequently transfer this
skill to the aid in place. Where appropriate, aids should be selected
according to the ease with which their controls can be felt and
manipulated, and if necessary, they can be modified by the addition of
extra knobs to facilitate operation. In some cases it may be appropriate to
fit a body-worn hearing aid or an aid with a stetoclip or headphone
attachment to overcome fitting and manipulation problems without
depriving the patient of independence. Hopefully the new generation of
remote-control hearing aids, which allow a head-worn aid to be adjusted
by manipulating a larger device kept in the pocket, will provide a more
elegant solution to these problems.

Sometimes a patient who has little or no problem fitting and using a
hearing aid may still have great difficulty caring for it adequately. A
patient with visual impairment may have the dexterity to use the aid and
change the batteries but be unable to see to clean the earmould, remove
wax or replace tubing. Problems can also arise due to impaired memory
or comprehension, even in a patient who uses a hearing aid regularly.
In the latter case, written instructions or diagrams may enable the
patient to cope alone, but it is probably preferable in most instances to
find a local person who can be taught to care for the aid as required,
providing the patient is happy with this arrangement.

(b) Comfort and compatibility of hearing aids

One of the most desirable things for successful hearing-aid use is for
patients to be able to forget that they are wearing the aid. This requires
that the aid and mould should fit comfortably and cause the patient
minimum inconvenience in daily activities. Some patients require a
great deal of help to achieve acceptable comfort and convenience.

When comfort is the main complaint, it is not always easy to elucidate
the origin of the problem from the patient's own description of
discomfort. It can be helpful if the patient is instructed to wear the aid
for a period immediately before seeing the audiologist, even if this
involves some pain, as a careful inspection of the auricle and meatus
may then reveal a reddened area, indicating where the mould or aid
needs modification. Some patients find that earmoulds made of soft
material that flex with movements of the ear are more comfortable than

rigid moulds, but soft moulds may have other disadvantages as indicated in Section 10.3.

A quite common problem is for the pinna to lie flat to the head so that the wearing of a postaural aid displaces the pinna. This can cause discomfort behind the pinna, the concha or sometimes down the side of the neck. It is clearly a situation where an intra-aural aid is preferable, but this may not be possible on financial grounds or when the patient needs more amplification than can be obtained from such an aid without producing acoustic feedback. In such cases the particular shape and size of the postaural hearing aid is important and this can be a critical factor in selection between different models. Modifications to the aid itself (e.g. rounding the corners or changing the angle of the earhook) may be required.

Similar considerations apply when the problem is one of compatibility, for example, with spectacles. The patient should be able to remove and replace spectacles without causing discomfort or dislodging the aid. Various models of hearing aids can be attached to or housed within a spectacle frame, but this is not necessarily desirable if it constrains the patient always to wear aid and spectacles together. Compatibility with any kind of head-worn apparel can present a major problem. Items of protective headgear or those worn for other occupational or religious reasons are obviously important, and it must be remembered that hats and wigs have a heat-conservation role as well as a social function for elderly or alopecic persons.

Despite careful selection or modification of the hearing-aid fitting, adaptations will sometimes have to be made to the other item in question, for example, by altering the shape of a spectacle arm or changing the style of a protective helmet. Some solutions may be innovative or even bizarre, but the simpler and less obtrusive the result, the more likely that the patient will be amenable to it, and the better the prognosis for successful hearing-aid use.

(c) Circumstances not conducive to hearing-aid use

Various practical problems arise from the inappropriateness of hearing-aid use in certain circumstances. Some patients, particularly if they live alone, may feel insecure being deprived of the environmental sounds and signals that normal-hearing people perceive, even when asleep. Such a patient may feel more secure sleeping in a room that is not completely dark, or if accompanied by a suitably trained dog, or even a cat. If there is some specific signal that needs to be detected, such as an alarm clock, a baby crying or an invalid calling, this can usually be achieved by use of an appropriate ancillary device.

A particularly unfortunate effect of not wearing hearing aids in bed can be the disruption of a patient's sexual or marital relationships because of the loss of intimate verbal communication, particularly when darkness removes the visual cues. As most patients are unlikely to volunteer the fact that sexual matters are becoming a problem, the audiologist should be prepared to ask about this and to provide or direct the patient to suitable counselling when appropriate. It can be particularly important to maintain the sexual bonds between patient and partner when their relationship is under pressure from the other compromises in social or employment status resulting from the hearing loss.

There is no simple solution to the limitations to hearing-aid use in the presence of water, such as when washing or swimming. Spoken communication is usually an integral part of activities such as attendance at the hairdresser's, a family day on the beach or participation in watersports. It is technically possible to manufacture waterproof hearing aids but there has been insufficient demand to warrant this, so there is currently little alternative than the learning of compensatory communication tactics. In certain kinds of employment, for example, if the person is a lifeguard or watersports instructor, an acquired hearing loss may then necessitate a change of job, for which suitable counselling and advice must be available.

10.3 MEDICAL PROBLEMS

One of the main disadvantages of regular hearing-aid use is that it involves sustained contact of man-made material with the skin in and around the ear. This can cause acute or chronic inflammation of the ear canal in patients prone to allergic reactions or ezcema. The ear fitting may also introduce bacterial or fungal infections that can be difficult to eradicate.

In all such cases, any obviously infected, inflamed or discharging ear should be referred for medical attention. Ear impressions should not be taken and it is preferable for the patient to avoid or minimize hearing-aid use until the condition has improved. If the reaction exhibits itself again within a short period of the patient using the earmould, alternative fittings or non-allergic or inert material should be produced. Wherever it is acoustically feasible, patients with a tendency to these conditions should have vented or unoccluding earmoulds and the moulds should be skeletonized so as to minimize the area of skin in the concha that is not in contact with the air. These problems are often worse with soft-textured earmoulds than with fittings with smooth hard surfaces.

Some patients maintain healthy external ears but are still bothered by excessive perspiration in the enclosed ear. Apart from being uncomfortable and likely to exacerbate any incipient infection, the perspiration condenses in the tube of postaural aids and can cause acoustic interference. Excessive condensation in the earhook may start to interfere with the function of the receiver. Vented and skeletonized moulds are again indicated and the patient can be educated to recognize the first signs of condensation and take remedial action. New types of hearing-aid tubing are now being manufactured that claim to eliminate condensation problems.

Patients suffering from infections, inflammation or excess perspiration should have binaural fittings wherever possible so that they can alternate hearing-aid use between ears to allow recovery of an ear or to reduce the frequency of the problems occurring. Where the use of vented or unoccluding earmoulds leads to feedback, the provision of 'CRIS-CROS' or 'HI-CROS' fittings allows the ears to remain unoccluded without feedback by physically separating microphone from aid output.

Advice on earmould care and hygiene should be given to all patients, remembering that these problems can be distressing and embarrassing to some people. If patients are forced to curtail hearing-aid use for any of these medical reasons, suitable counselling about their choice of when to use their aids and how to cope when they are not using them may be vital in minimizing the handicap caused.

10.4 ACOUSTIC PROBLEMS WITH HEARING AIDS

Many types of hearing loss are characterized by certain perceptual problems that limit the benefit that can be obtained from hearing aids, as discussed in the next section (section 10.5). Unfortunately, even the patient with none of these difficulties is unable to function as well with hearing aids as if he was normally hearing. This fact is not appreciated by those who regard straightforward conductive hearing losses as offering no particular rehabilitation problems. However, the performance of the hearing aid as perceived by the user is largely dependent on the nature of the listening environment, because of the effects of background noise and reverberation.

People suffering from a gradual or long-standing hearing loss have adapted to subjectively reduced levels of background sound. When these background sounds are suddenly reintroduced to the patient through amplification, a period of adjustment is required to relearn the identity of these 'new' sounds and mentally restore them to the auditory background where they can be ignored. However, to a degree, all background noises become more intrusive and more competitive with whatever the patient is trying to hear when wearing a hearing aid. This is largely due to the loss of fine judgement about the location of the different sounds around him/her. If a patient uses only one hearing aid and is impaired in the other ear, he/she will be deprived of binaural clues to localization. In addition, the loss of high-frequency hearing and the occlusion effect of the ear with an earmould reduces the localization function of the concha and prevents the listener from separating in space the various sound sources impinging on a single ear.

Poor localization can be a handicap in itself, both because the direction of a sound helps to identify it and because people often need to react to environmental sounds with respect to their direction. More importantly, the ability to localize different simultaneous sound sources appears to give the person a subjective improvement in signal-to-noise ratio, facilitating the discrimination of speech in noise. The mechanisms that allow a person to attend by choice to only one of many competing auditory signals are still not completely understood, but gross physical cues such as direction can be used to 'separate' one message from another for the purposes of selective attention. The effect of 'binaural release from masking' has also been clearly demonstrated in laboratory conditions (Carhart, Tillman and Johnson, 1967).

The problem of reverberation relates to the same underlying principles of 'separation' of signal from noise. Unless in completely anechoic test conditions, the listener receives numerous reflections of the original signal from the surrounding surfaces. The normal listener is usually only aware of these when they become very delayed in relation to the original signal, when they are perceived as echoes. In semi-reverberant conditions, the 'precedence effect' causes the signal and its immediate reflections to be integrated and localized in the direction of the original signal, so that the reverberations are not noticed. However, this effect seems to be strongly dependent upon binaural hearing and for many hearing-aid wearers, any reverberations constitute extra background noise with which the original signal must compete.

In practice, the degree to which these difficulties affect a patient will depend on the extent to which the person desires or needs to communicate in background noise or reverberant conditions. Theoretically, the problem may be reduced by improving the patient's ability to localize sounds by: (1) providing binaural amplification, (2) minimizing occlusion of the ear when the patient has sufficient residual hearing to use for natural localization, (3) optimizing the hearing at high frequencies, (4) providing aids with directional microphones, and (5) fitting the patient with intra-aural or in-the-canal aids that may preserve some of the external ear's localization function. Although some experiments have shown that binaural hearing aids can improve a patient's ability to discriminate speech-in-noise as an artificially controlled stimulus (e.g. Nabalek and Pickett, 1974), there is generally only circumstantial evidence of significant benefit from any of the above solutions in a generally noisy or reverberant environment. It is likely that the overall degree of benefit will depend on the patient's residual frequency and temporal resolution skills, which must be a critical part of the overall localization and discrimination process.

One recent development related to point (4), providing aids with directional microphones, is the use of small hand-held models in conjunction with direct-input hearing aids. The user directs the microphone towards whoever he/she wishes to hear, and thereby achieves a considerable increase in signal-to-noise ratio. Other ancillary devices such as the loop system are also essentially methods of improving signal-to-noise ratio and minimizing the effect of the acoustic environment (see Chapter 12).

Unfortunately, most of our everyday communication occurs in circumstances that are not amenable to use of ancillary aids. The greatest help available to the hearing-aid wearer when faced with an unfavourable acoustic environment is the adoption of suitable communication strategies. These would include obvious tactics to improve the signal-to-noise ratio such as removing or reducing competing sounds and moving closer to the speaker. Interference from reverberation can be reduced by moving away from a wall or into a more softly furnished environment, or by such simple measures as putting a cloth on a dining table or drawing curtains across a window. Speechreading is also important in helping a conversation to be picked out from background noise and reverberation. Some people seem to acquire such skills naturally and may not even be conscious of how much they are doing to improve their immediate environment. Other patients may require a considerable input in the way of education, counselling or more intensive training before they learn to exercise effectively these kinds of communication skills. Very elderly or handicapped patients may be unable to learn or execute such skills, in which case training should be directed towards the others involved.

Regrettably there will always be some situations, particularly in relation to employment conditions, where little can be done to improve an acoustically poor environment and where good use of communication skills still cannot compensate for the problems of hearing-aid use. The acoustics of classrooms, hospital wards, courtrooms and boardrooms can be so bad that the teacher, nurse, barrister or businessman with only a mild and theoretically 'correctable' hearing loss may get virtually no benefit from hearing-aid use in their workplace. The degree of handicap experience can thus seem out of all proportion to the level of hearing loss, which emphasizes the need for thorough assessment of the patient and his/her communication requirements before effective rehabilitation can begin. The only real solution to a patient's problems may be a change of work environment, which, in turn, could entail a complete change of career and hence of financial, social and even domestic lifestyle. In these cases such patients will probably need help to explore the possible alternatives facing them and the audiologist should ensure that suitable advice and counselling are available.

10.5 AUDITORY PROBLEMS

A hearing loss does not normally produce a uniform attenuation of all frequencies and all intensities of sound. Patients perceive signals that are mildly or grossly distorted in comparison with the original acoustic stimulus. Modern hearing-aid selection is based on the philosophy that an optimum fitting should more or less compensate for the configuration of each hearing impairment (apart from the acoustic problems already discussed), but there are still limitations to what can currently be achieved.

(a) Problems of frequency distortion

The majority of hearing impairments affect the high frequencies more than the low, with loss of important information for consonant discrimination. This is usually experienced as a lack of clarity of speech but not necessarily a lack of volume, frequently leading sufferers to blame other people's speech production for their own poor reception of the message.

Modern electroacoustic hearing aids tend to amplify high frequencies more than low, and a combination of aid selection and acoustic modification gives considerable scope for matching different configurations of hearing loss. However, problems still occur with steeply-sloping high-frequency hearing loss, with pronounced low-frequency loss, or where there is a combination of high- and low-frequency loss with good hearing at mid-frequencies. Most hearing aids are also unable to provide adequate amplification at very high frequencies (6–8 kHz) which appear to be important for speech discrimination in background noise. Even where an ideal fitting is theoretically attainable by use of an unconventional system such as a CROS aid, the patient may not receive sufficient additional benefit to compensate for the extra inconvenience or reduction in cosmetic status of the aid in question. The full implications of different hearing-aid fittings should therefore be discussed with the patient as part of the selection process.

When, for one of the above reasons, a hearing loss is to remain unaided or inadequately aided, such patients may require alternative help in the form of ancillary devices to alert them to important signals or to improve speech discrimination in certain situations. Counselling, education or additional communication training may all help to minimize discrimination problems.

Inadequate auditory input for accurate speech discrimination can also lead to distortion or omission of some elements in the patient's own speech production. This is one reason for selection of the optimum hearing-aid fitting and for encouraging the patient to use aids even if the overall improvement in received speech discrimination is minimal because of good speechreading skills. Communication training will sometimes be required to conserve the voice quality of certain patients if they are unable, even when aided, to monitor their own speech adequately.

(b) Problems of intensity distortion

Some hearing losses, originating from the cochlea, exhibit the phenomenon of recruitment of loudness, where the dynamic range between very quiet and very loud is reduced. The patient requires amplification of low-intensity sounds to make them perceptable, but may need little or no amplification of high-intensity sounds. This is why the level of amplification required by most patients is much less than that which would be predicted by a simple mirroring of their audiogram, as discussed in Chapter 4. In practice, a compromise is sought whereby speech at normal conversational level is amplified so as to be presented to the patient's ear at the most comfortable listening level (usually approximately halfway between the patient's threshold and loudness-discomfort level). This is intended to achieve maximum speech discrimination for normal conversation, but almost certainly means that the degree of amplification is not sufficient for very quiet environmental sounds to become audible. Therefore patients using an aid at a satisfactory level for conversation may not hear all the other significant sounds around them, such as a baby crying upstairs or a telephone ringing in another room. In this case ancillary devices may be needed in addition to hearing aids to alert patients to important events in their particular environment.

At the other extreme, the patient with severe recruitment may have a problem obtaining sufficient amplification for speech without other more intense sounds becoming unbearably loud. There are several methods by which the maximum output of amplification can be limited, but some can have a deleterious effect on speech discrimination and the better systems are more expensive. It is important that such patients appreciate the need to adjust the volume control of the hearing aid according to the sounds they are being exposed to, particularly if an aid with suitable output limiting has not been fitted. A hearing aid that regularly produces intolerably loud sounds will probably not be worn at all.

(c) Problems of frequency discrimination

Many sensorineural hearing losses are known to be accompanied by an impairment in the ear's ability to discriminate one frequency from an adjacent one, or to differentiate a signal from a background noise of similar frequencies. This is generally agreed to be related to the broadening or flattening of the tuning curves associated with individual cochlear neurones such that their response is no longer sharply specific to an individual frequency. In a mild form it is probably represented by the patient who has good unaided speech discrimination in quiet situations, but suffers an immediate degradation of discrimination in any degree of background noise. It is not yet routinely examined in the clinic and is certainly not indicated by performance on the normal speech-discrimination-in-quiet test. There is evidence that it varies considerably between patients with similar losses (Moore, 1985), but until appropriate psychoacoustic tests are introduced to rehabilitative assessment, it is not possible to judge the incidence of this problem in the population or its severity in the individual. Unfortunately, there is currently no satisfactory method of overcoming this problem in hearing-aid fitting, but tests of frequency resolution could be useful in determining the prognosis for hearing-aid fitting and the relative importance of alternative rehabilitative techniques.

In trying to fit a hearing aid to the patient with poor frequency resolution, the main priority is to give the patient realistic expectations of hearing-aid use, and to accept that in some cases, the perceived benefit may be so small that the patient will opt to remain unaided. With or without hearing aids, speechreading skills are likely to be of particular importance in trying to understand speech against competing signals or noise. Training in hearing tactics or conversation strategies may be necessary, particularly if the patient's work or social circumstances requires frequent communication in groups or background noise. The person with poor frequency resolution who uses hearing aids will obviously be particularly disadvantaged by the problems of background noise and reverberation described earlier in this chapter, and the benefit obtained from the aids will be even more dependent on the acoustic environment in which they are used.

(d) Other speech-processing problems

Small numbers of patients present with problems of distortion that fall outside the more typical patterns described above. Some are thought to suffer from poor temporal resolution in the form of decreased ability to detect intervals between successive signals and to discriminate between different durations of signal or interval. Temporal factors are known to be important in speech discrimination, but it has been suggested that temporal resolution problems only contribute significantly to discrimination difficulties in relatively severe hearing losses. It is not routine practice to test temporal resolution in the rehabilitation clinic, nor is it clear whether these problems could be overcome by either suitable hardware or appropriate training.

A few patients experience a gross distortion of sound whereby speech and music are made both unpleasant and unrecognizable, for example, in association with Menière's disorder. Some patients have, for shorter or longer periods, such poor speech discrimination in the affected ear as not to be helped by amplification, and may experience hyperacusis (undue sensitivity to loud sounds) or diplacusis (the same sound heard as a different pitch in the two ears). In unilateral cases, occlusion of the offending ear can relieve these latter symptoms, although it can be argued that this would inhibit any natural process of adaptation and desensitization that might otherwise occur while the ear is exposed to normal environmental and speech sounds. Interestingly, where such hearing losses are bilateral, one ear usually retains reasonably good speech discrimination and tolerance of amplification (Hood, 1984) suggesting that adaptation and desensitization to a distorted input can occur, but that the brain cannot resolve very discrepant inputs for the two ears.

There are also speech-discrimination problems that arise as a result of central disorders in the auditory-processing pathway. These are relatively uncommon, and are mainly seen following incidents such as skull injuries or cardiovascular accidents, when there is some indication that unusual problems may be involved. However, it is important for the prognosis of rehabilitation that such difficulties are recognized even if the exact nature of the central-processing problem cannot be identified.

Regardless of pathology or degree of distortion, hearing aids should always be tried if the patient is amenable, particularly if both ears are affected. Patients with very poor discrimination are effectively in the same situation as someone with a profound hearing loss, even though their auditory thresholds to pure tones may be quite good. Hearing aids may at least enable them to perceive when someone is speaking, even if they gain little benefit in the form of improved speech discrimination. They may also obtain important environmental clues from personal amplification, to a greater extent than can be provided by ancillary aids. However, training in supplementary or alternative communication skills will be vital to these patients, some of whom may also be able to utilize their residual hearing more effectively with the help of suitable auditory training techniques.

(e) Severe unilateral hearing loss

Severe unilateral hearing loss can be extremely disabling, particularly when of sudden onset. This is partly because of the loss of localization and resultant interference from background noise and reverberation discussed earlier. The patient will also have difficulty hearing in quiet situations if the speaker is positioned on the side of the bad ear because the head creates a shadow to high-frequency sound and only a degraded speech signal will reach the good ear. If this has normal or near-normal thresholds, the impaired ear cannot be helped by routine hearing-aid fitting because of cross-over via bone-conduction pathways to the good ear.

In such cases, depending on the situations where most problems are experienced, CROS or BI-CROS fittings can be extremely helpful in overcoming the head-shadow effect and restoring a sense of 3-dimensionality to the sound field. However, it can be difficult to predict exactly which patients will obtain significant benefit, and it is desirable for patients to have extended trials of such fittings, perhaps with some training, before any final evaluation and decision on fitting is made. Other patients with unilateral loss learn to manage very well without hearing aids by developing good hearing tactics and speechreading skills.

(f) Severe or profound bilateral-hearing loss

When a severe or profound hearing loss is bilateral, hearing-aid benefit will be limited, and it may not be possible to demonstrate any improvement in speech discrimination if the speech material is presented as an auditory signal alone. However, there is now considerable evidence to show that performance on a speechreading task can be considerably enhanced by the addition of even a very degraded auditory signal (Summerfield, 1983). Interest in this area has increased since the development of the cochlear implant because this prosthesis generally conveys only fairly fundamental information about voicing and some prosodic features of speech rather than sufficient frequency information to enable speech discrimination by purely auditory means. The patient with a cochlear implant is thus in a similar situation to the patient with profound hearing loss using a hearing aid. Cochlear implant programmes usually include a considerable period of training to help the patient make the best use of the available auditory input in complementing speechreading skills. A similar period of training may help the patient with severe hearing loss first trying to use a hearing aid, particularly if the loss is of recent onset. On the other hand, some patients with progressively deteriorating hearing losses prefer to give up hearing-aid use even while still able to perceive sounds through the aid, either because they find speechreading easier without the distorted auditory signal, or because of tinnitus exacerbated by auditory stimulation.

An alternative to hearing-aid use or cochlear implant in a profoundly deaf person is the vibrotactile aid, which converts auditory input to a vibrating stimulus from a transducer worn on the wrist or other sensitive part of the body. The information perceived by the wearer resembles that described above in relation to cochlear implants or poor residual hearing, giving mainly cues to voicing and some prosodic features of speech, and it is likely that similar training is necessary to achieve optimum improvement in speech discrimination. It remains to be seen whether profoundly deaf patients can learn to utilize vibrotactile cues as effectively as auditory ones.

Apart from the important consideration of speech discrimination, all these prostheses can play an important role in helping the user to maintain normal speech production, although additional voice-conversation measures may still be required. They can also help a profoundly deaf person to perceive environmental sounds. Lack of awareness of non-speech sounds can be extremely disorientating, whether it is the significant signals of environmental events that are missed, or the auditory background of body-noise, movement of people, weather, etc., of which we are not normally aware. For many profoundly deaf people, hearing aids or vibrotactile devices do little more than inform them of events immediately around them, but they still perform a vital role in keeping such persons in contact with their immediate surroundings in a way that vision alone cannot. For events somewhat removed from the person, other forms of visual or vibrotactile ancillary aid are necessary to help restore independent function. In the UK and USA, dogs are sometimes trained to act as 'alerting' companions for profoundly deaf people.

Whether or not any material support is used, patients with sudden, severe, hearing loss will require help to learn to make optimum use of whatever information is available to them in communication with their environment and the people in it. This training needs to be intensive and structured to the patient's particular needs. The communication skills required in order to function in a silent world are not likely to be naturally acquired as those that complement slightly degraded auditory input often are. Alternative communication techniques may need to be considered. Whatever the ultimate choice of communication strategies, deafened patients and their families will be in need of a great deal of information and support-counselling throughout the whole process of rehabilitation because of the severity and complexity of the likely effects on self-identity and life style. The process of adaptation and adjustment may take many years in a suddenly deafened adult, but he/she still represents a rehabilitative crisis deserving immediate and full attention, with the emphasis on good co-operation and collaboration, from all those professionals who have something to offer to the rehabilitation programme.

At the beginning of this chapter, stress was put on the need for correct assessment of the patient by 'the audiologist' to establish which kind of help the patient requires. However, in view of the diversity of problems and possible solutions, it must be recognized that no one profession or individual will necessarily possess the knowledge, skills and resources to provide all the required features of rehabilitation. The emphasis must be on co-operation between professionals and a team approach to solving the problems of each individual patient. Frequently, only one person will be involved in the initial evaluation, but that person must then accept a responsibility to assess the patient's need for any of the available services, and not just those that he/she can provide personally. He/she must be aware of all those services and resources in the community relating to employment, education, recreation and social interaction from which hearing-impaired people may benefit, but that are considered to be beyond the scope of this chapter. The audiologist must also recognize that each individual patient contributes skills, knowledge and resources to the rehabilitation process and so should share in all the planning, decision-making and referral activity that constitute the rehabilitation programme.

REFERENCES

Ashley, J. (1973) *Journey Into Silence*, The Bodley Head, London.
Blauert, J. (1983) *Spatial Hearing*, The MIT Press, Massachusetts.

Brooks, D.N. (1985) Factors relating to the underuse of postaural hearing aids. *Brit. J. Audiol.*, **19**, 211–17.

Carhart, R., Tillman, T. and Johnson, K. (1967) Release of masking for speech through interaural time delay. *J. Acoust. Soc. Amer.*, **42**, 124–38.

Hood, J.D. (1984) Speech discrimination in bilateral and unilateral hearing loss due to Menière's disease. *Brit. J. Audiol.*, **18**, 173–7.

Moore, B.C.J. (1985) Frequency selectivity and temporal resolution in normal and hearing-impaired listeners. *Brit. J. Audiol.*, **19**, 189–201.

Nabalek, A. and Pickett, J. (1974) Monaural and binaural speech perception through hearing aids under noise and reverberation with normal and hearing-impaired listeners. *J. Speech Hear. Res.*, **17**, 724–39.

Summerfield, Q. (1983) Audio-visual speech perception, lipreading and artificial stimulation. In *Hearing science and hearing disorders* (eds E. Lutman and M.H. Haggard), Academic Press, London.

Ward, P.R., Gowers, J.I. and Morgan, D.C. (1979) Problems with handling the BE10 Series hearing aids among elderly people. *Brit. J. Audiol.*, **13**, 31–6.

11

COMMUNICATION TRAINING

Denzil Brooks and Valerie Cleaver

Successful interpersonal communication involves a number of complementary processes depending on the medium in which the communication occurs. When a spoken message is received, the speaker's voice tone, facial expression, posture and gestures and the context can all contribute to the overall meaning. Normal verbal communication incorporates a range of expressive and receptive skills that are acquired as part of normal language development to help us to convey and receive information, ideas and feelings. In spoken English, gesture is generally less important than in certain other languages. However, the underlying psychology of interpersonal behaviour is sufficiently important that the overall interpretation of a conversation can be completely changed if different body language is used. To convey the same information in the absence of all the normal auditory and visual body-language clues requires a much broader vocabulary and subtler phraseology, as used by people who excel in the use of the written word. At the other extreme, indigenous manual communication, such as British Sign Language, has a smaller actual 'vocabulary' but uses facial expression and gestural cues to a much greater extent than an equivalent spoken language to express the same range of meaning. The dependence of successful communication on so many factors means that the impairment of any aspect of a person's expressive or receptive capability will affect the communication process. It also means that there are other channels that can be utilized to optimize communication when one function is impaired. The essence of communication training is the optimization of all the available expressive and receptive skills, making the best use of the residual impaired function and compensating where possible by enhancing other facets of communication.

Our concern here is with the person acquiring a hearing loss who therefore has difficulty receiving the spoken message. Such people may no longer be able to perceive all the phonetic contrasts that enable auditory word discrimination or to perceive by auditory means the physical location of the speaker. Some of the prosodic information that confers important differences in meaning, as well as information about the overall 'tone' of voice (implying the mood of the speaker) may be lost, as may the ability to monitor his/her own voice properly, which may cause changes in speech production affecting expressive communication skills. The training that is currently used to optimize the communication skills in hearing-impaired people falls into three broad areas. Firstly, training to facilitate reception of physical signals that can be utilized, which generally involves learning to make appropriate practical manipulations of the environment or the people in it. Secondly, training aimed at improving perceptual and cognitive skills to make the best interpretation of the information received. Thirdly, training in strategies to maintain communication even when failures occur, which involves patients in using their own verbal skills to manage the conversation to their advantage. The first and last of these areas are frequently described by the single term 'hearing tactics' (von der Lieth, 1972; 1973) and constitute a vital but often not formalized part of communication training. Instead, training has typically been focused on the improvement of perceptual and cognitive skills, under the title of speechreading instruction, auditory training and speech conservation. There are theoretical arguments against considering these communication skills in isolation from each other. Traditionally, however, speechreading has been largely taught as a group exercise, whereas adult auditory training and voice conservation have been more individually tailored. In practice, the methods of instruction employed also incorporate use of appropriate hearing tactics, although often not to the extent merited by their importance for successful communication.

11.1 HEARING TACTICS

(a) Optimizing the signal

The most commonly taught hearing tactics relate either to learning easy control of the hearing-aid (see Chapter 8), to improving the auditory signal-to-noise ratio for hearing-aid performance or to improving the reception of visual information. Listeners can do a lot to change their personal acoustic environment. They can move closer to the speaker, reduce or move away from sources of background noise, and avoid or reduce reverberation, for example, by moving from a corridor to a living room or by the increased use of soft furnishings. They can improve their visual reception by adjusting seating or lighting to their advantage. Loss of environmental signals can be partially compensated for by, for example, sitting with a view of the door to know if someone enters the room.

Some hearing tactics are directed at other people to facilitate communication from the speaker's point of view. It usually helps the hearing-impaired person if the speaker attracts the listener's attention before starting, speaks clearly but with a natural rhythm and avoids shouting, which distorts the face as well as the voice. Speaking slightly more slowly and using short simple sentences can greatly assist elderly listeners.

(b) Conversational strategies

There are also important hearing tactics that relate to the interactions between people that occur during the course of conversation (Suty, 1986). The hearing-impaired person may have arranged lighting and acoustics advantageously, but still have difficulty in understanding what is said. What happens then? Consider three possible scenarios:

1. The listener puts so much effort into hearing and understanding that he/she forgets to contribute the nods, smiles and 'mmmm's' that tell the speaker not only that he/she is being heard and understood, but also if the listener is generally in sympathy with what he/she is saying. The speaker, not receiving appropriate feedback, wonders what he/she is saying wrongly. Is the listener really listening, or simply bored and wishing he/she could get away from the conversation?
2. The listener mishears and makes an inappropriate response. The speaker indicates puzzlement or amusement and the listener does not know why. The speaker may then be reticent to clarify things, not knowing exactly what misunderstanding has occurred and not wishing to appear condescending.
3. The speaker changes the subject of the conversation and the listener completely loses track. He/she tries to bluff by nodding, smiling and pretending he/she is following, but sooner or later is expected to make an appropriate verbal response. He/she says 'pardon?' instead. The speaker looks (and is) nonplussed because he/she does not know how much of the conversation the listener has missed, or why.

In each example communication broke down due to absent or inappropriate feedback. Hearing-impaired persons need to develop skills as 'active listeners' so as to give appropriate feedback. (The term 'active listening' is typically used in discussion of counselling techniques, but is considered to be appropriate in the present context as well.) The individual has to remember to use normal encouraging body language if he/she is managing to follow the conversation. He/she has to learn how to handle the confusion that arises from mishearing, how to acknowledge when he/she has not heard, how to make it easy for the speaker to clarify things for him/her and to avoid giving the blank stare or puzzled look that discourages the speaker from continuing.

At the other extreme of poor listening is the person who totally dominates the conversation so that he/she does not have to listen at all. He/she avoids sustained eye contact, thereby ignoring the signals that normally indicate when someone else wishes to speak, and changes the subject of the conversation if he/she has difficulty in following what anybody else says. This person needs to understand what effect his/her communication style will have on other people, and how the success of his social interaction may be threatened nearly as much by such tactics as by withdrawal strategies. He/she needs to learn more socially acceptable ways of coping.

(c) Teaching hearing tactics

Since most of the general public are unaware of the subtle factors that can facilitate communication for hearing-impaired people, each individual has to accept responsibility for achieving whatever changes are possible, and for doing it in a tactful manner that will not draw attention to their own deficiency in hearing or to other people's deficiency in understanding their problems. It is easy to describe helpful environmental changes or good and bad conversational strategies and to suggest to hearing-impaired people what they might be doing wrong, but they have to perceive for themselves that there are alternatives to the way they are communicating and to feel comfortable that any changes they make are compatible with their life style and personality. The skills of a counsellor/therapist may therefore be required to assess each person's existing conversational strategies and to work with them and their family on improving their communication habits.

If a patient is very elderly or additionally handicapped, he/she may be unable, for mental or practical reasons, to execute some or any of the hearing tactics described here. In such cases, it is the other people in the patient's life – family, friends or care staff – who need to learn the appropriate hearing tactics, so that they can perceive and respond to the patient's needs, even when he/she is unable to communicate his requirements to them.

Whether training in hearing tactics is being aimed at the patient, at the family or carers, or both, individual counselling and group work can both help to develop the right skills. Patients and others usually benefit from sharing their problems and learning from each other's examples, although not all patients respond well to group situations. Programmes cannot be tailored to each individual's requirements, so that some people may spend a lot of time practising skills that they have already acquired or do not need. Another disadvantage of group work is that the poor performers in the class may tend to compare themselves unfavourably with the better communicators (when the difference between them may be only one of degree of hearing loss). They will not then necessarily acquire the enhanced confidence in their own communication ability, which is one of the overall aims of most communication training.

11.2 SPEECHREADING

(a) History

DeLand (1968) states that as early as 1500, it was observed that both hard-of-hearing adults and congenitally deaf children demonstrated extraordinary ability to 'read on the lips', but they were not specifically taught this art. Indeed, Bonet, one of the pioneers of deaf education in the latter part of the 16th century, said:

the reduction of the motions to a system to enable the deaf-mute to understand by the lips alone, as it is well known many of them have done, cannot be performed by teaching, but only by attention on their part and it is to this that their success is to be attributed, and not to the skill of the master.

Not everyone agreed. Then, as now, there were those who, despite the evidence, thought that the reading of lips was a skill that had to be taught by a specially gifted or trained person.

Formal classes for adults' lipreading instruction were commenced in the United States in the 1870s by Sarah Fuller who had previously been a teacher at the Clarke School, and by her assistant Mary True. Early teaching was analytic, each sound being treated as an individual contributor, firstly to the syllable, then to the word and so progressively to the meaning of the whole. Lillie Eginton Warren informed her pupils that the 'forty-odd' sounds of the English language were revealed in 16 'outward manifestations or facial expressions'. Once these had been learnt it was possible to break down any sentence into a string of words, each of which could be written in a coded form using the numbers 1 to 16.

Mrs Graham Bell, a one-time pupil of Mary True, was a highly skilled speechreader. She stated that the process was of a synthetic rather than an analytic nature. She identified the first step as selecting the right word from the pool of possible words, then grasping the meaning of the whole from the limited number of words recognized. Speechreading was not a phoneme-by-phoneme building up of a fully detailed structure, but the grasping of sense and meaning by integrating a number of salient parts. Mrs Bell was the inspiration for one of the best-known and respected proponents of speechreading, Edward B. Nitchie. He stressed that speechreading involved both eye and mind, first observing the appropriate facial movements and then interpreting these in the light of experience and knowledge of context – a type of Gestalt process.

Garstecki and O'Neill (1980) demonstrated that speechreading involved not merely the observation of the individual speaking, but also awareness of the environmental situation. Cues were obtained from the background that reinforced those obtained from the message.

A progression in the understanding of the mechanism of speechreading can be seen over three or four centuries. Bonet saw the process as essentially being related to the movement of the lips. Mrs Bell expanded the concept by stating that the mechanism was that of grasping meaning as a whole rather than trying to decipher each specific element. Jeffers and Barley (1971) indicated three steps within the process; first, the visual reception of motor or movement patterns; second, the perception of those patterns and third, the association of the perceived patterns with concepts. They postulate a fourth aspect related to the second and third steps, this being the filling-in of gaps in the information flow. Schow, Christensen, Hutchinson and Nerbonne (1978) describe speechreading as 'a process of being visually alert to all lip, facial, gestural and environmental clues: a skill which nearly all people have to some degree'.

(b) The limitations of visual speech reception

Markides (1977) reviewed the data on consonant identification by vision alone. This indicated that only 30–40% of initial and 20–30% of final consonants in words are accurately identifiable. However, for practical day-to-day interpretation of discourse, it is not absolutely essential to make faultless identification of consonants. In normal conversational speech there are contextual clues that significantly help in differentiating between sounds that are visually difficult to separate. Alexander Graham Bell called such sounds homophenes. Provided the speechreader has some knowledge of the topic under discussion, it will usually be possible to identify which of a number of homophenes is relevant. Binnie (1974) in a test with 34 normal-hearing persons, showed that although correct identification of phonemes by vision alone was only around 40%, when the responses were grouped according to homophenous categories, the overall correct score rose to 80%.

A factor to be considered in assessing the merits of combined auditory and visual input is the quality of the visual stimulus and the environmental situation in which speechreading is taking place. The tests, such as those described above, were performed under relatively good conditions for speechreading. Lighting was such as to obtain maximum benefit. The subjects tested were not reported as having any visual difficulties.

For the predominantly elderly population with hearing impairment, communicating in real-life situations, there may be a number of factors potentially capable of reducing the effectiveness of speechreading:

1. Lighting may be less than ideal. For best results, a good light on the face of the speaker, and not into the eyes of the speechreader, is desirable.
2. Reasonably good visual acuity is important. With diminished visual acuity, the broader aspects of body language, gesture, etc. will remain largely unaffected, but the more subtle aspects of lip, mouth and tongue movement will be lost. Markides (1977) suggests that at least 20/40 vision is necessary for adequate speechreading in normal situations.
3. An age-related decrement in speechreading performance in subjects over 60 years of age was observed by Farrimond (1959), the elderly only achieving about half the scores achieved by those aged 30–35 years. Simmons (1959) also noted a trend for older subjects to be poorer speechreaders, possibly due to a combination of poorer eyesight, reduced memory span and diminished powers of concentration. More recently Ewertsen and Birk-Nielsen (1971) reported a progressive deterioration in speechreading scores for words with increasing age.
4. A further complication is that not all speakers produce good clear, unambiguous movements of the facial structures. People smoke. They turn away while speaking. Some swallow their words or gabble them. Some barely move the lips while speaking, giving the appearance of a ventriloquist's dummy.

(c) Instruction in speechreading

In that speechreading appears to be an innate skill used by normal or hard-of-hearing individuals in circumstances when the auditory component of communication is difficult but the visual aspect is relatively clear and unambiguous, what need is there for specific instruction in speechreading? What is the role of the 'lipreading class'?

Some information relevant to the first question comes from experience in Sweden. In 1971, the Department of Audiology of the Sodersjukhuset distributed hearing aids to 3850 people (Lundborg, Linzander, Lindstrom et al., 1971). The need for, and success of, various rehabilitative procedures was examined relative to degree of hearing loss. For subjects with hearing levels between 40 and 60 dB (about 50% of the total case load) the recommendation centred primarily on amplification and the use of assistive listening devices. Speechreading and auditory training were only rarely deemed necessary, primarily in subjects where the hearing loss was of a steeply falling pattern. Likewise, for subjects in the 60 to 80 dBHL range (about 40% of the case load) the primary form of assistance was amplification and instrumentation. About 10% were found who required and benefited from speechreading and auditory training.

For the remaining 10% of subjects with losses over 80 dB, about 40% received help from a rehabilitation programme, the percentage being limited by factors such as age, additional handicap, etc. Overall, only about 10% of subjects were found to need and have benefit from speechreading.

Further information about the demand (which may be regarded as different from need) for lipreading has recently been obtained in a study in Manchester. Patients being reviewed one month after issue of a hearing aid were asked if they would be interested in attending speechreading classes. Of the 252 seen up to the time of the data analysis, 16 (8%) had visual difficulties such as to make speechreading impracticable; 24 (10%) suffered from major health problems that precluded their attendance at classes; 10 (4%) were working and unable to attend the classes. Of the 202 potential attenders, 155 (77%) indicated total satisfaction with their hearing aid(s) and declared that they did not wish to attend the free speechreading classes; 14 persons specifically indicated an unwillingness to attend speechreading classes. To each of the 33 who expressed interest, a personal invitation to attend the classes was sent by the speechreading teacher. Illness, travel difficulties, loss of interest, failure to respond, absence of perceived need and other factors reduced the actual number of participants to 12, that is, about 8% of those physically able to travel to the hospital, or 5% of the total population reviewed. These data suggest that the majority of those with hearing impairment who seek for treatment seem well satisfied with the assistance they obtain from well-fitted personal amplification. The demand for instruction in speechreading is limited to about 5–10% of the hearing-impaired population.

This low rate of demand/referral has been viewed with concern by the Association of Teachers of Lipreading to Adults (Levene and Sherren, 1985). These authors commented that many persons invited to attend classes did not do so, and that of those who did, very few continued to attend after one or two exploratory sessions. They therefore designed a new 12-week introductory lipreading course and prepared an information package for use at a hospital in London. Personal letters of invitation to a coffee morning were sent to selected patients, and all those who attended were given a package and an invitation to come to the classes. Approximately two-thirds joined and stayed on for the whole course.

To assess one aspect of the benefit obtained from such classes, Binnie (1977) enrolled 12 hearing-impaired adults in an intensive speech-reading course over a 12-week period. Tests of speechreading ability were administered before and after the course. They indicated no significant difference. McCormick (1980) also assessed lipreading skill in three groups of subjects. The first group consisted of 15 persons with normal hearing; the second of 15 hard-of-hearing individuals described by their tutors as either intermediate or advanced lipreaders having had, on average, over four years of lipreading tuition. The third group consisted of 24 first-time hearing-aid users. None had received any formal training in lipreading, but all participated in a rehabilitation programme totalling four hours spread over a two-month period. No significant difference was found between the lipreading skills of the experienced lipreaders and the normal-hearing persons. The hearing-aid users were significantly (5% level) poorer when first tested, but after the rehabilitation course, their scores were not significantly different from the other two groups. The relevant advice given during the course was to observe speakers' faces more closely.

Thus the findings of both Binnie (1977) and McCormick (1980) again suggest that the ability to use visual clues to supplement the (possibly deficient) auditory information is an ability possessed by the majority, and is not measurably improved by specific tuition in lipreading *per se*.

Reverting to the study by Binnie (1977), although no improvement in lipreading skill was measurable, the participants were positive about the benefits of the course, as were the patients of Levene and Sherren (1985). A major finding of both studies was a growth in self-assurance; a more assertive approach to communication difficulties. There was a better understanding of the nature of hearing impairment and hearing handicap. Benefits were obtained from shared experience, both in terms of understanding and of mutual support. One subject in the London group stated: 'I have learnt to wear my hearing aid and come to terms with my loss – before the class I suffered.' This supports the thesis that, probably because of inadequate guidance, hearing aids are frequently not giving the help of which they are capable. An overview of all the comments reported from the studies suggests that the main benefits from the 'speechreading' classes is not an improvement in the innate ability to interpret the visible aspects of human communication, but rather a better appreciation of the handicap; an increase in confidence through knowledge and sharing of experience; a greater awareness of other approaches to alleviating the effects of hearing loss, and possibly, a feeling of greater self-involvement in handling one's own rehabilitation.

In this we have a possible answer to the second question posed earlier regarding the benefits of lipreading classes. For some hearing-impaired individuals they are of unquestionable benefit in terms of improved self-esteem, confidence and morale. In the absence of any programme for hearing-aid rehabilitation – a situation common to many, indeed probably most, hospitals, the lipreading class may be the major factor in improving communication, not only through the improvement in non-auditory skills, but also with the hearing aid.

11.3 AUDITORY TRAINING

The term auditory training is used to describe the process whereby some hearing-impaired people can be trained to make better use of their residual hearing by repeated exposure to auditory stimuli, with or without amplification. It is generally agreed that auditory acuity *per se* cannot be improved by such training, but awareness and discrimination skills may be enhanced. Carhart (1961) described auditory training as '. . . the process of teaching the child or adult . . . to take full advantage of sound cues which are still available'. He suggests that the successive goals of a training programme are: to develop awareness of sound, to differentiate gross sounds, to practise discrimination of dissimilar speech sounds and eventually to achieve fine discrimination of acoustically similar phonemes. Other writers infer that auditory training involves the practice of good hearing tactics, with little reference to the development of new perceptual skills.

(a) The history of auditory training

As with speechreading, the origins of auditory training are largely based in early attempts to educate the prelingually deaf. According to Markides (1977) the use of loud sounds to stimulate the hearing of deaf people was first suggested as long ago as the sixth century AD and possibly even earlier. By the eighteenth and nineteenth centuries, systematic attempts were being made, with apparent success, to train hearing-impaired people to hear and differentiate words and speech sounds. With the development of more powerful hearing aids, greater attention was paid to the training of hearing-impaired children by auditory means (in addition to speechreading) and auditory training gradually became an accepted part of the education of children in schools for the deaf.

Not until the 1950s was the use of auditory training considered as a viable part of a rehabilitation programme for adults with acquired hearing loss. Subsequently, many clinicians, particularly in the USA have developed adult auditory-training programmes and reported success in qualitative terms. Quantitative benefits have been less well-researched (Bamford, 1981), as have the fundamental bases on which auditory training is based.

(b) The theoretical basis of auditory training

It is known that speech discrimination as an acquired skill in normal-hearing persons concentrates on those areas of phonetic distinction or contrasts that most meaningfully separate the different speech sounds of the native language. The phoneme, although often described in acoustic terms, is also a unit of meaning. A specific phoneme can occur in acoustically different forms (allophones) without the difference indicating a change of meaning. Different allophones of a phoneme are often used because of articulatory constraints imposed by adjacent speech elements, but the differences between allophones are not generally perceived by the speaker because they do not signify differences in meaning. In the learning of a foreign tongue it often becomes necessary to learn to differentiate between phonemes that are not differentiated in the native language.

Thus it is evident that people can learn to discriminate and reproduce auditory differences in a speech signal of which they were not previously aware. Hearing-impaired people may also be able to utilize different aspects of speech to improve discrimination skill. This process may occur naturally in someone with gradually progressive hearing loss, provided they have adequate exposure to conversation and receive the necessary feedback to reinforce the new discrimination features.

There is evidence from psychology literature of plasticity in speech discrimination, allowing subjects to be trained to improve their discrimination of artificially degraded speech. This is also reflected in the way those associated with a person with a speech impairment learn to interpret the distorted acoustical signals. Furthermore, there is evidence that hearing-impaired people with poor speech discrimination develop or maintain better discrimination in an ear that is being relied on than in one that is not (Hood, 1984). Speech discrimination is not therefore totally determined by the nature and degree of hearing loss, but can be influenced by the communication demands to which the ear is subjected.

These facts suggest that a mechanism exists that could enable hearing-impaired people to develop new speech-discrimination skills if they are able to receive any auditory information on which contrasts can be based. Two important questions remain to be answered. In which categories of patients is this likely to occur? Can it be facilitated or accelerated by training?

Unfortunately there is a dearth of scientific research in this area, as pointed out by Bamford (1981). Bode and Oyer (1970) and Watts and Pegg (1977) reported improvements in speech discrimination following auditory training, but quantitative studies are hampered by the extreme variability in individual responses to training. There is little indication of how to distinguish those persons who might benefit from those who will not. Markides (1977) suggests that a person with a relatively uniform hearing loss is easier to help through amplification and auditory training, but he does not distinguish the benefits of these two forms of help or give reasons for his conclusions. Freeman (1983) suggests benefit for those whose speech discrimination errors are 'bizarre' in relation to their pure-tone audiogram. Undoubtedly there is scope for research in this area, and the revival of interest in analytic speech audiometry may provide a useful foundation for future developments.

Two further groups of patients are now being taught using auditory training methods from whom more concrete evidence of benefit may be forthcoming. These are profoundly deaf patients with cochlear implants and those using vibrotactile aids.

Currently, great importance is placed by cochlear-implant teams on the post-implant training to enable th⁻ patient to make the best use of the limited 'auditory' stimulus he/she is receiving. Most of the current devices provide more than simple signal detection, giving some basis for differentiation between sounds, and extensive training is provided to maximize this ability.

The use of vibrotactile aids for speech discrimination is also receiving more attention with the development of sophisticated systems for extracting speech features. It can be argued that for some patients, such devices may give as much useful information as an implant and should be considered as a viable, or even a preferred non-invasive alternative (Summerfield, 1983). Significant improvements in audio-visual speech discrimination after training have been demonstrated with both types of device.

In both approaches, the emphasis in training has been on the use of auditory clues to supplement speechreading, as is also required by the patient with poor-quality residual hearing. For patients with less-severe hearing losses training may be carried out without visual clues, particularly if this represents their main area of need. The patient's life style should be considered in deciding the most appropriate mode of training, but in either case, the ultimate aim is to enable the person to detect and recognize differences between speech sounds that he/she has previously been confusing.

Discrimination can be considered as comprising two distinct processes. Firstly, perception of a difference between two sounds, and secondly correct identification of which sound is which. Training may involve a progression of repeated exposures to sounds that cannot initially be differentiated, with reinforcement of the identity of sounds that can be differentiated but not identified. For a person with sudden, severe hearing loss, the process may start with differentiation of grossly different sounds. For the less impaired, training may be with acoustically similar phonemes, words in running speech or in reverberent conditions.

Obviously, the training process can be greatly facilitated if the patient has a partner who is able and willing to assist with regular exercises. The involvement of family or friends, or the use of group work or recorded material all help to prevent benefit being limited to the voice of the therapist. For patients without access to formal programmes of rehabilitation, any optimization of their residual hearing may be entirely a self-taught skill, instruction manuals with exercises and advice of hearing tactics having been written for patients to use for practice with whoever is available (Scott, 1979). This requires a high degree of motivation and makes it more difficult for effective feedback to be given and for the training to be structured to patients' needs. The essence of good auditory training is probably the grading of the material used so that patients' confidence in their abilities can be developed. They need to be shown the discriminations that they can already make, while at the same time working on exercises that progressively extend their skills. As with any adult-education programme, it is also important that the training is presented in as interesting and stimulating a format as possible, particularly for severely impaired persons who may have little other satisfactory opportunity for conversation and discussion.

11.4 SPEECH CONSERVATION

Significant problems of speech production related to hearing loss are normally associated with prelingual hearing impairment because of the difficulties involved in speech and language development when the child has poor auditory speech discrimination. However, severe acquired hearing loss can also lead to speech problems. These are most likely to affect the quality of speech, rather than rendering it unintelligible, but for a person whose ability to communicate is already impaired and whose confidence in interpersonal relationships is fragile, there is a great need to maintain good expressive skills.

(a) Problems connected with hearing-aid use

Concern may be expressed by patients in the audiology clinic about their own voices when first using hearing aids. Wearing an aid will amplify the patient's own voice both by air conduction and because of the occlusion effect of the earmould in the ear canal. Most patients will benefit from the reassurance that they are unlikely to shout or talk unnecessarily loudly when they are using the hearing aid, even though it may (at first) seem that way to them. Indeed, family or friends may notice and comment on the reduction in level of the voice and the better modulation that occurs when the aid is worn.

(b) Problems related to profound hearing loss

If patients are completely deprived of the ability to monitor their own speech or the environment around them, their first problem is likely to be one of knowing the level at which to pitch the voice. To help overcome this, training can be given in tactics that can provide information about the different background-noise levels that the person is experiencing. Environmental context is obviously important, in that noise levels are likely, for example, to be higher at a crowded party than on a hospital ward. However, there is still an element of unpredictability about this, and useful information can be derived from observing other people speaking; are they all chatting simultaneously, or are they giving the impression of confiding in quiet intimate conversations. Even if patients misjudge the environment and speak at an inappropriate level, they will often get unintentional feedback from those listening, as the latter are likely to move closer and concentrate harder if the voice is too quiet, and to move away if it is too loud. An overloud voice may also cause other people not involved in the conversation to turn and look. In learning these skills, it is also helpful if the patients' close associates are prepared to give unobtrusive signals about their voice level, both to reinforce the correct judgements they are learning to make, and to help them to adjust appropriately when they have misjudged the environment. There will always be those occasions when noise levels change abruptly (e.g. at a noisy social gathering when someone is about to make an announcement) when it helps the patients to be cued to the change, although there are some subtle visual clues to such occurrences if patients can develop sufficient sensitivity to them. Other problems arise when the severely or profoundly impaired person develops changes in speech production resulting from the inability to monitor the voice normally. The needs of these patients with acquired hearing loss, where the essence is on preserving the person's normal breath control, intonation and articulation, etc., are very different from those of the person with prelingual hearing loss. There is evidence that the degree of deterioration of speech production occurring after acquired profound hearing loss relates to the age of onset of the loss (Cowie, Douglas-Cowie and Kerr, 1982), and there are certainly some totally deafened persons who maintain essentially normal voices. However, those patients with severe or suddenly acquired hearing loss should at least have their speech regularly monitored, and high-quality tape recordings of a suitably structured interview are recommended to provide a permanent record for subsequent assessment by a speech therapist or speech pathologist (Parker, 1983).

11.5 ALTERNATIVE COMMUNICATION

There are individuals with severe or profound hearing loss who need, or prefer to use, alternative forms of communication to supplement or substitute oral means. For some, the strain of speechreading with little auditory or vibrotactile information is considerably alleviated if some form of manual communication is used by the speaker. In those countries where phoneme–manual systems are widely used (e.g. Denmark with the mouth–hand system) this is the natural means of supporting speechreading. In the United Kingdom, the manual alphabet is easily learnt and can be particularly helpful if used on a discretionary basis mainly to cue the first letter of a word when this is ambiguous or not visible by speechreading alone. A few patients, finding their ability to integrate with the normally hearing world drastically reduced, chose to learn the indigenous sign language and mix with the prelingually deaf community.

   In all these cases, hearing-impaired people make a choice that will be at least partly dependent on the willingness or ability of those around them to use the appropriate communication methods. The use of natural gesture and occasional finger spelling should certainly be encouraged in the close family if the patient finds this acceptable. Children, in particular, can respond very well to such techniques to improve communication with a parent, providing all the family enter into the spirit of the learning process and see communication as a challenging and rewarding objective. For some, writing may be a more acceptable alternative. Ideally, the writer should seek to communicate not only the essential information, but also the thoughts and feelings that are part of the message.

   Finally, mention should be made of those with multiple handicaps, who are often in care situations. Optimizing communication should help the carers as well as maintaining some quality of life for the sufferers. The use of writing, communication boards, signs or symbols are all possible approaches where the reception of oral information is poor or non-existent. Elderly people suffering from loss of vision and hearing are unlikely to cope with learning the normal deaf–blind alphabet, but spelling words on the palm of the hand can be effective and requires no special skills on the part of the communicator. It is also important that all patients are given adequate opportunity for self-expression, allowing the two-way element that is the key to inter-personal communication to be maintained.

REFERENCES

Bamford, J. (1981) Auditory training. What is it? What is it supposed to do, and does it do it? *Brit. J. Audiol.*, **15**, 75–8.

Binnie, C.A. (1974) Auditory and visual contributions to the perception of selected English consonants for normally hearing and hearing-impaired listeners. In 'Visual and audio-visual perception of speech' (ed. H. Birk-Nielsen and E. Kampp) *Scand. Audiol.*, suppl. 4, 182–20.

Binnie, C.A. (1977) Attitude changes following speechreading training. *Scand. Audiol.*, **6**, 13–19.

Bode, D.L. and Oyer, H.J. (1970) Auditory training and speech discrimination. *J. Speech Hear. Res.*, **13**, 839–58.

Bonet, J.P. (1620) *Reduccion De Las Letras Y Arte Para Enseñar A Hablar Los Mudos.* Madrid.

Carhart, R. (1961) Auditory training. In *Hearing and deafness* (ed. H. Davis), Holt, Rinehart and Winston, New York.

Cowie, R., Douglas-Cowie, E. and Kerr, A.G. (1982) A study of speech deterioration in post-lingually deafened adults. *J. Laryngol. Otol.*, **96**, 101–12.

DeLand, F. (1968) *The story of lipreading*, A.G. Bell Assn. for the Deaf Inc., Washington, D.C.

Ewertsen, H.W. and Birk-Nielsen, H. (1971) A comparative analysis of the audio-visual, auditive and visual perception of speech. *Acta Otolaryngol.*, **72**, 201–5.

Farrimond, T. (1959) Age differences in the ability to use visual clues in auditory communication. *Lang. and Speech*, **2**, 179–92.

Freeman, G. (1983) The basis of practical auditory training. In *Rehabilitation and acquired deafness* (ed. W.J. Watts), Croom Helm, London.

Garstecki, D.C. and O'Neill, J.J. (1980) Situational cue and strategy influence on speechreading. *Scand. Audiol.*, **9**, 147–51.

Hood, J.D. (1984) Speech discrimination in bilateral and unilateral hearing loss due to Menière's disease. *Brit. J. Audiol.*, **18**, 173–7.

Jeffers, J. and Barley, M. (1971) *Speechreading (lipreading)*, Chas. C. Thomas, Springfield, Ill.

Levene, J.C. and Sherren, P. (1985) Lipreading teachers and hearing therapists working together. *Hearing Therapy No. 5*, 3–5.

Lundborg, T., Linzander, S., Lindstrom, B., Sward, I. and Fransson, A. (1971) Special devices for the hearing handicapped patient. *Nordisk Audiologi.*, **3/4**, 96–132.

Markides, A. (1977) Rehabilitation of people with acquired deafness in adulthood. *Brit. J. Audiol.*, suppl. 1.

McCormick, B. (1980) The assessment of audio-visual speech discrimination skills in aural rehabilitation programmes. In *Disorders of auditory function* (eds I.G. Taylor and A. Markides, Academic Press, London, pp. 305–20.

Parker, A. (1983) Speech conversation. In *Rehabilitation and acquired deafness* (ed. W.J. Watts), Croom Helm, London.

Schow, R.L., Christensen, J.M., Hutchinson, J.M. and Nerbonne, M.A. (1978) *Communication disorders of the aged*. Univ. Park Press, Baltimore.

Scott, D. (1979) *Learning to listen again*. The Canadian Hearing Society, Toronto.

Simmons, A.A. (1959) Factors related to speechreading. *J. Speech Hear. Res.*, **2**, 340–52.

Summerfield, Q. (1983) Audio-visual speech perception, lipreading and artificial stimulation. In *Hearing science and hearing disorders* (eds M.E. Lutman and M.H. Haggard). Academic Press, London.

Suty, K.A. (1986) Communication strategies for hearing-impaired people. *Hearing. Rehab. Quarterly*, **11**, 4–20.

Watts, W.J. and Pegg, K.S. (1977) The rehabilitation of adults with acquired hearing loss. *Brit. J. Audiol.*, **11**, 103–10.

von der Lieth, L. (1972) Hearing tactics. *Scand. Audiol.*, **1**, 155–60.

von der Lieth, L. (1973) Hearing tactics II. *Scand. Audiol.*, **2**, 209–14.

12

ANCILLARY AIDS FOR THE HEARING IMPAIRED

Geoff Plant

Many of the problems that confront hearing-impaired persons in everyday life cannot be solved merely by the fitting of appropriate hearing aids and providing counselling in their use. There remain many situations where the hearing aid provides only limited assistance and the hearing-impaired person is placed at a serious disadvantage. Persons with acquired hearing losses quite often find themselves avoiding situations that were previously of great importance to them. The effects of distance, noise and reverberation either singly or in combination conspire to greatly lower the ability of the hearing impaired to adequately cope in such settings as restaurants, churches and theatres.

Even a simple activity such as watching television or listening to the radio can place almost intolerable strain on many hearing-aid users. As a result, the hearing-impaired person is deprived of a rich potential source of entertainment and information. Quite often this is rationalized by statements such as 'Oh, there's nothing worth watching anyway'. In many cases, unfortunately, the decision is not based on free choice. Rather, the hearing-impaired person has been forced to adopt this position because of the limitations imposed by the hearing loss and the failure of hearing aids to overcome these limitations. Other seemingly trivial activities may also cause significant difficulties. Many hearing-impaired persons, for example, are unable to hear the ring of an alarm clock. Hearing-impaired parents may be seriously disadvantaged by being unable to hear their infant's cry. For others the problem may stem from an inability to hear the telephone ring or a visitor knocking on the front door. The most extreme problem is faced by the small group of profoundly deaf persons who derive little or no benefit from hearing-aid usage.

A growing awareness of these problems has resulted in many audiologists and therapists investigating the use of supplementary aids for the hearing-impaired. In most countries interest in the wide range of supplementary aids that may assist the hearing impaired is a relatively recent phenomenon. A noteworthy exception, however, has been the Swedish Hearing Health Care System, which has provided supplementary aids as part of their regular service since 1964 (Lundborg, 1977). As a result of this long-term involvement, the provision of supplementary aids is now seen as part of a standard audiological service. Some idea of the scope of this service can be gained from Fagerberg's (1977) report that 'the total costs for auxiliary aids approximately equal those for hearing aids in Sweden'. The Department of Audiology at Sodersjukhuset in Stockholm reported in 1984 that on average, two to three supplementary devices were provided with every hearing-aid fitting. The range of supplementary aids provided included signalling devices (60% of cases), aids to telephone use (50% of cases) and television/radio aids (50% of cases). It is unfortunate that much of the knowledge gained by these workers is not readily available outside Sweden. Although a number of papers by Swedish workers in the area have been published in English (Lundborg, Lindzander, Lindstrom *et al.*, 1971, 1972; Lundborg, 1977; Fagerberg, 1977; Johansson, 1977) these tend only to give a brief outline of the work undertaken. Detailed descriptions of the aids provided are available (Handikappinstitutet, 1972; 1982) but unfortunately, these are written only in Swedish. It is to be hoped that similar materials will eventually be made available in English. A detailed description of the Swedish experience would be of great assistance to those organizations and individuals considering implementation of a service that includes the provision of supplementary aids for the hearing-impaired.

The aim of this chapter is to provide a general overview of the range of supplementary aids available for use by hearing-impaired persons. The aids available can be divided into the following broad categories:

1. Assistive listening devices and systems.
2. Aids to telephone use.
3. Signalling and alarm systems.
4. Television and radio aids.
5. Alternative communication aids for the profoundly deaf.

12.1 ASSISTIVE LISTENING DEVICES AND SYSTEMS

Noise is an enemy of both listeners and talkers. Noise and reverberation often adversely affect interpersonal and large area communication. Most of the interference can be overcome by providing a favorable signal-to-noise ratio through the use of assistive listening devices. (Vaughn, 1986)

Audiologists and others working with the adult hearing-impaired are familiar with the great problems created for hearing-aid users by noise and reverberation. Quite often, new hearing-aid users will complain that although their aids function very well in the acoustically pristine environment of the clinic, they provide much reduced benefit in many everyday listening situations. This is not surprising when the effects on the hearing-impaired listener of a poor signal-to-noise ratio are considered. Gengel (1971) for example, found that a signal-to-noise ratio (S/N) of less than +15 dB led to a decline in the speech-discrimination abilities of hearing-impaired subjects. Similarly Bankoski and Ross (1984) report that hearing-impaired persons 'require a signal-to-noise ratio (S/N) of +10 to 15 dB to achieve the same speech-discrimination score, which a normal hearing person can achieve at zero S/N'. The effects of reverberation on hearing-impaired listeners also need to be considered. Finitzo-Hieber and Tillman (1978) found that the speech-discrimination scores of a group of hard-of-hearing children declined with increasing reverberation times. Harris and Reitz (1985) reported similar results for a group of elderly hearing-impaired subjects. The situation becomes even more difficult when the hearing-aid user is faced with the combined effects of an adverse S/N ratio and reverberation. Harris and Reitz (1985) concluded that the speech-discrimination performance of the elderly hearing-impaired was 'drastically reduced under the adverse conditions of reverberation plus noise'. Similarly, Nabelek and Mason found that 'the combined effects are greater than the effect of reverberation and noise measured separately' (Nabelek and Mason, 1981).

There are many situations in everyday life where the hearing-aid user is forced to attempt speech communication in less than optimal acoustic conditions. Many hearing-aid users find speech understanding so difficult under these circumstances that they avoid such situations wherever possible. There are, however, a number of other possible solutions to the problem. Some hearing aids offer the possibility of plugging in an external microphone, which can be held or worn by the speaker or placed nearby. In group conversations the use of a plug-in conference microphone may also prove of greater assistance. Such an approach represents an effective solution for many of the situations involving either one-to-one or small-group interactions. The reduction of the distance between the speaker and the microphone results in a more acceptable signal with reduced noise and reverberation effects.

At greater distances, however, there is a need for a remote microphone that is not physically attached to the hearing-aid user. Audiofrequency induction loop systems have been used to accomplish this for many years. With this system, the amplified signal from the microphone(s) is directed into a wired loop, which creates a field of electromagnetic energy with the audio signal superimposed upon it. This signal is picked up by the telecoil of the hearing-aid, amplified and delivered via the hearing-aid's earphone. Induction loop systems do have a number of advantages. They are relatively cheap, easy to install and allow freedom of movement within the looped area. The hearing-impaired person requires no special equipment other than a hearing aid fitted with a telecoil. In many situations such as churches and auditoriums, induction-loop systems offer a real solution to the problems created by poor acoustic conditions. The system can also be used in theatres with the sound system directly connected to the loop amplifier. Unfortunately there are also a number of disadvantages with induction-loop systems. The most obvious is that they require the installation of a wired loop. Although it is theoretically possible to transport an induction loop from situation to situation, this can require a great deal of preparation before the loop is ready for use. As a result, most induction-loop systems are permanently situated in specific areas. Another problem with such systems is that they are prone to variations in signal strength within the looped area. This can range from a minimal change in the signal to 'dead spots' where no signal at all is received.

Radio frequency systems represent a more acceptable, albeit more expensive, solution to the problems of speech reception at distance and in noise. These systems usually utilize frequency modulated (FM) transmission and consist of a relatively lightweight microphone/transmitter worn by the speaker and a receiver worn by the hearing-impaired person. The microphone/transmitter picks up the speaker's voice and transmits it in much the same way as a radio station. This signal is picked up by the receiver and presented to the hearing-impaired person via her/his hearing aids or alternatively, through headphones or earphones. Reception is not restricted to a particular area defined for example by a wired loop. Depending upon the particular system, reception may be possible over distances ranging from 10–100 metres or even further. Radio frequency systems are truly portable and enable the user to receive an optimal auditory signal in a wide variety of environments.

The effectiveness of such systems has been demonstrated in a study by Bankoski and Ross (1984). They found that it was 'possible to significantly improve the speech perception abilities of hearing-impaired adults through the use of FM systems'. In their study, speech materials were presented to hearing-impaired listeners in an auditorium via either the auditorium's sound system or one of two FM systems. The subjects' performance using either of the radio systems was significantly better than the results obtained when they were forced to rely upon the signal provided by the auditorium's sound system. A more recent innovation has been the introduction of short-range wireless systems, which employ infra-red transmission. The infra-red light with the audio signal modulated onto it is emitted from transmission diodes, picked up by light-sensitive diodes on a wearable receiver and converted into an audio signal. The signal is then presented either through a stethoscope headset, headphones or, via direct electrical coupling or the use of the telecoil position, the user's personal hearing-aid(s). A transmission range of up to 30 m^2 is possible using a lightweight microphone/ transmitter worn by the speaker. A larger non-wearable panel of light-emitting diodes is needed for larger area transmission. In this case, the speaker uses either a wireless microphone or a microphone that is physically connected to the infra-red transmitter.

Infra-red transmission offers the user a high-quality auditory signal free of the problems imposed by distance, noise and reverberation. The signal is confined within a well-defined area as 'infra-red light cannot penetrate opaque walls' (Vaughn, 1983). This offers users confidentiality and also enables these systems to operate in adjacent rooms without any problems of 'spillover'. This feature, however, restricts infra-red equipment to indoor use as reception is subject to interference from the infra-red components of sunlight.

Of the systems reviewed in this section, radio systems appear to be the most versatile. They offer the hearing-impaired user the opportunity of optimizing the audio signal in a wide variety of situations ranging from one-to-one communication to large-group meetings. They can also be used without any fixed installations and operate effectively both indoors and outdoors.

12.2 AIDS TO TELEPHONE USE

Alexander Graham Bell, the inventor of the telephone, devoted much of his life to the development of the oral communication skills of deaf persons. It is, therefore, ironic that telephone conversations represent one of the most frustrating communication situations for many hearing-impaired people. For example, Barcham and Stephens (1980) asked 500 hearing-impaired persons to list the difficulties they experienced because of their hearing loss. Almost 20% of their respondents reported difficulties with telephone conversations. Even greater problems were found by Thomas, Lamont and Harris (1982) in a study of the vocational problems of persons with average sensorineural hearing losses of 60 dB or more. Of their sample, 60% reported difficulties with the telephone. Birk-Nielsen and Gilberg (1978) attempted to relate telephone difficulties to the 'speech-reception threshold' (SRT) in the better ear. They found that subjects with either a slight (SRT: 0–25 dB) or a moderate (SRT: 30–45 dB) hearing impairment were in most cases 'able to use the telephone without special devices'. Subjects with more severe losses, however, required additional assistance in the form of a telephone amplifier or by coupling of the hearing-aid and the telephone.

Assistive devices for the telephone vary greatly in their complexity. The simplest is probably the use of a telephone with an adjustable volume control. This allows users to increase the telephone signal to their preferred level. Although this system is used successfully by many hearing-impaired persons, it does suffer the disadvantage of requiring a specially adapted telephone. For this reason the use of a portable inductive coupler represents a more flexible system, as it can be used with any telephone. The coupler is attached to the earpiece of the telephone and produces a magnetic field, which is picked up by the hearing aid's telecoil, amplified and presented through the hearing aid's earphone. The use of an inductive coupler enables the hearing-impaired person to receive the telephone signal at an appropriate level. In most cases, switching the hearing aid to the telecoil position involves shutting off the aid's microphone. As a result, the aid user receives the telephone signal free of amplified ambient noise. Telephones are also available that have an inductive coupler fitted in the ear piece. These offer the advantages of portable couplers but restrict the hearing-impaired user to that specific telephone. It should be noted that persons with mild hearing losses, especially those with vented earmoulds, may still pick up ambient noise even when the hearing-aid microphone is turned off. It should also be recognized that problems created by trans-mission variations and interference on the telephone line will still be present with the use of a telephone coupler.

Many profoundly deaf persons are unable to use telephones because they lack the ability to understand speech via audition, even with appropriate amplification. Many congenitally deaf persons also find conventional telephone communication impossible because they have unintelligible speech. For such persons, the use of a text-telephone provides an opportunity to use telephone communication. The system 'converts electric signals from a teletypewriter into acoustic signals that can be transmitted over a standard telephone and reconverted into a printed signal by a similar coupling at the other end of the transmission' (Riko, Cummings and Alberti, 1979). The obvious disadvantage of text-telephone systems is that calls can only be made to persons who also possess the system. Recently, attempts have been made to overcome this problem by the establishment of intermediary exchanges that relay messages to or from hearing persons using conventional telephones (Taylor, 1980). It is also possible that in the future text-to-speech,

speech-synthesis and speech-recognition systems may enable at least limited direct telephone communication between profoundly deaf and hearing persons (Stevens-Carlson and Bernstein, 1986; Stoker, 1982).

Problems related to telephone use also include the inability to detect the phone ringing for incoming calls. A number of possible solutions exist for this problem. Visual alerting systems such as a flashing light activated by the telephone ring may be suitable for those with more severe hearing losses. An alternative system involves the use of a transmitter placed beside the telephone that sends a radio signal that activates a tactile receiver, worn by the hearing-impaired person, whenever the telephone rings. This allows full freedom of movement within the transmission range of the system – usually around 30 metres. For persons with mild-to-moderate hearing losses a simpler solution may involve the use of an acoustic signal that encompasses the frequency range where they have better hearing. For persons with a high-frequency hearing loss, for example, a signal in the range 500–1000 Hz may be suitable.

12.3 SIGNAL AND WARNING SYSTEMS

There are a number of auditory alerting or warning signals that can create difficulties. In Barcham and Stephen's (1980) study for example, 24% of respondents reported difficulties hearing the door bell, while 11% had problems detecting warning signals such as alarms and sirens. In many cases the alternative solutions offered to enable detection of a telephone ring may be used. For example, a visual or tactile signal may be activated when the door bell is pushed or a fire alarm sounds. Baby-cry alarm systems are also available that provide a visual or tactual signal whenever the infant makes a noise. Such systems are currently unable to differentiate between the baby's cry, coo or babble and are triggered by all sounds made by the baby. A baby alarm that enables at least partial discrimination between these sounds has recently been described (Lundh, 1986) and may in time become commercially available.

The inability to hear the alarm clock in the morning may create very real difficulties for many hearing-impaired persons. Fortunately, alarm clocks are available that provide either a tactual or visual signal. The visual systems usually consist of a flashing-light indicator. Tactile systems involve the use of a small vibrating pad that can be placed under the pillow. These systems are usually battery powered, thus offering the advantage of being easily portable and able to be used in any situation.

12.4 AIDS FOR TELEVISION AND RADIO

Many hearing-impaired people experience great difficulty in listening to the radio or television. The previously mentioned problems posed by distance, noise and reverberation may also affect the understanding and enjoyment of radio and television programmes. As a result of these factors, many hearing-impaired people require the volume at a level that is uncomfortably loud for other family members. The hearing-impaired member may also have to insist on absolute quiet if he/she is to follow the programme. This can greatly disrupt normal family activities and lead to long-term resentment of what may be perceived as unrealistic demands made by the hearing-impaired family member.

The assistive listening devices and systems previously described may also be used as radio and television aids. The microphone/transmitter of a radio-frequency or infra-red system may be placed beside the speaker of the radio or television, enabling the hearing-impaired person to receive an audio signal free of the problems created by distance, noise and reverberation. Many systems also have an auxiliary input allowing the user to electrically couple the transmitter and the sound source. This removes the possibility of the system picking up any ambient noise and transmitting it along with the desired signal. The use of the system in this mode will allow other family members to carry on conversations without disturbing the hearing-impaired person's listening.

Induction-loop systems represent a relatively inexpensive alternative for use with the TV or radio. The loop can be connected to take the place of a loudspeaker '. . . thereby enabling the hearing-aid wearer to listen without anyone hearing a sound. Alternatively, the loop can be installed so as to provide normal sound through the loudspeaker to other persons in the room while the hearing-aid wearer enjoys uninterrupted listening using the telecoil facility' (Gore, 1985). The wired loop may be placed around an entire room, a portion of the room or can even be located in a small cushion placed beside the hearing aid.

Some hearing aids also offer the possibility of using a cord to directly couple the sound source and the hearing aid. The user can adjust the volume control of her/his hearing aid to the desired level and receive a signal unaffected by distance, ambient noise and reverberation. Other hearing-impaired persons prefer to use either a small insert earphone or headphones for listening to the radio or television. The output of these may be determined by the volume control of the radio or television or there may be an independent volume control. The major disadvantage of these latter systems is that they involve the use of trailing cords, which may represent a danger to many elderly people.

12.5 ALTERNATIVE COMMUNICATION AIDS FOR THE PROFOUNDLY DEAF

Most of the devices described in this chapter have been designed for use by persons with at least some residual hearing capacity. There is, however, a small group of hearing-impaired persons who derive little or no benefit from amplification. Lind (1973 cited in Risberg, 1978), for example, found that 40% of a group of Swedish hearing-impaired adolescents reported receiving little or no help from conventional hearing aids. For those students with average losses greater than 105 dB HTL, this figure rose to 60%. This finding is in agreement with the belief of a number of researchers (Nober, 1970; Ericson and Risberg, 1977; Erber, 1979) that many profoundly deaf persons do not have true hearing but rather perceive amplified sound via tactile receptors in their ears. The information available to such cases is extremely limited providing only temporal and intensity cues. As a result, the past decade has seen greatly heightened interest in the development of cochlear implants and tactile aids for the profoundly deaf.

Cochlear implants seek to overcome the problems created by profound deafness by electrically stimulating the auditory nerve directly. A number of different approaches have been adopted by research groups around the world. In some cases only one electrode is used (House, 1976; Fourcin, Rosen, Moore et al., 1979; Hochmair-Desoyer, Hochmair and Burian, 1985) while others provide information via a number of implanted electrodes (Tong, Clark, Seligman and Patrick, 1980; Rebscher, Kessler and Calvert, 1985; Dankowski, 1985). With most systems, the electrode is implanted within the cochlear but at least two devices (Fourcin, et al., 1979; Hochmair-Desoyer et al., 1985) utilize extra-cochlear electrode placement. The processing of the speech signal also varies from system to system. Some devices attempt to present the full speech signal (House, 1976; Rebscher et al., 1985; Dankowski, 1985), others present selected speech parameters such as voice fundamental frequency (Fourcin et al., 1979) or vowel formant frequency (Tong et al., 1980). The results reported indicate that even single-channel implant systems provide useful speech information for most users. Robbins, Osberger and Miyamoto et al. (1985) evaluated the ability of 20 adults to understand connected discourse via lipreading alone and lipreading supplemented by a single-channel cochlear implant. Of the subjects, 16 showed improved performance in the lipreading-plus-implant condition. Subjects using single-channel implants also report that the devices provide an awareness of environmental sounds and assist in the control of their own speech level and rate (House, 1976).

The improvements in lipreading that occur when the visual signal is supplemented by multi-channel electrical stimulation are overall greater than those obtained with single-channel systems (Dowell, Martin, Clarke and Brown, 1985). Multi-channel systems also offer the possibility of speech understanding by listening alone. Dowell, Clarke, Seligman and Brown (1986), for example, report that four of 13 subjects implanted with the Nucleus multi-channel system 'were able to understand connected discourse without lipreading or other visual cues' (Dowell, *et al.*, 1986). Mecklenburg and Brimacombe (1985) also report that around 80% of subjects using the Nucleus implant 'have demonstrated the ability to carry on interactive telephone conversations without the use of a telephone code'.

Tactile aids represent an alternative approach aimed at providing speech information for profoundly deaf persons. Approaches adopted include both single- (Spens and Plant, 1983; Franklin, 1984; Summers, Peake and Martin, 1981) and multi-channel (Engelmann and Rosov, 1975; Saunders and Franklin, 1982; Brooks, Frost, Mason and Chung, 1985; Grant, Ardell, Kuhl and Sparks, 1986) devices, which utilize either vibrotactile (Engelmann and Rosov, 1975; Summers *et al.*, 1981; Spens and Plant, 1983; Franklin, 1984; Brooks *et al.*, 1985) or electrotactile stimulation (Saunders and Franklin, 1982; Grant *et al.*, 1986). Single-channel devices that present information only on the syllabic rhythm of speech have been shown to provide a useful supplement to lipreading performance (Spens and Plant, 1983). More complex aids presenting either selected speech features (Grant *et al.*, 1986; Plant, 1986) or the broad-band speech signal (Brooks, Frost, Mason and Gibson, 1986a,b; Saunders and Franklin, 1982) offer improved performance for both speech perception and production tasks. Multi-channel tactile aids also offer the potential for speech understanding via the tactual sense alone. Research undertaken with deaf-blind users of Tadoma, a manual form of lipreading 'in which the listener receives speech information by placing his hand on the talker's face and monitoring the articulation process' (Durlach, Reed, Braida, *et al.*, 1982) has shown that tactual speech perception is possible (Reed, Rabinowitz, Durlack, *et al.*, 1985). Results reported by Brooks *et al.* (1986a) show that a subject with only 200 hours' exposure to their tactile display was able to identify some unknown words presented tactually alone. Multi-channel tactile aids also offer information that greatly assists the development of speech production with profoundly deaf children. Oller, Eilers, Vergara and La Voie (1986) have reported substantial gains in speech communication for children fitted with multi-channel electrotactile and vibrotactile aids.

Both cochlear implants and tactile aids offer benefits for many profoundly deaf persons currently receiving little assistance from conventional amplification systems. The decision as to which system should be used with individual cases is extremely complex. Factors such as the subject's age, etiology, current audiological and medical status and the number of years since the onset of profound deafness all need to be considered. Of equal importance are the subject's perceived needs and goals and potential to attain these with the available systems. Careful counselling and a clear, logical explanation of the advantages, disadvantages and potential of the various systems should be a major priority for clinician's dealing with profoundly hearing-impaired persons.

The devices and systems outlined in this chapter offer many benefits for hearing-impaired persons. Centres providing audiological services need to be aware of the full range of assistive devices that can be used to overcome specific problems that confront the hearing impaired. The clinician needs to be aware of the requirements of individual cases so that advice can be offered as to the most appropriate systems. The use of interviews and questionnaires offers the clinician the best opportunity to determine the needs of each individual case. Wherever possible, the clinician should have access to a range of devices for demonstration purposes.The opportunity to compare various systems in a structured environment should provide hearing-impaired persons with the opportunity to select those systems most appropriate to their needs.

The clinician with a knowledge of and access to a wide range of supplementary aids and devices is an invaluable resource for all hearing-impaired persons. The effects of supplementary aids on the quality of life of many hearing-impaired persons makes this an area warranting special attention by all clinicians.

REFERENCES

Bankoski, S. and Ross, M. (1984) FM system's effect on speech discrimination in an auditorium. *Hear. Instrum.*, **7**, 8–12.

Barcham, L.J. and Stephens, S.D.G. (1980) The use of an open-ended problems questionnaire in auditory rehabilitation. *Brit. J. Audiol.*, **14**, 49–58.

Birk-Nielsen, H. and Gilberg, L. (1978) Telecommunication performance of persons with hearing handicap in relation to speech reception threshold. *Scand. Audiol.*, **7**, 3–10.

Brooks, P.L., Frost, B.J., Mason, J.L. and Chung, K. (1985) Acquisition of a 250-word vocabulary through a tactile vocoder. *J. Acoust. Soc. Amer.*, **77**, 1576–9.

Brooks, P.L., Frost, B.J. , Mason, J.L. and Gibson, D.M. (1986a) Continuing evaluation of the Queen's University tactile vocoder. 1: identification of open set words. *J. Rehab. Res. and Dev.*, **23**, 119–128.

Brooks, P.L., Frost, B.J., Mason, J.L. and Gibson, D.M. (1986b) Continuing evaluation of the Queen's University tactile vocoder II: identification of open set sentences and tracking narrative. *J. Rehab. Res. and Dev.*, **23**, 129–38.

Dankowski, K. (1985) INERAID artificial multichannel cochlear implant. *Hear. Instrum.*, **36**, 43–4.

Dowell, R.C., Martin, L.F.A., Clark, G.M. and Brown, A.M. (1985) Results of a preliminary clinical trial of a multiple-channel cochlear prosthesis. *Ann. Otol. Rhinol. and Laryngol.*, **94**, 244–50.

Dowell, R.C., Clark, G.M., Seligman, P.M. and Brown, A.M. (1986) Perception of connected speech without lipreading, using a multi-channel hearing prosthesis. *Acta Otolaryngol.*, **102**, 7–11.

Durlach, N.I., Reed, C.M., Braida, L.D., Schultz, M.C. and Norton, S.J. (1982) Research strategy for the study of tactile speech communication. In Pickett, J.M. (ed) *Papers from the Research Conference on Speech-Processing Aids for the Deaf.* Gallaudet College, Washington.

Engelmann, S. and Rosov, R.J. (1975) Tactual hearing experiment with deaf and hearing children. *J. Exceptional Children*, **41**, 243–53.

Erber, N.P. (1979) Speech perception by profoundly hearing-impaired children. *J. Speech Hear. Dis.*, **44**, 255–70.

Ericson, L. and Risberg, A. (1977) Threshold of hearing, vibration and discomfort in a group of severely hard of hearing and profoundly deaf students. *STL-QPSR 4/1977*, 22–8.

Fagerberg, G. (1977) Auxiliary aids for the hearing-handicapped in Sweden: problems and actions. *Scand. Audiol.*, suppl. 8, 82–6.

Finitzo-Hieber, T. and Tillman, T.W. (1978) Room acoustics effects on monosyllabic word discrimination ability for normal and hearing-impaired children. *J. Speech Hear. Res.*, **21**, 440–58.

Fourcin, A.J., Rosen, S.M., Moore, B.C.J., Douek, E.E., Clarke, G.P., Dodson, H. and Bannister, L.H. (1979) External electrical stimulation of the cochlea: Clinical, psychophysical, speech-perceptual and histological findings. *Brit. J. Audiol.* **13**, 85–107.

Franklin, D. (1984) Tactile aids. New help for the profoundly deaf. *Hear. J.*, **37**, 20–4.

Gengel, R.W. (1971) Acceptable speech-to-noise ratios for aided speech discrimination by the hearing-impaired. *J. Aud. Res.*, **XI**, 219–22.

Gore, G.B. (1985) User and installation notes on audio frequency loop systems for use with hearing aids. NAL Report No. 110.

Grant, K.W., Ardell, L.H., Kuhl, P.K. and Sparks, D.S. (1986) The transmission of prosodic information via an electrotactile speech reading aid. *Ear Hear.*, **7**, 328–35.

Handikappinstitutet (1972) Horseltekniska Hjalpmedel *Rapport* **3**, 1–35.

Handikappinstitutet (1982) Horseltekniska Hjalpmedel *Rapport* **13**.

Harris, R.W. and Reitz, M.L. (1985) Effects of room reverberation and noise on speech discrimination by the elderly. *Audiol.* **24**, 319–24.

Hochmair-Desoyer, I.J., Hochmair, E.S. and Burian, K. (1985) The Vienna extra- and intra-cochlear prosthesis: speech-coding and speech understanding in *New dimensions in otorhinolaryngology – head and neck surgery* (ed. E. Myers) Elsevier, Amsterdam, Vol 2.

House, W.F. (1976) Cochlear Implants. *Ann. Otol. Rhinol. Laryngol.*, suppl. 27.

Johansson, B. (1977) Technical supplement to the hearing aid. *Scand. Audiol.*, suppl. 8, 87–91.

Lundborg, T. (1977) Communication devices in addition to hearing aids. *Scand. Audiol.*, suppl. 8, 71–81.

Lundborg, T., Linzander, S., Lindstrom, B., Sward, I. and Fransson, A. (1971) Special devices for the hearing handicapped patient. *Nordisk Audiology*, **3/4**, 96–132.

Lundborg, T., Linzander, S., Lindstrom, B., Sward, I. and Fransson, A. (1972) Special devices for the hearing-handicapped patient. *J. Audiol. Tech.*, **11**, 82–105.

Lundh, P. (1986) A new baby alarm based on tenseness of the cry signal. *Scand. Audiol.*, **15**, 191–6.

Mecklenburg, D.J. and Brimacombe, J.A. (1985) The Nucleus 22-channel cochlear implant system. *Hear. Instrum.*, **36**, 35–8, (46).

Nabelek, A.N. and Mason, D. (1981) Effect of noise and reverberation on binaural and monaural word identification by subjects with various audiograms. *J. Speech Hear., Res.*, **24**, 375–83.

Nober, E.H. (1970) Cutile air and bone conduction thresholds of the deaf. *Except. Child.*, **56**, 571–9.

Oller, D.K., Eilers, R., Vergara, K. and La Voie, E. (1986) Tactual vocoders in a multisensory program training speech production and reception. *Volta Rev.*, **88**, 21–36.

Plant, G. (1986) A single transducer vibrotactile aid to lipreading. *STL-QPSR*, 1/1986, 41–63.

Rebscher, S.J., Kessler, D.K. and Calvert, D.M. (1985) The UCSF/Storz cochlear implant project. *Hear. Instrum.*, **36**, 39–40.

Reed, C.M., Rabinowitz, W.M., Durlack, N.I., Braida, L.D., Conway-Fithian, S. and Schultz, M.C. (1985) Research on the Tadoma method of speech communication. *J. Acoust. Soc. Amer.* **77**, 247–57.

Riko, K., Cummings, F. and Alberti, P.W. (1979) The role of communication aids in the rehabilitation of hearing impairment. *J. Otolaryngol.*, **8**, 10–23.

Risberg, A. (1978) Requirements on speech processing aids for the profoundly deaf. Some preliminary results. *Scand. Audiol.*, suppl. 6, 179–98.

Robbins, A.M., Osberger, M.J., Miyamoto, R.T., Kienle, M.L. and Myres, W.A. (1985) Speech tracking performance in single-channel cochlear implants subjects. *J. Speech Hear. Res.*, **28**, 565–78.

Saunders, F.A. and Franklin, B. (1982) Transmission of information via electro-tactile display. Paper presented at the Tactual Communications Conference, Witchita, Kansas.

Spens, K.-E. and Plant, G.L. (1983) A 'tactual' hearing-aid for the deaf. *STL-QPSR* **1**, 52–6.

Stevens-Carlson, G. and Bernstein, J. (1986) A system for telephone communication between hearing-impaired and normal-hearing people. *Volta Rev.* **88**, 367–73.

Stoker, R.G. (1982) Telecommunications technology and the hearing-impaired: recent research trends and a look in the future. *Volta Rev.*, **84**, 147–55.

Summers, I.R., Peake, M.A. and Martin, M.C. (1981) Field trials of a tactile acoustic monitor for the profoundly deaf. *Brit. J. Audiol.*, **15**, 195–9.

Taylor, K. (1980) Intermediary communication centre for text telephones. In *Project deafened adults* (ed. A. Fransson), Grafiska, Stockholm, pp. 36–40.

Thomas, A., Lamont, M. and Harris, M. (1982) Problems encountered at work by people with severe acquired hearing loss. *Brit. J. Audiol.*, **16**, 39–43.

Tong, Y.C., Clark, G.M., Seligman, P.M. and Patrick, J.F. (1980) Speech processing for a multiple-electrode cochlear implant hearing prosthesis. *J. Acoust. Soc. Amer.*, **68**, 1897–9.

Vaughn, G.R. (1986) Assistive listening devices and systems (ALDS) come of age. *Hear. Instrum.*, **37**, 12–16.

Vaughn, G.R. (1983) Assistive listening devices . . . Part II, large area sound systems. *ASHA* **25**, 25–30.

13

TINNITUS

Anthony Corcoran

This chapter will describe briefly the mechanisms and causes behind tinnitus, its effect on the people who experience it and some possible treatments. A more detailed description is available in Slater and Terry (1987). Readers requiring even more detail are recommended to consult McFadden (1982).

Tinnitus can be simply defined as 'Unwanted sounds appearing to originate within the patient's head'. The sounds are usually variations on a high-pitched hiss but can include drumming, banging, pulsing wooshes and pure tones. The distress caused can vary from mild annoyance to active consideration of suicide. The following extract from a referral letter gives an idea of the range of sounds and distress that can be experienced by one patient:

> The worst tinnitus is in the left ear and takes the form of multiple sounds which are hissing, screaming, squealing and pulsating and are at their very lowest at the same intensity as his own voice. Despite this he manages to sleep quite well, but they have affected his concentration and he is unable at the moment to carry on with his work. The most severe problem, for which he originally came to see you, was the sudden onset of a very loud sound in his head like a referee's whistle. This has continued non-stop since then and at one time he thought he was going quite mad. (Slater and Terry, 1987)

It is conventional to describe tinnitus as either 'objective' or 'subjective', depending on whether it can be heard by someone other than the patient. These terms are unfortunate as they imply that only tinnitus sounds that can be heard by the clinician are real (objective) and those sounds that the patient alone can hear (subjective) are unreal. This distinction clouds the point that it is the patient's *perception* of the tinnitus that is important. Virtually all tinnitus investigations and treatments are aimed at assessing and then modifying that perception.

13.1 'OBJECTIVE' TINNITUS

There are a small group of tinnitus mechanisms that are obvious acoustic events within the patient's head. These 'objective tinniti' fall into two groups: those due to muscle activity and those due to blood flow.

If tensor tympani or stapedius muscles develop a tonic/clonic contraction/relaxation cycle then the resulting 'drumming' sound will be easily transmitted via the ossicles both into the cochlea and out through the eardrum. A similar activity in parts of the palatal musculature may cause repeated opening and closing of the lower end of the Eustachian tube. This can generate a 'clicking' sound. These mechanisms are unlikely to be due to sinister pathology and the tinnitus they produce is not usually very distressing. Simple relaxation techniques are usually very effective in reducing the underlying muscle tension.

Blood flow in smooth-walled, elastic arteries is fairly quiet. However, where turbulence occurs, the sound may be transmitted through tissue to the cochlea and maybe even to the eardrum. The internal carotid artery undergoes a marked direction change close to the middle ear. The turbulence this causes may be heard as a pulsing 'woosh' sound by normal-hearing patients in a quiet place. This is not normally an indication of a sinister pathology. However, if the sound is sufficiently loud to be heard by another person, it suggests a greater degree of turbulence in the blood vessel and warrants further investigation by a physician.

13.2 'SUBJECTIVE' OR CONVENTIONAL TINNITUS

As this is the most common form of tinnitus, the descriptor 'subjective' will be taken as read for the remainder of the chapter.

Tinnitus usually presents as one or more high-pitched whistles or hisses. Institute of Hearing Research data (IHR, 1981) suggest that 5% of the adult population experience severe tinnitus and 0.5% have tinnitus that has a severe effect on their lives.

As a complaint, tinnitus has a long history. This does not imply a complete understanding of its causes or mechanisms. It is useful to distinguish between events or conditions that cause tinnitus (*causes*) and the manner in which these causes actually produce the tinnitus (*mechanisms*). There does not appear to be a consistent link between causes and mechanisms. This is not really surprising when one considers the poor state of our knowledge of tinnitus mechanisms.

13.3 CAUSES OF TINNITUS

A condition or event can be regarded as a cause of tinnitus if there is a close link between its appearance and that of the tinnitus. In this respect there are a large number of accepted causes of tinnitus. Not surprisingly, virtually every cause of hearing loss has also been linked to tinnitus. There is strong evidence implicating the following causes: noise, drugs (some diuretics, antibiotics and anti-inflammatory agents; aspirin causes temporary tinnitus); metabolic disorders including Menière's syndrome and diabetes and auditory nerve tumours.

13.4 MECHANISMS OF TINNITUS PRODUCTION

McFadden (1982) makes the important point that the tinnitus experienced by a patient may have more than one mechanism. This is not unexpected when we consider the variety of sounds that can make up a patient's perception of his tinnitus. McFadden suggests that single-tone tinnitus corresponds to a single-point source of dysfunction within the auditory pathway and broad-band noise or multiple sounds indicate dysfunction at multiple points along the auditory pathway.

There are three current hypotheses for the mechanisms of subjective tinnitus at different locations in the auditory pathway. All have some points to recommend them but none provides a complete explanation of the phenomenon.

(a) Decoupling of stereocilia

The stereocilia (hairs) of hair cells in the cochlea are known to have some form of physical connection with the jellylike tectorial membrane. Relative movement between the basilar membrane (supporting the hair cells) and the tectorial membrane leads to deformation of the stereocilia and in turn to depolarization of the hair cells and the start of neural signals up the auditory pathway. Interestingly, the single row of inner hair cells has far more afferent (sensory) nerve fibres than the three rows of outer hair cells, which have many more efferent (motor) nerve fibres.

There is some speculation that efferent signals to outer hair cells change the stiffness of their stereocilia and thus influence the mobility of the tectorial membrane and its subsequent ability to deform stereocilia on the inner hair cells (which are richly supplied with afferent fibres). This implies a hypersensitivity of inner hair cells to stereocilia deformation. If the tectorial membrane is no longer connected to the inner hair cell stereocilia, they would be free to move under the Brownian motion within the endolymph surrounding them. This could be expected to produce a 'noiselike' signal.

An obvious cause of this 'decoupling' could be Menière's syndrome where raised endolymph pressure can cause gross deformations within the cochlea.

(b) Changes in spontaneous firing rate of nVIII fibres

These nerve fibres have 'resting' firing rates of 0–100 pulses per second. It is natural to consider that tinnitus may be due to abnormalities in these spontaneous firing rates.

Kiang, Moxon and Levine (1970) administered kanamycin to cats. This drug is known to produce hearing loss and tinnitus in humans. Using microelectrodes in nVIII fibres, they found reduced sensitivity and almost total absence of spontaneous firings in fibres with high characteristic frequencies (i.e. from the basal end of the cochlea where the ototoxic effects of the kanamycin were most severe). They suggested that the tinnitus from this cause experienced by humans is due to an 'edge effect' i.e. the presence of markedly different spontaneous firing rates in adjacent nerve fibres might lead to the sensation of sound at higher brain centres. This suggestion is supported by the observation that tinnitus frequencies can occur in the transition region between normal and impaired hearing on the audiogram (Penner, Brauth and Hood, 1981). In contrast, Dallos and Harris (1978) found no change in chinchilla nVIII spontaneous firing rates following kanamycin adminis-tration. However Schmiedt, Zwislocki and Hamernick (1980) did find reduced spontaneous activity in gerbil nVIII fibres after kanamycin. There may be significant species differences in the response to this drug.

Evans, Wilson and Borerwe (1981) recorded from cat nVIII fibres before and after salicylate (aspirin) administration. They found no change in spontaneous firing rates of fibres with low initial rates. However, fibres with high spontaneous firing rates had significantly increased rates after the salicylate administration. They did not find any frequency-specific effects, which is difficult to reconcile with the high-frequency tinnitus reported by humans after salicylate treatment.

Thus the evidence for changes in spontaneous neural activity as a mechanism of tinnitus is equivocal to say the least.

(c) Abnormalities in 'central' auditory pathways

There is some evidence for this in those unfortunate patients who have had nVIII sectioned to relieve their tinnitus and found it had no effect (Hazell, 1979). Melding and Goodey (1979) suggested that tinnitus was similar to epilepsy, i.e. overactivity in central parts of the auditory pathway. Based on this hypothesis there have been several trials of anticonvulsants but with equivocal results.

It is important to note that (1) the tinnitus experienced by the patient is a *real* sensation even though it cannot be measured directly, and (2) the distress caused is not necessarily linked in any way to the cause, mechanism or indeed, the loudness of the tinnitus.

13.5 EFFECTS OF TINNITUS

Earlier in this chapter a referral letter described one patient's tinnitus and the distress it caused him. We have already noted that the quality of the tinnitus and the distress it causes are not consistently linked. For example, a person with a quiet tinnitus may experience more of distress than someone else with a louder tinnitus. Thus, if we are to help someone, we need to assess the 'effects' of the tinnitus as well as the tinnitus itself.

A recent questionnaire survey (Stephens, 1987) asked 58 tinnitus sufferers to list the difficulties the tinnitus caused them.

1. Description of tinnitus . . .   40%
2. Getting to sleep . . .   36%
3. Hearing problems . . .   28%
4. Inability to concentrate . . .   24%
5. Sensitivity to loud noises . . . 18%

Interestingly, a description of the tinnitus itself turns up as the most commonly quoted 'difficulty'. This may be due to subjects misreading the questionnaire instruction but it underlines the central point of tinnitus. It is annoying of itself.

Tinnitus is unlike other background sounds. It is difficult to ignore or suppress. This is partly due to its quality (pitch, location) and partly to the effects it has on the sufferer (loss of sleep, fatigue, anxiety, etc.). It is easy to build up a vicious circle between these two areas and often it is difficult to sort out how much of the patient's distress is directly due to the tinnitus itself and how much to the effects of the tinnitus.

(a) Tinnitus annoyance

The main complaint of tinnitus sufferers is quite simply that of a sound that will not go away. This is because the sufferer cannot suppress it in the same way as an annoying background sound, for example, the hum of a fluorescent tube. Imagine a mechanism in the brain that 'filters out' or 'suppresses' background noises at an early stage in the analysis of neural code from the ears. To do this the 'noise suppressor' would have to recognize the background sounds before consigning them to some mental wastepaper basket. The recognition could depend on acoustic and spatial clues.

As I write this paragraph I am dimly aware of a noisy fluorescent tube on the ceiling of my office. The noise suppressor has recognized the quiet humming and localized its position by comparing the sound in my left and right ears. Each time I move my head, this left–right difference changes a little, so adding to the 'noise suppressor's' information and confirming the location of the tube about 5 ft above me and slightly to my right. Once the humming has been recognized as a harmless background sound, the noise suppressor can direct attention away from it. However, if the humming started to move, the noise suppressor would detect this from the changes in the spatial acoustic clues and would direct my attention towards the sound.

If the humming above me was replaced by a hissing at my feet, my awareness level would rise dramatically. The noise suppressor decides that 50 Hz humming sounds from above are probably noisy fluorescent tubes and warrant little attention, whereas a hissing sound from underneath the desk needs investigation. If I was not able to determine the cause of that hissing I would be a little concerned – what if it was a snake?

Tinnitus fits into the 'raised awareness' group of sounds for two reasons, both connected with its location within the hearing system. First it appears to move or rather the tinnitus sound moves with the sufferer's head movements. External sounds (like the fluorescent tube) are usually in a fixed position. Head movements produce changes in the left–right difference of the sound and aid localization. Tinnitus sounds do *not* change with head movements because they are generated within the head. Thus every time the tinnitus sufferer moves his/her head, that 'noise suppressor' is a reminder that the tinnitus is still there.

This leads on to the second reason for raised awareness of tinnitus. Its location *inside* the sufferer is cause for anxiety. 'What is making this noise? Is it something serious? Is it a brain tumour? Am I going mad? Will it be like this for the rest of my life?' Once the sufferer associates the tinnitus with these questions, especially the last, it is very difficult for him/her (or the noise suppressor) to direct attention away from it.

(b) Sleep problems

This is the most common effect of distressing tinnitus. Typically, sufferers will describe 'getting off to sleep' as more of a problem than remaining asleep. This is not surprising when we consider that we try getting to sleep when we are tired and when we are tired we are less able to suppress unpleasant sensations such as tinnitus. The noise suppressor works best when we are awake and alert. Once asleep, of course, there is a general suppression of information reaching the cortex. However, it is not unusual for people to wake for very short periods during the night and then drop off again. If the sufferer becomes aware of tinnitus during one of these periods, it will be difficult to get back to sleep.

The sufferer may lose significant amounts of sleep because of the tinnitus. This leads to fatigue, which in turn, makes the noise suppressor less effective and so the sufferer becomes more aware of the tinnitus. Thus a vicious circle builds up.

(c) Hearing problems

Earlier in the chapter we saw how causes of tinnitus were also causes of hearing loss. However, a tinnitus sufferer may experience greater handicap from the hearing loss than someone without the tinnitus. First, the tinnitus may partially mask out speech sounds and second, the anxiety caused by the tinnitus may make the 'noise suppressor' less effective. This would make it more difficult for the sufferer to suppress the external background sounds as well as the tinnitus. Again the increased effort that has to be put into listening causes fatigue and so decreases the noise suppressor's effectiveness making the sufferer more aware of the tinnitus – another vicious circle!

13.6 INVESTIGATION OF TINNITUS

Tinnitus investigations fall into two groups: those done to exclude any treatable or sinister cause and those done to find the best treatment for the patient's tinnitus.

The first requirement is best met by using the same investigation tools as for a hearing loss. There are very few measures of the tinnitus itself that will give reliable information as to its cause (Hazell et al., 1985). However, if the patient also has a hearing loss, it is likely that the hearing loss and tinnitus share the same cause. The second requirement to determine the best treatment for the patient, is more complex. We need to have information about the tinnitus and the ways it distresses the patient. We also need to find out a little more information about the patient.,

The best way to obtain this information is in an interview. A questionnaire may provide some of the information but should not be used to replace an interview. It is this contact with a professional who takes the tinnitus seriously, who is reasonably well informed and is prepared to listen that is the basis of tinnitus counselling. This is an essential part of any treatment for tinnitus (Hazell *et al.*, 1985).

In addition to the interview, it is useful to make *some* measures on the patient's tinnitus.

(a) Interview topics

Quality: what does the tinnitus sound like?

Get the patient to describe all the sounds, then rank them in descending order of annoyance. The purpose of this question is not just to obtain information but to get the patient to start thinking analytically about his tinnitus. In particular, what is it that is most annoying about the tinnitus?

Location: where is the sound located?

There may be multiple locations, again rank them in descending order of annoyance. Note any discrepancies in the rankings between sounds and locations.

Onset: when did the tinnitus first start?

Also, what else happened when the tinnitus first started? For example, was there an injury, an illness, major stress, etc? If there is more than one onset date for different tinnitus sounds, note them in rank order of descending annoyance.

Long-term time course: how has the tinnitus changed since onset?

The obvious point here is to ask whether the tinnitus is worse or better than at onset, or, did the tinnitus get quieter and recently come back to its present level of annoyance? Were any changes gradual or relatively sudden and was anything associated with the changes.

Short-term time course: how much does the tinnitus change day to day?

Does the tinnitus change at different times of the day? How does it change? Does it change at different times of the week or month, or is it linked with the menstrual cycle?

Modifying factors: what makes the tinnitus worse or better?

Ask the patient if he/she knows what things or events can make the tinnitus worse? What things make it better? This is important as obviously, the patient should avoid the things that worsen the tinnitus and exploit those that ameliorate it.

(b) Tinnitus measures

Measures of tinnitus are notoriously variable and should not alone be used to assess severity or treatment details. However, there is significant clinical value in both tinnitus-match and tinnitus-mask measures in that they can be used as part of the counselling process. Many patients find it beneficial to be able to match their tinnitus to a synthesized sound. Being able to say 'Yes, that's what it sounds like.' is valuable as it reinforces the idea that the tinnitus is a 'real' sound and that they are not imagining it. It is also useful to try simple tinnitus masking with an audiometer set to WBN. If the patient's tinnitus is easily masked, it suggests the tinnitus can be suppressed with a masker. Simple match and masking procedures are described in Hazell (1979).

(c) Information counselling

Once all the investigations, interview and hearing/tinnitus measures are complete we start to have a picture of the patient's tinnitus. This is a good time to recap and ensure that the patient is fully briefed on the following topics.

Good prognosis for people with tinnitus

Most people with tinnitus report an initial bad period lasting three to 12 months, followed by a gradual reduction in annoyance and distress. The tinnitus may not disappear completely and may indeed return to its previous 'bad' level for short periods. These are usually associated with periods of stress.

The non-sinister nature of the tinnitus

Obviously this can only be done after suspected sinister pathologies (especially auditory nerve tumours), have been excluded. However, this is a major worry to some tinnitus sufferers and it may be worth wheeling out a senior consultant to pronounce the 'all clear'.

The possible cause and mechanism of the tinnitus

Tailor this to suit the tinnitus sufferer's understanding.

Details of the patient's own tinnitus, especially modifying factors

This is important. The tinnitus sufferer needs to understand and accept that tinnitus is *not* all-powerful. Breaking the tinnitus down into its components and especially seeing how *he/she* can modify *it* is a valuable part of the tinnitus-counselling process.

The nature of the 'noise suppressor'

This is important. If the tinnitus sufferer can understand and accept how this mechanism works he/she has a weapon with which to fight the tinnitus. The patient is no longer a victim.

13.7 TREATMENT OF TINNITUS

Tinnitus treatments fall into four main groups, surgical, medical and audiological/psychological.

(a) Surgical treatments

The aim here is to prevent 'tinnitus signals' reaching the brain by cutting the auditory nerve or destroying the cochlea. This assumes that the tinnitus mechanism is not at a higher centre in the auditory pathway. The surgical procedures are complex and the side effects can be severe. Apart from the obvious one of total deafness on the operated side, there will almost always be a period of severe vertigo before the vestibular centres adapt. Hazell (1979) reported tinnitus relief in only about 50% of patients undergoing surgery.

(b) Medical treatments

The aim here is more subtle. The emphasis is on treating the tinnitus wherever its mechanism lies and if that fails, treating the effects of the tinnitus.

Lignocaine, a local anaesthetic has been widely reported as providing short-term benefit to many tinnitus sufferers. However, it is not yet possible to get the same effect over the long term. In addition, its mode of action is not fully understood though it is thought to act on the auditory nerve directly (Majumdar, Mason and Gibbin, 1983).

Anti-convulsants such as Tegretol have been tried with varying degrees of success. Their use presupposes that the tinnitus is of central origin working in a similar manner to epilepsy. Donaldson (1987) reported a recent study where Tegretol produced less benefit than the placebo.

Anti-depressants, tranquillizers and sleeping tablets have all been prescribed to help tinnitus sufferers cope with the effects of tinnitus. There is little evidence that they work directly on the tinnitus itself.

(c) Audiological treatments

With these treatments, the aim is to give the patient some control over tinnitus. There are two parts to the process: (1) investigation and information, (2) hardware and skillbuilding. These are held together with a 'cement' of (3) counselling, for it is important that the patient comes to terms with the tinnitus and is actively involved in working out coping strategies.

Investigation and information

These have been covered earlier in this chapter (see section 13.6).

Hardware and skillbuilding

The choice is between hearing aid, tinnitus masker and a combination unit (combined hearing aid and masker). If the patient has a communication problem *even if he does not admit to it* he should try a hearing aid. The extra stress produced by poor hearing will exacerbate the tinnitus by reducing the effectiveness of the 'noise suppressor'. A properly fitted and used hearing aid (or aids) will reduce this significant area of stress. In addition, the aid will 'exercise' the noise suppressor. However, this exercise is in the suppression of external sounds and as we have already seen, these are usually less annoying than the internal tinnitus. If the hearing aid does not reduce the tinnitus annoyance, then a combination unit may help.

Tinnitus maskers

Tinnitus maskers look like hearing aids and have the same components but with one important difference. The hearing aid's microphone is replaced in the masker by a small noise generator. The output of the masker is broad-band noise. The spectrum of this noise can be modified in the same way as a hearing aid's frequency response, with the tone control(s) and by changing the earmould acoustics. The user can adjust the level of this 'masker noise' with a volume control.

Tinnitus maskers work in two ways. First, they provide immediate relief from the tinnitus by masking it with the masker noise. Second, they act as a training aid to exercise the noise suppressor within the patient's hearing system.

Initial relief

The obvious question regarding tinnitus maskers is 'Don't they just replace one noise, the tinnitus, with another, the masker noise?' This is true, but it is the nature of the masker noise that is important. First the fact that the user has control over the masker noise and knows that it comes from outside means his/her noise suppressor is more prepared to suppress it. Second, it is possible to make the masker noise genuinely less annoying by modifying its spectrum. There are no definite rules in this respect but a rough consensus suggests the masker-noise spectrum: (1) should contain the main tinnitus frequency if possible and (2) should have a narrow rather than very broad bandwidth. The user should be advised to adjust the volume control until the masker noise just covers the tinnitus.

Some sufferers experience a 'residual inhibition' of their tinnitus when they remove their masker after having worn it for some time. This can range from a mild reduction in tinnitus level for a few seconds to complete abolition for several hours. Prior to trial there is no way of predicting which tinnitus sufferers will experience residual inhibition, so it may be better not to mention it for fear of raising false hopes.

Sufferers will get benefit from maskers even if the masker only reduces the tinnitus level and does not mask it completely. This is because the 'inevitability' of the tinnitus has been broken. The patients realize that they are not powerless in the face of the tinnitus, they now have some control over it. This is an important point. If patients can accept this, they are well on the way to developing effective suppression skills. However, if audiologist and patient spend too long in a search for the 'perfect' tinnitus masker, the patient may become discouraged and reinforced in the belief that there is nothing the sufferer can do personally to combat the tinnitus.

Long-term relief

The major characteristic of tinnitus that makes it difficult to ignore is its location within the sufferer's head. This means that it does not have the usual spatial clues of a background noise and so the 'noise suppressor' in the tinnitus sufferer's hearing system is not prepared to ignore it. The masker noise has the same spatial characteristics as tinnitus. There is none of the expected change in level or spectrum with head movements. Thus, as the masker users learn to ignore the masker noise (because they have control over it) they are building up a suppression skill that the noise suppressor can use on the tinnitus. It is not unusual to find tinnitus sufferers who gradually taper off their use of the masker over a period of a few months (Stephens and Corcoran, 1985).

(d) Psychological treatments

These fall into two main groups: those that work on the sufferer's ability to cope with the tinnitus and those that work directly on his perception of the tinnitus.

Self-help groups

Slater (1987), gave a useful description of the role of self-help groups such as local Tinnitus Associations. He listed seven areas where these groups were valuable:

1. Help and advice from people who have the same experience.
2. A pragmatic approach to coping with tinnitus.
3. Beneficial effects of the 'helpers'.
4. Achieving control over the tinnitus.
5. Encouraging people to 'experience' the tinnitus rather than 'suffer' it.
6. De-mystifying professional approaches to tinnitus.
7. Avoiding isolation.

There is a slight risk that joining a self-help group would encourage morbid fascination with tinnitus but this is worth taking as the benefits can be considerable. The British Tinnitus Association (c/o RNID) are happy to provide addresses of local associations or to help in setting up a new one.

Relaxation exercises and biofeedback

These are aimed at reducing the overall level of resting muscle tension in the tinnitus sufferer's body. Long-term mild stress encourages a permanent 'state of readiness' in the muscles. This increase in resting muscle tension is fed back to the brain and encourages a mild level of anxiety. This can continue after the original cause of stress has been removed. Relaxation exercises and biofeedback are designed to break this vicious circle. Further details can be found in Slater and Terry (1987).

Cognitive therapy

This works directly on the tinnitus sufferer's perception of his tinnitus. It usually involves several sessions with a psychologist, either one to one or in a group. The aim is to change the negative thoughts that produce the distress associated with tinnitus. Hallam and Jakes (1987) describe the technique in more detail.

Tinnitus is a distressing condition. Its causes and mechanisms are not fully understood. However, there are a number of treatments available that will reduce the distress experienced by a tinnitus sufferer. It is not possible to predict which will be best for an individual patient. Apart from surgical intervention and some radical drug therapies it is possible to try different treatments until an effective one is found. This contributor's preference is for counselling together with a tinnitus masker as it encourages the tinnitus sufferer to take an active part in his/her own treatment.

REFERENCES

Dallos, P. and Harris, D. (1978) Properties of auditory nerve response in the absence of outer hair cells. *J. Neurophysiol.*, **41**, 365–83.

Donaldson, I. (1987) Drug therapy. Paper presented at British Tinnitus Association AGM, Westminster.

Evans, E.F., Wilson, J.P. and Borerwe, T.A. (1981) Animal models of tinnitus in *CIBA Foundation Symposium 85, Tinnitus*, London, Pitman, pp. 108–29.

Hallam, R. and Jakes, S. (1987) Can one learn to tolerate tinnitus? Paper presented at British Tinnitus Association AGM, Westminster.

Hazell, J.W.P. (1979) Tinnitus. In *Scott-Browne's diseases of the ear, nose and throat* (eds J. Ballantyne and J. Groves), Butterworths, London, Vol. 2.

Hazell, J.W.P., Wood, S.M., Cooper, H.R. *et al.* (1985) A clinical study of tinnitus maskers. *Brit. J. Audiol.*, **19**, 65–146.

Institute of Hearing Research (1981) Epidemiology of tinnitus in *CIBA Foundation Symposium 85, Tinnitus*, Pitman, London, pp. 16–25.

Kiang, N.Y.S., Moxon, E.C. and Levine, R.A. (1970) Auditory nerve activity in cats with normal and abnormal cochleas. In *Sensorineural hearing loss* (eds J.E.W. Wolstenholme and J. Knight), Churchill, London.

Majumdar, B., Mason, S.M. and Gibbin, K.P. (1983) An electrocochleographic study of the effects of lignocaine on patients with tinnitus. *Clin. Otolaryngol.*, **8** (3), 175–80.

McFadden, D. (1982) *Tinnitus: facts, theories and treatments*, National Academy Press, Washington D.C.

Melding, P.S. and Goodey, R.J. (1979) The treatment of tinnitus with oral anticonvulsants. *J. Laryngol. Otol.*, **93**, 111–22.

Penner, M.J., Brauth, S. and Hood, L. (1981) The temporal course of the masking of tinnitus as a basis for inferring its origin. *J. Speech Hear. Res.*, **24**, 257–61.

Slater, R. and Terry, M. (1987) *Tinnitus: a guide for sufferers and professionals*. Croom Helm, London.

Schmiedt, R.A., Zwislocki, J.J. and Hamernik, R.P. (1980) Effects of hair cell lesions on responses of cochlea nerve fibres. *J. Neurophysiol.*, **43**, 16–30.

Slater, R. (1987) On helping people with tinnitus to help themselves. *Brit. J. Audiol.*, **21**, 87–90.

Stephens, S.D.G. (1987) The Complaints of Tinnitus Sufferers. Paper presented at British Tinnitus Association AGM, Westminster.

Stephens, S.D.G. and Corcoran, A.L. (1985) A controlled study of tinnitus masking. *Brit. J. Audiol.*, **19** (2), 159–67.

14

PREVENTION OF HEARING LOSS

Susan Bellman

Hearing loss is a very common problem throughout the world and in developed countries the prevalence of hearing loss increases with age, with 80% being sensorineural in nature. This form of hearing loss is very rarely, if ever, reversible and the only way to reduce the number of hearing-impaired individuals in the future is by preventive measures. In less-developed countries, the majority of those with hearing loss have middle-ear disease. This may be theoretically correctable but again, prevention would have a far greater effect on the numbers of those affected. Preventive audiology will be most effective if aimed at disorders that are common and potentially avoidable, so the emphasis of this chapter will be in this area.

In the younger child hearing loss has greater effects on communication skills and the development of psycho-social problems, so although prelingually deafened individuals only make up a very small proportion of the total hearing-impaired population, prevention takes on an even greater importance in this group.

One of the most important factors in the causation of hearing loss is trauma. This may affect the ear in a variety of ways, including trauma caused by noise, direct physical injury, dysbarisms and iatrogenic trauma.

14.1 TRAUMA

(a) Noise and the ear

It has been shown that once the 'age' effect had been allowed for, the most important factor influencing the hearing level of an individual is the degree of past exposure to noise (Davis, 1983). Isolated groups, for example the Kalahari bushmen, enjoy good hearing into old age while leading their nomadic existence although admittedly, also escaping the other 'diseases of the developed countries' (Jarvis and Heerden, 1967).

The two effects of continuous noise exposure on the ear are first, a direct effect on the hair cells and the second, an indirect effect on the blood supply to the inner ear. The result on the hearing is first a temporary threshold shift with the effect on the fine-tuning mechanisms of the hair cells persisting longer. However, with continual exposure to this type of noise the hearing loss becomes permanent. The extent of the hearing impairment depends on both the intensity of the sound reaching the ear and the duration of the exposure, the total effect following the so-called equal energy principle (Burns and Robinson, 1970).

Preventive audiology could have a major impact by reducing exposure to continuous noise, which in practice is mainly industrial in origin. There are three possible approaches to this problem. These are reduction in noise at source, hearing protection and limiting unnecessary exposure. The last two approaches are cheaper to implement and may be the only methods available using existing technology. However, problems are found in the use of all types of hearing protection, and the benefits can be lost with a relatively brief exposure to high-level sounds. Noise reduction at source involves the use of less noisy equipment or modification of existing equipment. This approach to noise reduction, with automation of processes where this is not possible, offers the main prospect of progress in this field.

Despite the fact that industrial hearing loss has been recognized for very many years, noise reduction at source was felt to be too expensive to implement. The main spur to developments in this field in the UK has been the recognition of noise-induced hearing loss as an occupational disease in 1974, with resulting financial compensation. The Code of Practice sets a maximum acceptable level for continuous exposure of 90 dB(A) for an eight-hour day. Despite pressure from the EEC to reduce the maximum exposure levels to 85 dB(A) the higher level has been retained in the UK.

There is considerable variability in any individual's susceptibility to noise-induced hearing loss, the reasons for this being uncertain, although there may be a genetic component. An effective hearing-conservation programme should be able to identify those at greater risk before their hearing is substantially damaged. This predisposes an ongoing screening programme with counselling for those affected. A positive approach to health education of workers, including the importance of hearing protection, is essential to maximize the acceptability of the programme.

The effects of recreational noise have also to be considered, including exposure to the sound of motorbikes, loud music and power tools, as well as gunfire. The equal energy principle means that all these sounds contribute to the overall noise exposure.

Impulsive noise also causes hearing impairment and the most common causes are repeated firing of guns and certain industrial processes such as riveting. However, impulsive noise damage can also be caused by single events such as explosions, when there may be the additional effect of blast, causing damage to the tympanic membrane and a superimposed conductive component to the hearing loss.

Exposure to impulse noise, particularly from gunfire, can be reduced by the wearing of hearing protection, and this is widely implemented in military and club situations. However, recent evidence suggests that some earmuffs used in military service may be inadequate protection against rifle fire and, in particular, cannon fire and further improvements in this field are still needed (Ylikaski, Pekkarinen and Starck, 1987). In addition, there are still individuals who think it unmanly to use protection and only good health education and good example is going to improve the situation. The most effective approach again is to reduce total exposure.

An additional form of noise exposure suggested by some workers is that of the use of powerful hearing aids for the hearing impaired. Present evidence would not support the supposition that these lead to a deterioration in hearing, except for the very occasional patient where this may be an additional factor in a progressive hearing loss.

It has also been suggested that the sound levels of incubators may cause damage to the immature hearing mechanisms of neonates. The sound levels recorded are around 60–70 dB(A) and the vast majority of babies passing through these units have normal hearing. However, noise cannot be excluded as a minor factor playing a part in the causation of hearing loss in a few sick babies in whom other factors present play a far more important role.

(b) Accidental trauma

Direct trauma to the external and middle ear is most likely to be seen in the young or mentally disturbed, the most common problem being the insertion of small objects into the external meatus by the individual concerned. These may become lodged causing local inflammation and obstruction of the meatus leading to a conductive hearing loss. Attempts may be made by a parent or other inexperienced person to remove the object using unsuitable instruments and this can then lead to damage of the tympanic membrane and middle ear with the possibility of permanent hearing impairment. Direct trauma can also be caused by attempts at aural hygiene, in particular, using cotton wool on sticks.

This occasionally has disastrous results but more frequently leads to a build-up of compressed wax, which causes hearing problems and needs to be removed by syringing. Health education is the only effective way to reduce hearing loss from these causes.

Head injuries may also affect the ear, causing both hearing loss and vestibular problems. Damage can occur at any point on the auditory pathway from the external meatus to the cortex. The most severe effect is from a fracture of the temporal bone severing the eighth nerve or traversing the cochlea, leading to a total loss of auditory and vestibular function on the affected side. There is a marked difference between the occurrence of hearing problems following severe head injury associated with unconsciousness, and that following more minor head injury (Browning, Swan and Gatehouse, 1982). However, although temporal bone fractures are most likely to occur as a result of severe head injuries, hearing loss can occur following more minor injury, particularly when associated with bleeding from the external meatus.

This form of hearing loss will only be prevented by measures that reduce the possibility of head injury. More effective crime prevention and restriction of damaging activities such as boxing could reduce deliberate head injuries. Accident prevention, including wearing of seat belts and crash helmets, and general health education at work and home may reduce accidental head injury.

(c) Dysbarisms

Changes in atmospheric pressure may cause hearing problems in several ways. Individuals exposed to reduced atmospheric pressure in inadequately pressurized aircraft may suffer from middle-ear problems and otalgia and effusions can occur. This is particularly likely if Eustachian-tube function is poor, for example, in young children with intermittent middle-ear problems and adults with upper respiratory tract infections, and under these circumstances problems may occur in commercial aircraft.

Middle-ear problems also occur in divers, who are exposed to a raised atmospheric pressure if middle-ear pressures are not deliberately equalized during descent. However a more serious problem in divers is decompression sickness (bends). This can lead to cochlear and brain-stem lesions caused by bubbles of nitrogen or helium in the tissues, leading to necrosis.

In addition to the effects on individuals with normal auditory systems, pressure changes may provoke perilymph leaks in individuals with congenital abnormalities of the round or oval windows. This is also a possibility following stapes surgery.

Barotrauma may be reduced by preventing individuals with hearing difficulties and/or middle-ear disease from undertaking underwater activities or flying in aircraft that are insufficiently well-pressurized. This already occurs in reputable military and club situations.

(d) Iatrogenic trauma

Hearing loss continues to occur unexpectedly following instrumentation in two main situations. The first is inadequately controlled ear syringing by primary physicians and their assistants, sometimes using poor techniques. This can lead to injury and infection of the external ear canal, perforation of the tympanic membrane, exacerbation of chronic middle-ear disease and occasionally damage to the ossicular chain. The greatest risk is in patients with a history of middle-ear infection.

The second situation is following middle-ear surgery and may arise from unexpected malformations of the middle and inner ear, and inexperience on the part of the surgeon. Malformations may give rise to abnormalities of the scala vestibuli with excessive loss of perilymph at operation, leading to hair-cell damage. This is a recognized problem in certain syndromes and surgery is avoided in affected individuals. However, most litigation has been in respect of stapes surgery, where the expectation is for a good result and a deterioration in hearing is a disaster for the patient.

Iatrogenic trauma to the ear is best prevented by avoiding potentially damaging medical intervention unless essential. In the case of more mundane procedures, such as removal of wax, the equipment used should minimize any possible risk and the person performing the procedure should be well trained and willing to refer on, to more specialized centres, patients in whom difficulties are expected or encountered. In the case of middle-ear surgery, techniques that are less hazardous to cochlear function should be regarded as methods of choice (Smyth, 1982). There is also a very strong case for such procedures to be carried out in a few specialized units, where sufficient numbers are operated on for surgeons to develop and maintain the advanced skills necessary, thus further reducing the risks.

14.2 INFECTION AND THE EAR

Another major cause of hearing impairment is infection and there are many different types that have been implicated. Only the most important will be covered in this chapter.

(a) Prenatal infections

Rubella

The association between maternal rubella and congenital defects, including deafness, cataracts and cardiac lesions, was first noted in Australia, with confirmation rapidly following from other countries. Since then, the incidence of congenital rubella infection has been reduced by preventive measures but figures still show that approximately 50% of those children known to be infected have a hearing loss.

It is possible to eradicate congenital rubella as a cause of hearing loss by appropriate immunization, first introduced in 1970, and this should be a global aim. The effectiveness of an immunization programme depends on the rate of uptake in the community and the persistence of immunity. Different policies regarding the target community and age at immunization are in use in various countries.

In the USA, vaccine is recommended for children of both sexes between one year and puberty, commonly being given to preschool children in combination with measles and mumps vaccines (see pp. 222–3). This is not compulsory but children may well not be admitted to school without immunization in the absence of a valid medical reason for exemption. Immunization is also available to all susceptible males and females, the aim being eradication of the disease in the community.

In the UK, immunization has been offered to females between the ages of 11 and 14 years, whilst at school, and to susceptible adult females of child-bearing age. In the latter group, it is customary to combine this with contraceptive advice, because of the risk of the vaccine causing rubella embryopathy, although this may be less than anticipated.

In circumstances where rubella infection during early pregnancy has been confirmed, a few countries allow termination of the pregnancy to prevent the birth of a child who is likely to be severely handicapped. Legalized abortion where there is a substantial risk of the child being born abnormal was introduced in the UK in 1968, and suspected rubella infection has been one of the more common reasons for termination of pregnancy under this clause, accounting for approximately 500–1000 cases per year. Termination of pregnancy following rubella infection is not legally available in many countries, and women continue to produce affected children. In the long run there is no doubt that an effective immunization programme should eliminate the need for women to be faced with this distressing situation.

Ideally all women should be screened for rubella antibodies prior to pregnancy, for example, during contraceptive clinics, so that immunity can be confirmed. Where this has not been possible, they should be screened as early as possible during pregnancy. This will aid the recognition of congenital infection and should also ensure that all rubella-negative mothers are immunized following delivery. In women who have been exposed to rubella but would not wish to consider termination, gamma-globulin can be used in an attempt to prevent infection.

Cytomegalovirus (CMV)

Congenital cytomegalovirus infection is now recognized to be the most common intrauterine infection. In the UK the prevalence is 3–4 per 1000 live births, with about 10% of these having some handicap, including hearing loss in about a quarter (Preece, Pearl and Peckham, 1984). It was at first assumed that congenital infection could only follow primary maternal infection, but congenital infection has now been recognized in siblings, and can follow reactivation of the virus. This is reported to be the more common mode of transmission in those infected children who developed hearing loss (Harris, Ahifors, Ivarsson *et al.*, 1984). Where there is a sensorineural hearing loss, this may be progressive in nature.

Prevention of congenital cytomegalovirus infection is a more complicated problem than that of congenital rubella. Acquired CMV infection is common, for example 20% of infants become infected within the first year of life (Peckham, Johnson, Ades *et al.*, 1987). For those still susceptible, live CMV vaccine is available and can give good antibody levels with few side effects. However, it is mainly used at this time on adults whose immunity is compromised by disease or drugs. The possibility that the live virus may persist with reactivation in pregnancy has led to caution in its more widespread use. At the moment, killed virus is difficult to produce and immunologically poor, so that long-term immunity is uncertain. In the long term, a reliable vaccine will be the most effective way to reduce hearing impairment and other handicapping conditions due to congenital CMV infection.

Termination of affected pregnancies is not appropriate in confirmed antenatal CMV infection. Infection is asymptomatic and widespread so that screening would be essential for identification of cases. The number of affected children following maternal infection is much smaller than in the case of rubella. Infection is as likely to cause damage during the later stages of pregnancy, when the foetus is viable, as in the earlier stages and, unlike rubella, it is not possible to be sure that subsequent pregnancies will be unaffected.

(b) Postnatal systemic infections

Meningitis

This remains a major cause of sensorineural hearing loss in many countries. In developed countries, meningitis is reported to be the cause of hearing loss in 6–10% of those children with severe impairment (Martin and Moore, 1979). In developing countries the proportion is higher, with meningitis accounting for up to a quarter of schoolchildren with sensorineural hearing loss.

Hearing loss can follow meningitis due to a variety of organisms, with an overall incidence of 12–13%. However, the incidence depends on the organism, the highest figures follow pneumococcal meningitis, where <44% of survivors have a hearing loss, with 6–10% having a hearing loss following *H. influenza* and meningococcal meningitis (Jadavgi, Biggar, Gold and Prober, 1986). An improvement in hearing with time has been reported in a small proportion of those with post-meningitic deafness but the incidence of impaired hearing overall, following bacterial meningitis is probably underestimated.

The incidence of meningitis may be reduced by improving social conditions and nutrition, as with many other infectious diseases. Early identification and treatment of infected individuals should cause a reduction in the long-term sequelae seen, but will not completely eradicate hearing impairment, as this can still follow minor infections with prompt and effective treatment. On some occasions, ototoxic drugs may have to be used, particularly in gram negative or tuberculous infections, and in these cases, it may be difficult to separate the effects of the drug and infection.

Meningitis tends to show seasonal peaks in incidence in many countries with superimposed severe epidemics, particularly of meningococcal meningitis, leaving a large number of hearing-impaired individuals in a particular area or country. Where there is a seasonal pattern or epidemic of meningitis, the incidence could be reduced by immunization. This would need to be repeated regularly where meningitis is common because of the short period of protection conferred by the relevant vaccines. The local population could also be screened to identify possible carriers of the infection. A suitable immunization programme and earlier chemotherapy for affected individuals should cause a substantial fall in the incidence of the profound hearing impairment, particularly in developing countries.

Measles

This infection can lead to both sensorineural and conductive hearing losses, destructive middle-ear disease being found particularly where there is poor nutrition and inadequate medical care. Measles can be prevented effectively by immunization in infancy, particularly when uptake is high within the community. The occasional infection following immunization is usually very mild. Measles immunization is already part of the WHO's Expanded Program of Immunization, with at least 139 developed and developing countries involved. It is dependent on the production of cheap, stable vaccine, but present storage facilities can be inadequate. However, solar-powered refrigerators are now available and research continues into improved and more heat-stable vaccines.

Mumps

Sensorineural hearing loss of some degree occurs in 5–25% of cases of mumps with partial recovery in 50–90% of cases (Vuori, Lahikainen and Peltonen, 1962). Fortunately this hearing loss is usually unilateral. A vaccine is available against mumps but has not been widely used in isolation. In the USA and Scandinavia, a triple vaccine against measles/mumps/rubella has been introduced prior to school entrance, and this has led to a noticeable drop in the incidence of the disease. In the UK, a trial of this triple vaccine has started in some districts, although the uptake is unfortunately likely to be much lower. Immunization will hopefully lead to a fall in hearing loss due to these diseases.

(c) Localized infections

Acute otitis media

This commonly occurs with upper respiratory infections and can lead to complications that remain a major cause of hearing impairment throughout the world. In developed countries, such as the UK, the rate of complications started to decline rapidly as living conditions improved, falling further following the introduction of antibiotics.

There is no evidence that the incidence of acute otitis media itself has dropped. It is particularly common in children in day nurseries, and recurrent infection is more likely when a child has several siblings, is exposed to passive smoking at home or has persistent rhinorrhoea (Pukander, Luotonen, Timonen and Skarma, 1985). There is also some evidence that early treatment of uncomplicated otitis media with antibiotics may increase the rate of recurrent infection, possibly due to the prevention of development of immunity as well as the emergence of resistant organisms. However, with good socioeconomic conditions more than 90% of cases heal spontaneously without any treatment.

The most effective way to prevent hearing loss caused by acute otitis media is to raise the general living standards of the population. This is as relevant to deprived areas of developed countries as to the developing countries. Personnel are needed capable of recognizing and monitoring ear infections so that treatment with antibiotics can be given to anyone whose infection has not rapidly resolved spontaneously or who may be developing other more serious complications. Some populations seem to be far more affected by otitis media than others, for example the Australian aborigines, and need a more intensive programme.

Where facilities are available, the additional treatment of other infected foci in the upper respiratory tract, e.g. tonsils or sinuses, may help to prevent recurrent infection. Some surgeons also believe that grommet insertion may aid in the prevention of recurrent infection.

Chronic suppurative otitis media

This complication of acute otitis media has become less common in developed countries, but the number of older adults with mastoid cavities reflects the importance of chronic ear disease in the past. It remains one of the most important causes of hearing impairment in the developing countries, as well as a source of potentially life-threatening disease. There is also evidence that the incidence of sensorineural hearing loss is 7–10% higher in individuals with chronic otitis media, than in the general population, and prevention should hopefully also limit this complication (Paparella, Morizono, Chap, *et al.*, 1984).

Prevention of chronic ear disease depends first on reducing the effects of acute otitis media as described previously, and secondly, on active treatment of middle-ear disease in its early stages. The most effective measure is aural toilet but antibiotics may be helpful and surgical intervention may be needed to control active disease, including cholesteotoma, thus limiting the damage occurring.

There has been a suggestion that grommet insertion in otitis media with effusion (see following section) may prevent chronic ear disease by restoring middle-ear pressures to normal and preventing the occurrence of retraction pockets and cholesteotoma. This seems a simplistic approach as the division of the middle ear into compartments can lead to attic disease in the presence of normal middle-ear pressures behind the pars tensa. However, the high incidence of chronic middle-ear disease in adult life found in those born with cleft palates, many of whom have had long-standing, middle-ear effusions, demonstrates the importance of adequate ventilation of the middle ear.

When chronic middle-ear infection has occurred, some restoration of hearing may be possible by tympanoplasty/ossiculoplasty as long as there is no active disease remaining. This surgical correction of hearing loss should be included in any programme designed to prevent hearing impairment due to middle-ear disease.

Otitis media with effusion

This condition has been recognized with increasing frequency over the past two decades and is a cause of mild to moderate, usually temporary hearing impairment in childhood. Its importance is related to the fact that it affects children at the age of learning language and other skills. Its effects are particularly noticeable in children with a pre-existing sensorineural hearing loss or other handicapping condition, and it is in these children that prevention of hearing loss (or additional hearing loss) is most important.

Various aetiologies have been implicated in the production of a middle-ear effusion, including recurrent infection, allergy and the mechanical effects of large adenoid size or the muscular abnormalities of a cleft palate. Most medical treatments, e.g. antihistamines and vasoconstrictor nasal drops, have been found to be no more effective than a placebo, but there is some evidence that antibiotics may be of benefit in preventing recurrence of effusions following operative treatment. It has also been suggested that when allergic factors are present, the condition may respond to exclusion diets.

In the short term, the only method of restoring normal hearing, apart from the use of hearing aids is myringotomy, and grommet insertion where necessary. The immediate effect of grommet insertion on restoration of hearing is well documented but in older children, it has been found that by one year post-operatively, adenoidectomy alone is associated with improvement in hearing to virtually the same level. However, without either grommet insertion or adenoidectomy the hearing at one year remained poor (Maw and Herod, 1986).

In the long term the condition is usually self-limiting, and there is still controversy regarding the effects of ventilation tubes on the tympanic membrane. There is occasional ottorhoea in <20% cases following insertion of grommets, with 1% needing tube removal. Persistent perforations occur in 4% but there are very few reports of cholesteotoma. Tympanosclerosis has been reported by many authors to be present in 40–50% ears following grommet insertion, although the clinical significance is still uncertain.

Until a more satisfactory method of preventing this condition is found, grommets and adenoidectomy remain the treatment of choice to restore the hearing in children with persistent problems and/or other handicaps. In individuals with long-term problems, such as a cleft palate, a more permanent tympanostomy tube can be used.

14.3 GENETIC HEARING LOSS

Genetic hearing loss occurs both in isolation and as one of the features in many syndromes. It is very difficult to estimate the prevalence of genetic hearing loss overall, because in the absence of a positive family history or recognized syndrome, the genetic aetiology of many cases is not identified. However, genetic hearing loss accounts for approximately 50% of prelingual hearing loss and it has been suggested that a genetic aetiology should be assumed in children where no other cause can be found on full investigation (Taylor, Hine, Brasier *et al.*, 1975). This would usually be autosomal recessive inheritance with some new mutations. Although the onset of hearing loss may be congenital, it may also be delayed and can manifest itself at any time from infancy to old age. There also appears to be a genetic susceptibility to hearing loss caused by other factors, such as ototoxic drugs and noise, and also possibly to the effects of congenital rubella infection (Barr, 1982). Genetic hearing loss is often sensorineural, but it can also be conductive or mixed, and the severity varies considerably, with many individuals having a progressive impairment.

The factors to be considered in programmes to reduce the prevalence of genetic hearing loss are firstly the accuracy with which affected individuals can be identified and then the acceptability of genetic counselling and its possible effectiveness in leading to a drop in the number of hearing-impaired.

Autosomal dominant hearing loss could theoretically be eliminated, apart from new mutations, if all affected individuals were identified and did not produce children. This would reduce the incidence of genetic hearing loss by 10–15%. However, partial penetrance and variable expressivity are marked features of autosomal dominant hearing loss and the less severely affected carriers of the gene may be difficult to identify, even in syndromal hearing loss.

Autosomal recessive hearing loss is more common, but affected siblings account for less than 15% of the genetically deaf population. Thus any reduction in the number of hearing impaired by appropriate identification and counselling would be small. The number of gene loci responsible for autosomal recessive hearing loss has been estimated as at least 10 (Rose, Conneally and Nance, 1977). The chance of two people carrying the same gene is difficult to estimate, but certainly new cases of hearing loss will continue to occur unexpectedly.

Given these problems in identification of genetic hearing loss, counselling will have a limited affect on the prevalence of hearing loss, although it could obviously be of great value to individual families.

Two factors would improve the effectiveness of genetic counselling – identification of carriers and antenatal diagnosis. The latter may be of value in the identification of some of the rarer forms of deafness e.g. mucopolysaccharidoses and chromosomal abnormalities, but the need for prenatal diagnosis is based on the poor prognosis of the general condition and not the possible hearing loss.

14.4 NEOPLASIA

Neoplasms affecting the middle ear, cochlea and cochlear nerves are fortunately rare, as the damage to hearing produced is usually permanent.

The middle ear may be affected by histiocytosis X in childhood and by carcinoma in the adult. Treatment is directed to the tumour and the earlier this is detected and treated the greater the chance of some middle-ear function remaining. Carcinoma of the middle ear is more likely to occur where there is squamous metaplasia associated with chronic infection so that procedures designed to reduce or eliminate chronic middle-ear infection should reduce the prevalence of this tumour.

The cochlea can be involved in systemic conditions such as leukaemia. Some neoplastic conditions may affect the inner ear at an early stage, whereas other conditions, if treated early, may respond before there is permanent inner-ear damage. Thus, although the aim of early treatment is to improve the overall condition of the patient, it does have a role in prevention of hearing loss.

The cochlear nerve can be affected by benign Schwannomata, epidermoids, meningiomata or metastases affecting the cerebello-pontine angle. There is little that can be done to prevent these rare neoplasms occurring in any individual, although inherited neurofibromatosis, associated with some of these tumours could, theoretically, be reduced by genetic counselling. For there to be any preservation of hearing the tumour has to be detected and surgery performed at a very early stage and facilities for this are essential. The results are disappointing overall, even in the case of acoustic neuromas, which almost invariably arise on the vestibular section of the eighth nerve.

14.5 OTOTOXICITY

A wide range of drugs produce damage to hearing and vestibular function as a side effect. Many drugs such as quinine and salicylates have long been known to cause a drop in hearing which is usually reversible. More recently, drugs causing a permanent hearing loss have been developed. The most important of these are the aminoglycoside antibiotics, e.g. streptomycin and gentamicin. These may be potentiated by loop diuretics, e.g. furosemide, which normally cause a reversible hearing loss (West, Brummett and Himes, 1973). Other drugs that are known to be ototoxic include antimetabolic drugs used to treat cancer, e.g. cisplatinum, and some of the beta-blockers. Noise exposure may also potentiate the effects of some of these drugs (Humes, 1984).

Potentially ototoxic drugs should be used with care and in the case of aminoglycosides, blood levels should be monitored. This is particularly important if renal function is poor and the drugs cannot be excreted normally. Eardrops containing ototoxic drugs rarely cause hearing loss, but again it is wise to avoid their use wherever possible, particularly for long-term use in chronic middle-ear disease.

14.6 METABOLIC PROBLEMS AND THE EAR

A wide range of disorders that can affect the ear are here very loosely classified together as metabolic.

(a) Perinatal problems

Two main factors used to be implicated in the causation of hearing impairment in neonates. The first of these was hypoxia/anoxia. Some children are known to be affected by prolonged anoxic episodes, but prenatal hypoxia may also be important. The second factor was hyperbilirubinaemia or kernicterus, which was most likely to follow rhesus incompatibility. In developed countries, both of these are rarely seen now because of better prenatal and perinatal care. In particular, the incidence of kernicterus has been reduced by a number of factors. These include the monitoring of rhesus status and antibodies, with intra-uterine transfusion and premature delivery when necessary. Anti-D immunization eliminates antibodies present postpartum or post-abortion in affected mothers, reducing the risk to future pregnancies. Exchange transfusions reduce the bilirubin levels when very high and more recently, ultraviolet-light therapy breaks down the damaging pigment.

Good perinatal care is the best means of preventing hearing loss in neonates and has been very effective in babies over 30 weeks' gestation. However, hearing loss continues to be a problem as smaller and younger babies are surviving. In these cases, a combination of factors seems to be responsible for any hearing impairment. Intracranial haemorrhages, hypoxia and prolonged gentamicin therapy seem to be the important statistically.

(b) Thyroid dysfunction

Childhood hypothyroidism (cretinism) is still a major cause of hearing impairment throughout the world. This is particularly so in developing countries where iodine intake is low and goitre is endemic, e.g. sub-Himalayan regions. This form of hypothyroidism could be prevented by the addition of iodine to the diet, with iodized oil administered during pregnancy. Although the hearing loss was not thought to be affected by the age at which replacement therapy was started, it is now apparent that very early replacement therapy following neonatal screening in combination with the Guthrie test has led to a greatly improved prognosis for hearing loss and general development.

Adult hypothyroidism (myxoedema) is also thought to be associated with hearing loss, found in up to 85% of affected individuals. As clinical features can be misleading, screening is necessary to identify this. Early treatment may prevent or partially reverse the hearing loss, although recent studies have shown more disappointing results (Parving, Parving and Lyngsoe, 1982). In addition, many of these individuals have multiple medical problems and the contribution of the thyroid dysfunction to the hearing loss may be difficult to ascertain.

(c) Diabetes mellitus

An increase in hearing loss has been noted in this condition, which is relatively common, particularly among the elderly. Because such individuals frequently have multiple medical problems, it is again difficult to define the contribution of the diabetes to this loss. However, it appears to potentiate the effects of aging on the cochlear by its effect on the vascular supply (Axelsson, Sigroth and Vertes, 1978). More subtle central dysfunction has also been noted. The incidence of diabetes is related to diet and could be reduced by effective health education. The effects of diabetes, including those on the hearing, could be reduced by screening and appropriate therapy.

(d) Dyslipoprotenaemia

This condition may be associated with hearing loss by reducing the blood supply in the small vessels of the cochlea. Except in severe hereditary forms, it can only be identified by screening. Any other condition that narrows the arteries or increases the blood viscosity may potentiate the problem. It also appears that this condition may potentiate the hearing loss produced by noise exposure, with obvious implications for preventive audiology (Axelsson, 1985). It responds well to diet and medication and the early reports of this on auditory symptoms has been encouraging.

(e) Paget's disease

This disease again occurs in a significant number of the elderly, being associated with a mixed hearing loss. Sudden sensorineural loss may occur but in the majority, the sensorineural component may be no more than found in the general population. The conductive loss is related to abnormal bone overgrowing the stapes and oval window and at the moment there is no preventive measure available. There is a high complication rate on surgery and no effective medical treatment.

(f) Renal disease

As more patients survive renal failure due to dialysis and transplants, the extent of hearing loss in renal disease has become clearer. The potentiating effects of aminoglycosides and loop diuretics have already been mentioned, but one in six patients with chronic renal failure have hearing impairment without taking these drugs, and there seems to be some relationship to the number of dialyses or transplants. Hearing impairment has been recorded as occurring during and being reversed by dialysis, so osmotic changes in the blood may be responsible (Sittoni, Colletti, Bonanni and Vigili, 1985). Prevention of hearing loss involves the avoidance as far as possible of any factor, particularly drugs, which could contribute to cochlear damage, because of the way many factors potentiate each other.

14.7 MULTIFACTORIAL CAUSATION OF HEARING LOSS

Deterioration in hearing is related to both loss of hair cells and primary neurones in the spiral ganglion, neither of which regenerate. Thus each insult to the ear will have an additive effect on auditory function. Also pre-existing cochlea damage may increase susceptibility to other factors such as ototoxic drugs. There may also be genetic influence on susceptibility to ototoxic drugs, particularly aminoglycosides, and possibly to the effects of noise and congenital infections. Thus from a preventive point of view, any possible source of damage to the ear should be avoided, as each factor may contribute to the overall degree of impairment and its resulting disability.

REFERENCES

Axelsson, A., Sigroth, K. and Vertes, D. (1978) Hearing in diabetes. *Acta Otolaryngol.*, suppl. 256.

Barr, B. (1982) Teratogenic hearing loss. *Audiology*, **21**, 111–27.

Browning, G.G., Swan, I.R.C. and Gatehouse, S. (1982) Hearing loss in minor head injury. *Arch. Otolaryngol.*, **108**, 474–7.

Burns, W. and Robinson, D.W. (1970) *Hearing and noise in industry*, HMSO, London.

Davis, A. (1983) Prevalence of hearing disorders in *Hearing science and hearing disorders* (ed. M.E. Lutman and M.P. Haggard), Academic Press, London.

Harris, S., Ahlfors, L., Ivarsson, S., Lernmark, B. and Svanberg, L. (1984) Congenital cytomegalovirus infection and sensorineural hearing loss. *Ear Hear.*, **5**, 352–5.

Humes, L.E. (1984) Noise induced hearing loss as influenced by other agents and by some physical characteristics of the individual. *J. Acoust. Soc. Amer.* **76**, 1318–29.

Jadavgi, T., Biggar, W.D., Gold, R. and Prober, C.G. (1986) Sequelae of acute bacterial meningitis treated for seven days. *Pediatrics*, **78**, 21–5.

Jarvis, J.F. and Heerden, H.G. (1967) The acuity of hearing in the Kalahari bushmen. A pilot study. *J. Laryngol. Otol.*, **81**, 63–8.

Martin, J.A.M. and Moore, W.J. (1979) *Childhood deafness in the European Community*, Commission of the European Communities, EUR 6413.

Maw, A.R. and Herod, F. (1986) Otoscopic, impedance and audiometric findings in glue ear treated by adenoidectomy and tonsillectomy. *Lancet* 21 June, 1399–1402.

Paparella, M.M., Morizono, T., Chap, T. Le, Mancini, F., Sipila, P., Choo, M.B., Lider, G. and Kim, C.S. (1984) Sensorineural hearing loss in otitis media. *Ann. Otol. Rhinol. Laryngol.*, **93**, 623–9.

Parving, A., Parving, H.-H. and Lyngsoe, J. (1982) Hearing sensitivity in patients with myxoedema before and after treatment with l-thyroxine. *Acta Otolaryngol.*, **95**, 315–21.

Peckham, C.S., Johnson, C., Ades, A., Pearl, K. and Chin, K.S. (1987) Early aquisition of cytomegalovirus infection. *Arch. Dis. Child*, **62**, 780–5.

Preece, P., Pearl, K. and Peckham, C. (1984) Congenital cytomegalovirus. *Arch. Dis. Child* **59**, 1120–6.

Pukander, J., Luotonen, J., Timonen, M. and Skarma, P. (1985) Risk factors affecting the occurrence of acute otitis media among 2–3 year old urban children. *Acta Otolaryngol.*, **100**, 260–5.

Rose, S.P., Conneally, P.M., Nance, W.E. (1977) Genetic analysis of childhood deafness. In *Childhood deafness, causation, assessment and management* (ed. F.H. Bess), Grune and Stratton, New York.

Sittoni, V., Colletti, V., Bonanni, G. and Vigili, M.G. (1985) Hearing loss in renal disease and the problem of haemodialysis. In *Disorders with defective hearing* (eds V. Colletti and S.D.G. Stephens), Karger, Basel.

Smyth, G.D.L. (1982) Recent and future trends in the management of otosclerotic conductive hearing loss. *Clin. Otolaryngol.*, **7**, 153–60.

Taylor, I.G., Hine, W.D., Brasier, V.J., Chiveralls, K. and Morris, T. (1975) A study of the causes of hearing loss in a population of children with special reference to genetic factors. *J. Laryngol. Otol.*, **89**, 899–914.

Vuori, M., Lahikainen, E.A., Peltonen, T. (1962) Perceptive deafness in connection with mumps. *Acta Otolaryngol.*, **55**, 231–6.

West, B.A., Brummett, R.E. Himes, D.L. (1973) Interaction of kanamycin and ethacrynic acid. *Arch. Otolaryngol.*, **98**, 32–7.

Ylikaski, J., Pekkarinen, J. and Starck, J. (1987) The efficiency of earmuffs against impulse noise from firearms. *Scand. Audiol.*, **16**, 85–8.

15

FUTURE TRENDS

David Preves

15.1 STATUS OF CURRENT HEARING-AID FITTINGS

Hearing aids have recently been enjoying a comparatively widespread market acceptance due to improvements in component design and miniaturization, advanced production techniques and increased public awareness of the potential benefits that may be derived from amplification. Statistics published by the Hearing Industries Association show that over 1 268 000 hearing aids were sold in the United States in 1985 (Mahon, 1987). Worldwide about 3.4 million aids were supplied in 1984 (Skadegard, 1985). While the overall market grew from 1986 to 1987 by only 11% in the US, sales of in-the-ear (ITE) aids were about 19% ahead of their 1986 total, accounting for about 64% of the total hearing-aid sales. Included within the statistics for ITE-type aids are sales figures for in-the-canal (ITC) aids, which made up about 11% of total sales in 1986 and 14% in 1987. Postauricular aid sales were down about 16% from 1986 to 1987, accounting for 21% of US hearing aid sales. Worldwide, ITE aids are gaining in popularity but are not the dominant type in any other country besides the United States.

The popularity of ITE and ITC aids in the United States stems from both acoustic and cosmetic advantages. The relatively weak high-frequency components of speech contain the most important energy for good speech intelligibility – the second and third formants or energy peaks that are produced by the vocal tract configurations of the speaker, and their temporal transitions to other frequencies. Studies of diffraction caused by the head using probe microphones have shown that the head, pinna and external meatus provide a natural preamplifier, having almost 20 dB gain in the 2500 to 4000 Hz frequency region (Wiener and Ross, 1946; Wiener, 1947; Berland and Nielsen, 1968; Shaw, 1966). Hence, one of the easiest ways of improving the signal-to-noise ratio of hearing-aid-processed speech signals is to maximize the high-frequency signal incident to the hearing-aid microphone by placing it at a location within the concha where head diffraction is most favourable. The results of using an ITE microphone inlet location can be an improvement in intelligibility for hearing-aid wearers (Jervall *et al.*, 1983; Randolph, Gierela and Ross, 1977; Freedman, 1970).

Studies comparing the subjective opinions of patients wearing ITE aids and postauricular hearing aids with comparable electroacoustic performance have shown a preference for ITE aids thought to be due to improved cosmetics and ease of handling the hearing aids (e.g. Murphy, 1981). A result of this trend toward ITE aids and to the even smaller ITC aids in the United States, is that these hearing-aid types are being requested for fitting a wider variety of hearing-impairment configurations.

Fitting severe hearing losses has led to the development of higher gain and high maximum output capability for ITE and ITC aids. Providing higher gain has usually resulted in greater susceptibility to feedback problems.

Some ITE fittings have utilized push–pull circuits that can simultaneously drive two receivers whose diaphragms operate in phase opposition. This provides higher gain and higher maximum-output sound-pressure level, while partially cancelling the acoustical and mechanical feedback signals that might have otherwise led to oscillation.

On the other end of the spectrum, fitting mildly hearing-impaired individuals who have normal hearing through 2 kHz or even through 3 kHz has required larger venting capability in ITE and ITC aids, both for acoustic considerations and to avoid the feeling of occlusion. In response, half-concha ITE aids have been developed that leave the lower half of the concha totally unoccluded, thus forming a very large vent. Through the refinement of component placement, it has been possible to put larger and larger vents into tiny ITC aids in order to provide assistance to those hearing-impaired persons having sharply sloping audiometric configurations.

From a sampling of hearing-aid fittings in the United States, 27% were binaural in 1983 rising to about 37% in 1987 (Cranmer, 1983; Cranmer, 1987). Thus the percentage of binaural fittings does not appear to be growing in the last few years.

Although the effectiveness of current hearing-aid fittings continues to improve as the technology of designing and building hearing aids advances, several major problems still exist. Subjective assessments of the quality of hearing-aid fittings by hearing-aid wearers and hearing-aid dispensers usually reflect the same problem areas to be improved on: suppression of environmental noise, minimization of acoustical feedback oscillation and improving the sound quality of hearing-aid-processed signals (Tyler, Baker and Armstrong-Bednall, 1983; Berger *et al.*, 1982; Nielsen, 1979).

Today, the effectiveness of most hearing aids is still regarded as somewhat limited because of the inability of the hearing-aid amplifier to separate out undesired noise from desired speech. Recent Hearing Industries Association statistics indicate that 13.5% of 3.9 million hearing-aid owners in the USA do not use their aids and that background noise interference was cited as a major problem by 32% of those who rejected their hearing aids (HIA, 1984). In a more recent study by the Federal Trade Commission, of the 10% of those expressing dissatisfaction with their hearing aids, 74% complained of problems of unwanted noise (FTC, 1985). Background noise, which has power spectral energy that is usually greatest in the low frequencies, may mask out the relatively important but weaker high-frequency components of speech for hearing-impaired listeners.

The problem of persons with cochlear pathology having more difficulty discriminating in noisy backgrounds than normal-hearing persons is caused perhaps, in part, by the abnormal widening of the critical bands of their damaged auditory systems (Scharf, 1978). This phenomenon may result in more upward spread of masking than occurs for normally functioning auditory systems (Martin and Picket, 1970; Nabelek, 1982; Plomp, 1978). The inability of most hearing aids to deal effectively with difficult message-to-competition situations becomes especially problematic for hearing-impaired individuals trying to listen in large gatherings that occur, for example, in reverberant church basements, cafeterias and at parties (Giolas *et al.*, 1979). Hearing aids in use today generally have significant amounts of undesirable environmental noise amplified together with the desired stimuli (Surr, Schuchman and Montgomery, 1978).

To solve these problems, recent innovations in new hearing aids include a trend towards more sophisticated circuitry to improve signal-processing capability. In the past, such efforts were fraught with difficulties of inadequate component miniaturization, as well as low-voltage and low-current requirements imposed by currently marketed hearing-aid batteries. However, recent advances in reducing the spacing between components on low-current integrated circuits have made it possible to package circuits having considerable signal-processing capability in a very small size that allow operation from a single 1.3 volt miniature battery.

These circuitry innovations, made possible by technological advances in the semiconductor industry, should help to solve the noise and feedback problems cited above that make many of today's hearing-aid fittings less than optimal.

15.2 ATTEMPTS TO REDUCE NOISE
AND THE RESULTING ACOUSTIC-FEEDBACK
OSCILLATION PROBLEM

In an effort to minimize the amplification of environmental noises, hearing-aid fittings usually emphasize the high frequencies and attenuate the low frequencies with high-pass filters. Implicit in this everyday practice is the assumption that background noise is mainly low-frequency weighted. One of the most effective methods of implementing a low-frequency filter, from the subjective viewpoint of hearing-aid wearers, is the earmould vent, which acts as a high-pass filter (Studebaker and Zachman, 1970) attenuating low-frequency gain and reducing amplification of environmental noise. There is another reason for including vents in earmoulds: the top curve on Figure 15.1(a) depicts the gain derived primarily from the resonance of an unaided real ear, as measured with a probe-tube microphone. This gain becomes partially obliterated by occluding the ear as shown on the bottom curve of Figure 15.1(a). The result is an insertion loss in the higher frequencies above 2 kHz as shown on Figure 15.1(b). It is possible to counteract the insertion loss by utilizing as much as possible of the gain that is provided by the physiology of the ear canal. For these reasons, and for eliminating the feeling of occlusion, many hearing aids are fitted utilizing the largest possible vents in the earmould.

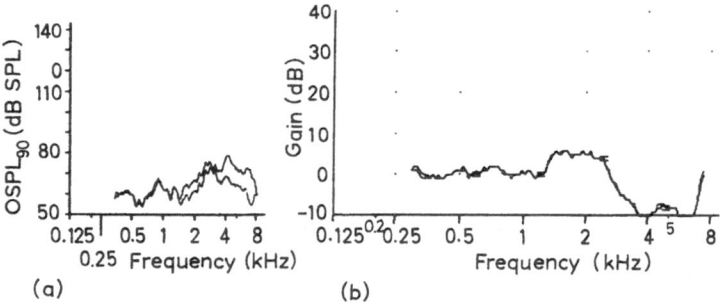

Figure 15.1 Probe microphone response in a real ear: (a) unoccluded (top curve) and with an IROS ITE aid with power turned off (bottom curve). (b) The resulting insertion gain/loss.

A major problem with hearing aids using venting is their propensity to produce a squealing oscillation due to acoustical feedback before adequate gain is achieved (Nielsen, 1979; Berger and Hagberg, 1982). This problem is caused when high-frequency amplified signals 'leak out' from the ear canal and get back into the hearing-aid microphone inlet. The acoustic leakage may be caused by an unintentional vent created by a poorly fitting, non-sealing earmould or via an intended earmould vent (Egolf, 1982; Veit, 1981). The probability of acoustic-feedback oscillation is particularly of concern for subminiature hearing aids such as ITE and ITC aids where microphone and receiver are in close proximity. As a general rule, the higher the gain provided by a hearing aid, the smaller the earmould vent must be because of the risk of acoustic-feedback oscillation.

The frequency response and the transient response of a hearing-aid fitting close to the onset of acoustic instability are known to be severely degraded (Preves, Ruzicka and Peterson, 1985). Hearing-aid wearers who use their aids near the point of acoustic-feedback oscillation may be receiving severely distorted speech in both the spectral and temporal domain (Yanick, 1977). Speech from a particular speaker may be characterized by resonances of the talker's vocal tract. The vocal tract changes shape during production of various utterances and hence the resonant frequency peaks or formant frequencies also change. If a hearing aid has a large peak in its frequency response, as shown in Figure 15.2, due to being near the onset of acoustical-feedback oscillation, a formant transition (caused by movement of the speaker's vocal tract) occurring in the spectral vicinity of the frequency-response peak, may be distorted severely enough as it passes through the peak to detract from its perception by hearing-impaired persons.

It would be of value to have a method for determining how severe this

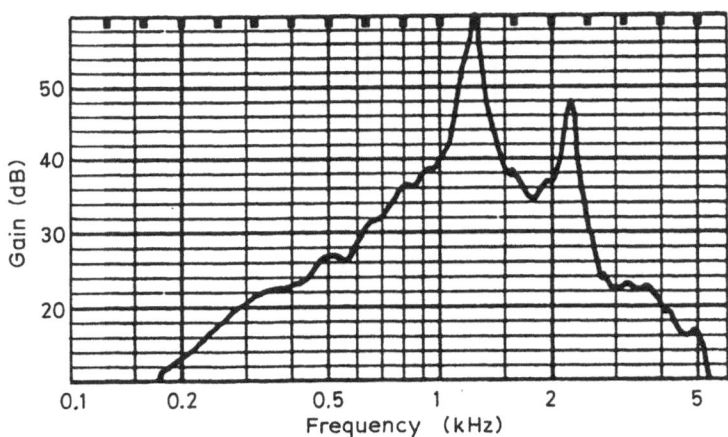

Figure 15.2 Insertion gain on Kemar for a vented hearing aid near acoustic-feedback oscillation.

degradation is on the speech materials employed during speech discrimination tests of hearing-impaired persons wearing hearing aids that are near the onset of acoustic-feedback oscillation.

15.3 THE NATURE OF ACOUSTIC-FEEDBACK OSCILLATION

The technique of characterizing a hearing-aid fitting as a feedback control system may be employed for determining the proximity of hearing-aid fittings to acoustic-feedback oscillation (Veit, 1981; Egolf, 1982; Preves, 1985). The exact nature of the feedback-produced oscillation depends on several factors including the physical characteristics of the hearing aid, the geometry of the wearer's ear, the volume-control setting, the size of the earmould vent and the physical fit of the hearing aid and earmould in combination. These parameters combine in various ways for different hearing-aid fittings to form widely varying magnitude and phase characteristics for the acoustical feedback that originates from the receiver/earmould outlet. The combination of the magnitude and phase of this acoustical-feedback signal, when measured in an open-loop condition as shown in Figure 15.3, determines whether a hearing aid worn *in situ* will oscillate or not. Ignoring for the moment the phase shifter in Figure 15.3, note that the loop has been opened between the hearing-aid microphone and amplifier.

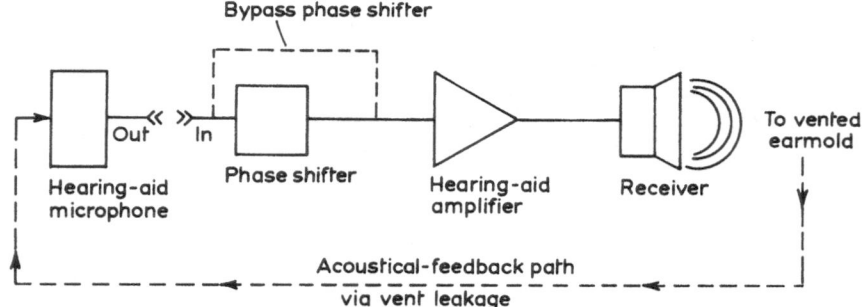

Figure 15.3 Measurement of open-loop transfer-function to determine proximity of hearing-aid fitting *in situ* to onset of acoustic-feedback oscillation. Optional phase shifter is used to stabilize loop and prevent oscillation. Out/in = feedback loop transfer function.

Feedback in produced as a result of a loop created when a part of the hearing-aid receiver output is transmitted through the air via earmould vent and around the periphery of the earmould to the microphone input. This signal may be amplified again and again, possibly resulting in continuous oscillation. At a particular frequency (usually at or very near a peak in the hearing-aid-frequency response) the acoustic-feedback-leakage component adds in-phase or, in a positive sense, with an incoming signal to the hearing-aid microphone (Figure 15.4(a)).

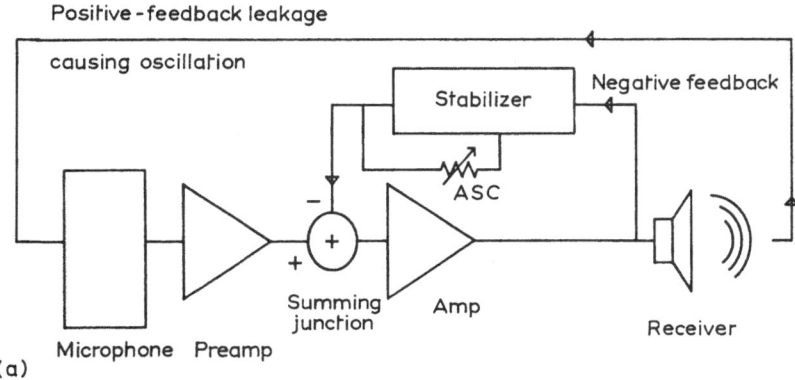

(a)

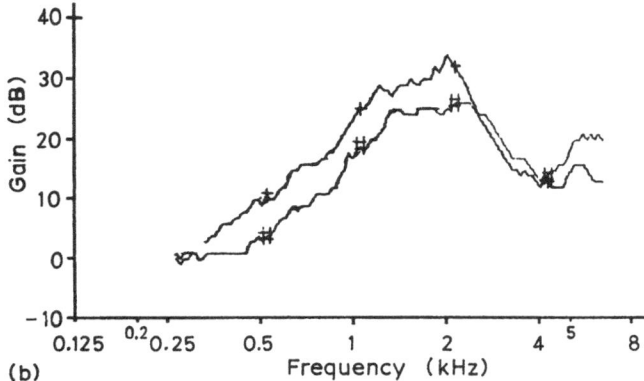

(b)

Figure 15.4 (a) Block diagram of a hearing-aid fitting showing positive feedback created by acoustic leakage. Negative feedback is provided by a stabilizing circuit to cancel the positive feedback at the summing junction. Adjustable stabilizer control (ASC) adjusts the amount of negative feedback provided. (b) Maximum insertion gain before feedback oscillation provided in a real ear by an IROS ITE hearing aid with (top line up to 3 kHz) and without (bottom line up to 3 kHz) stabilizer circuit.

15.4 PREVENTING ACOUSTIC-FEEDBACK OSCILLATION

Among the electronic means evaluated for acoustic-feedback-oscillation elimination are (1) high-frequency attenuation (low-pass filtering), (2) notch filtering to reduce gain at the feedback frequency, (3) phase-shifting the signal, (4) providing negative feedback to counteract the positive feedback from the earmould leakage and (5) frequency shifting the signal (Veit, 1981; Egolf, 1982; Preves, 1984b). Purely acoustic means may also be used to reduce the tendency for oscillation by modifying the earmould or earhook sound bore (Macrae, 1982; Killion, 1980; Killion and Wilson, 1985).

(a) Low-pass filtering

Of the methods currently employed to prevent the acoustic-feedback oscillation, the most common practice is to electrically or acoustically attenuate high-frequency gain with a low-pass filter. Unfortunately, these procedures often have an undesirable side effect – that of providing inadequate high-frequency gain for some hearing-impaired persons.

(b) Notch filtering

Notch filtering to eliminate acoustic feedback is based on the theory that if the feedback frequency can be determined, the gain at that frequency can be attenuated sufficiently to eliminate oscillation. This method of feedback suppression for hearing aids is commonly used in the audio industry for suppressing oscillation in public-address systems (Boner and Boner, 1965). A problem with notch filtering is that feedback may occur at more than one frequency so that more than one notch filter may be required (Beex, 1980). By carefully controlling the phase characteristic of the notch filter, feedback components at nearby frequencies can have a phase characteristic so as to not cause oscillation. In addition to electrical notch-filtering (Figure 15.5(a)), an acoustical notch filter may be implemented by constructing the vent and main bore in earmoulds to certain prescribed dimensions (Macrae, 1982). However, this approach results in a relatively wide notch, which leaves a large gap in the frequency response in the critical high-frequency region (Figure 15.5(b)).

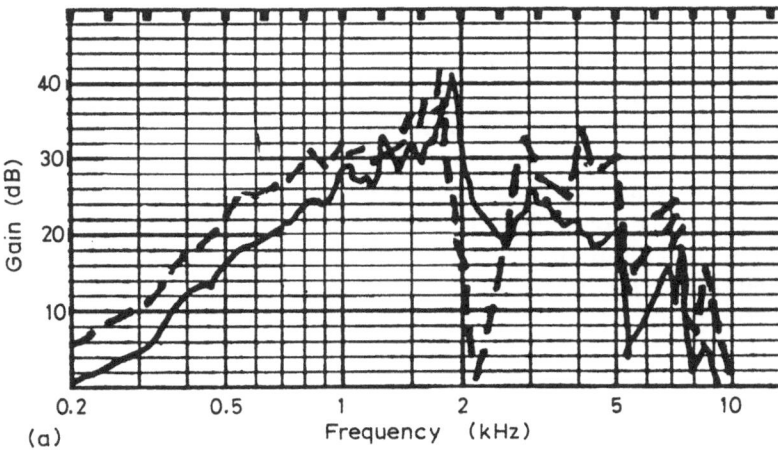

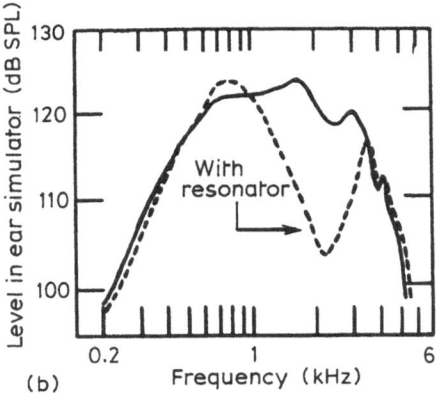

Figure 15.5 (a) Maximum insertion gain achievable before onset of acoustic-feedback oscillation for an ITE aid on KEMAR with (- - - -) and without (———) an electrical notch filter. (b) Ear simulator response of a hearing-aid with Helmholtz resonator notch filter in the sound channel. After Macrae 1982; reprinted with permission.

(c) Phase shifting

Incorporating a phase compensator in the hearing-aid amplifier (Figure 15.3) has been utilized for suppressing acoustic feedback and improving the transient response of a vented hearing-aid (Preves, 1982, 1983; Preves, Ruzicka and Peterson, 1985). In a study to determine whether the addition of a phase-shifting network to a conventional hearing-aid amplifier provided more insertion gain before onset of acoustic-feedback oscillation, custom in-the-ear earmould modules were made for 10 ears. Each earmould module contained a hearing-aid microphone and receiver and a 3 mm-diameter vent (Preves, 1984). An external amplifier, connected to each module via cords, had 120 dB peak SSPL90, 50 dB peak gain and a frequency response slope of 10 dB between 500 Hz and the frequency of peak gain, as measured on an HA-1 2 cc coupler. Maximum insertion gain before onset of acoustic-feedback oscillation was obtained with a probe microphone for each of the ears for two conditions – first, amplifier alone and second, phase compensator

MAXIMUM INSERTION GAIN WITH A 120–50–10 SAV FULL OPEN
BEFORE ACOUSTICAL FEEDBACK OSCILLATION OCCURS ON
REAL EARS AS MEASURED WITH PROBE MICROPHONE AND
60dB INPUT SPL.

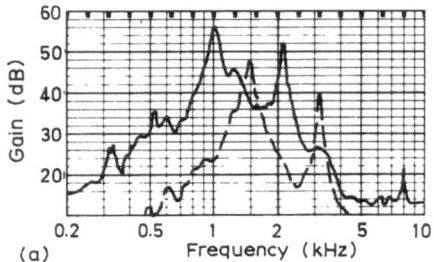

	FEEDBACK FREQUENCY
W/O PHASE SHIFTER – – –	3.1KHz
WITH PHASE SHIFTER ——	2KHz

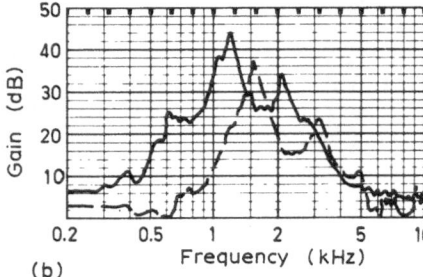

	FEEDBACK FREQUENCY
W/O PHASE SHIFTER – – – –	1 5 KHz
WITH PHASE SHIFTER ——	2KHz

Figure 15.6 (a) Maximum insertion gain response obtained before acoustic-feedback oscillation with probe-microphone measurements for two real ears with (——) and without (- - - -) phase compensation added to the amplifier of an ITE aid. (b) Oscillation frequencies with (——) and without (- - - -) phase compensation after volume control was turned up.

added to the amplifier. Maximum real-ear-insertion gain-frequency response for two of the ears from the study is shown in Figure 15.6. Figure 15.7 shows the mean increase in achievable insertion gain before onset of acoustic-feedback oscillation of 12, 13 and 18 dB, for the condition with phase compensator added, as compared to the amplifier alone at 250, 500 and 1000 Hz, respectively. Less increase in insertion gain was obtained at higher frequencies.

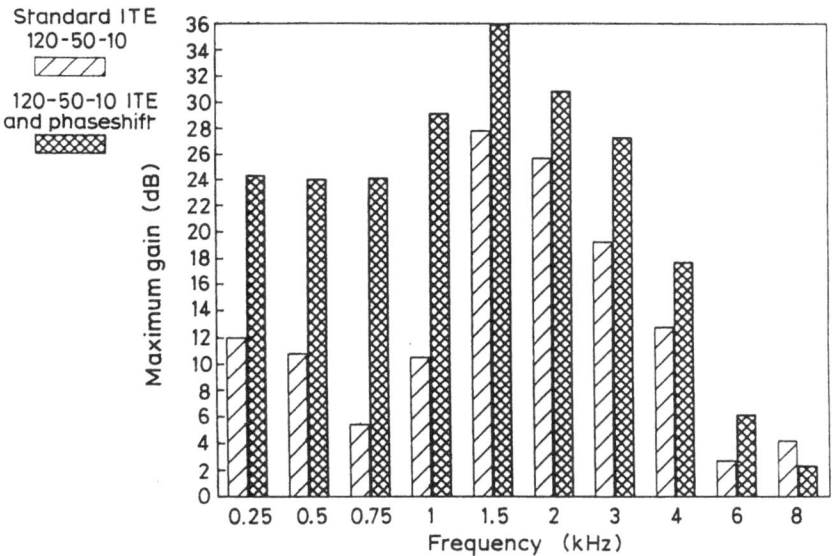

Figure 15.7 Mean maximum insertion gain obtained before onset of acoustic-feedback oscillation with probe-microphone measurements for ten real ears with and without phase compensation added to the amplifier of an ITE aid. Amplifier had 50 dB peak gain, 10 dB peak SSPL90 and difference between peak gain and 5000 Hz gain of 10 dB in a 2 cc coupler.

(d) Negative feedback

A technique for preventing acoustic-feedback oscillation that is similar to phase compensation is shown in Figure 15.4(a). Here, a portion of the electrical output signal to the receiver is fed back in a negative phase to incoming signals from the hearing-aid microphone. The resultant is a cancellation of some of the positive acoustic feedback leaking out of the earmould (Preves, Sigelman and Le May, 1986). Figure 15.4(b) shows the maximum insertion gain possible, as measured with a probe microphone, before onset of acoustic-feedback oscillation provided in a real ear by an IROS ITE hearing-aid with the negative-feedback circuit switched into and out of the circuit. With the negative feedback circuit activated, the volume control could be turned up about 7 dB higher before onset of oscillation than with it deactivated.

(e) Frequency shifting

Frequency shifting has been recommended for cancelling acoustic-feedback oscillation in public-address systems (Schroeder, 1961) and has also been recommended for minimizing acoustic feedback in hearing aids (Bennett, Srikandan and Browne, 1980). With this technique, the frequency of the input signal is shifted to a slightly lower or higher frequency before it reaches the hearing-aid receiver in amplified form. After repeating several cycles of this frequency shifting process, the frequency of the feedback leakage component would be sufficiently different from the frequency of a peak in the hearing-aid-frequency response to avoid oscillation.

Although electronic notch-filtering, phase compensation and frequency-shifting techniques for preventing acoustic-feedback oscillation are viable, none of these approaches have generally found their way into routine hearing-aid-production hearing instruments as yet. The main reason for this apparent lack of incorporating such promising technology seems to be the problem of inadequate component miniaturization.

15.5 SUPPRESSING ENVIRONMENTAL NOISE

Among methods currently employed in hearing aids to improve signal-to-noise ratio by suppressing environmental noise are fitting binaural hearing aids, employing directional microphones, incorporating fixed or adaptively changing electronic high-pass-filtering, high-pass filtering with earmould venting and utilizing single- or dual-channel compression (automatic gain control).

Since environmental noise often has a long-term spectrum that is predominantly low-frequency weighted, simply providing less low-frequency gain with a fixed or manually adjustable high-pass filter is a method commonly used to improve the signal-to-noise ratio. There are numerous studies examining the benefits in speech intelligibility resulting from high-pass filtering with various filter cut-off frequencies and various slopes (Thomas and Pfannebecker, 1974; Thomas and Ohley, 1972). With this technique, although speech-vowel information is severely attenuated, most of the studies show intelligibility improvement with even extreme amounts of high-pass filtering. This is particularly the case if the high-pass filter is followed by peak clipping (Thomas and Sparks, 1971). Methods of implementing high-pass filters in hearing aids include a low-cut microphone response, appropriate selection of resistors and/or capacitors in the amplifier, modifying the earhook for a postauricular hearing aid and by venting the earmould.

(a) Peak clipping and compression

For transforming the dynamic range of speech and other environmental signals into the limited dynamic range of a recruiting pathological auditory system, compression or automatic gain control (AGC) amplifiers have been utilized. These methods may also have application for reducing environmental noise in hearing aids. Limiting the maximum-output sound pressure to a point below the loudness-discomfort level may also be accomplished with a peak-clipping circuit. This produces harmonic distortion, as also happens when a hearing-aid reaches saturation. However, speech intelligibility may not be adversely affected if the peak clipping is symmetrical. In fact, there have been studies suggesting that high-pass filtering prior to a symmetrical peak clipper can significantly improve the intelligibility of speech in the presence of white noise (Thomas and Niederjohn, 1970; Licklider and Pollack, 1948). The rationale is based on the zero-axis crossings of unfiltered clipped speech being largely representative of first-formants, thus containing relatively little consonant information.

With simple differentiation by a high-pass filter prior to the symmetrical peak clipping, which has been called 'whitening speech', more emphasis is placed on the higher frequency consonant information, the result being more intelligible speech in competing noise. In real-world situations, the noise is frequently one or more competing talkers rather than white noise as in the laboratory studies, and high-pass filtering together with symmetrically peak clipping the signal may not improve intelligibility (Young and Goodman, 1977). Of course, none of the results of the laboratory studies mentioned above would be applicable to peak clippers used in hearing aids unless their circuits also perform infinite, symmetrical peak-clipping. Many hearing aids currently in the marketplace employ asymmetrical peak-clipping circuitry.

An alternative form of peak clipping called 'carrier clipping' has been proposed (Drysdale and Gregory, 1979), but subsequent studies have shown that this type of peak clipping actually reduces signal-to-noise ratio and may lower speech intelligibility more than either a linear circuit or compression circuit for listening in high levels of environmental noise (Troscianko and Gregory, 1984).

There has been considerable controversy as to whether a compression hearing aid improves signal-to-noise ratio (Rutherford, 1957; Krebs, 1964). Several studies have examined the issue of whether the compression ratio of an AGC circuit makes a difference in speech discrimination with hearing aids (Caraway and Carhart, 1967; Vargo, 1972; Burchfield, 1970; Yanick, 1973; Yanick, 1975; Sung and Sung, 1982). In these studies, compression ratios evaluated by speech-discrimination tests were 2:1, 3:1 and 5:1 with the speech materials delivered at several presentation levels. The results were inconsistent, with some subjects showing significant improvement resulting from using compression as compared to linear amplification, and some showing no significant improvement. In retrospect, some of these studies may have suffered from the inability of speech-discrimination tests to viably differentiate hearing-aid performance. It appears that a compression ratio of at least 10:1 would be best for compression-limiting hearing aids worn by persons with extremely limited dynamic ranges in noisy environments (Walker and Dillon, 1982).

For single-channel compression aids, the time constants of the AGC circuit going into and out of compression can be, in some cases, easily perceived by the wearer. This problem is frequently caused by the AGC circuit reducing the gain across the entire frequency range in reaction to low-frequency noises. Additionally, the time constants of the AGC circuit may distort the temporal characteristics of the speech signal itself. The effect of the attack and recovery times of the AGC circuits on speech intelligibility has been a frequently studied subject (Lynn and Carhart, 1963; Burnett and Schweitzer, 1977; Schweitzer and Causey, 1977; Sung and Sung, 1982). These studies generally agree that attack times should be as short as possible in order to avoid overshoots of sound pressure reaching or exceeding the loudness-discomfort level of the aid wearer. Additionally, a very short attack time would presumably cause minimum disturbance of the temporal features of speech. No clear agreement exists for the recovery time. Studies have shown that the optimum recovery time depends on auditory-system pathology. For example, a 200–400 millisecond recovery time increased speech intelligibility for persons with endolymphatic hydrops and presbycusis (Lynn and Carhart, 1963). In other studies, a maximum of 150 milliseconds for recovery time provided the best speech intelligibility for hearing-impaired persons (Schweitzer and Causey, 1977; Johansson, 1973). After an extensive literature review, a recovery time of between 60 and 150 milliseconds has been recommended as most desirable for compression limiters (Walker and Dillon, 1982).

Frequency-dependent compression is a term used to describe a single-channel AGC circuit having some form of low-frequency gain reduction via a tone control located prior to the AGC sensor. The net result is to elevate the low-frequency AGC kneepoint, or the signal-level threshold required for low-frequency signals to exceed before compression can occur. Thus, frequency-dependent compression with its frequency-dependent AGC kneepoint may somewhat prevent the activation of the compression circuit by low-frequency environmental noise. In actuality, the majority of AGC hearing aids have some kind of low-frequency gain-regulating circuit prior to the AGC-level sensor.

(b) Multi-channel compression

To more effectively eliminate the problem in single-channel compressors of having the gain across the entire frequency range reduced by low-frequency environmental noises, a multi-band compressor having independent AGC circuits for each frequency band has been proposed as being superior, especially for severely hearing-impaired persons with extreme loudness recruitment (Villchur, 1973). With multi-band compression, an increase in low-frequency noise causes a gain reduction only in the low-frequency band as shown in Figure 15.8. In theory, the weaker high-frequency content of speech, critical for good intelligibility, would then continue to be maximally amplified (Linear Technology, 1983; Kates, 1986). Additionally, severe loudness recruitment in the high frequencies may be compensated for by a separate high-frequency-band compressor (Goldberg, 1982). One important issue for multi-band compressors is whether the hearing aid should react to and correct for

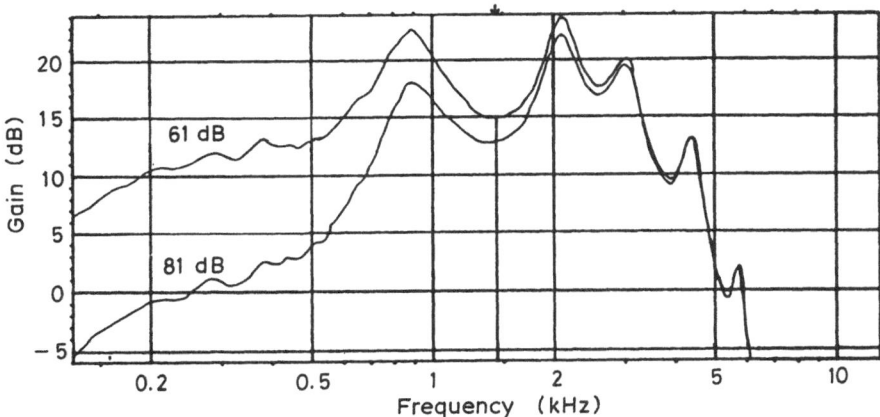

Figure 15.8 Change in frequency response on a 2 cc coupler of a 2-channel postauricular hearing aid (Siemens 283) caused by varying input level of random noise having a flat spectrum from 61–81 dB total RMS SPL.

the rapid level changes of speech – a deliberate distortion of the speech signal in itself – or whether the natural temporal and spectral cues of speech should be preserved (Braida *et al.*, 1982).

Some studies have documented the benefits of multi-channel over single-channel-compression and linear-circuit hearing aids (Yanick, 1976; Mangold and Leijon, 1981; Goldberg, 1982; Laurence, Moore and Glasberg, 1983; Moore and Glasberg, 1986). However, there are also studies that have generally failed to demonstrate significant improvements in speech intelligibility (Barfod, 1976; Abramovitz, 1980; O'Loughlin, 1980; Lippman, Braida and Durlach, 1981; Walker and Byrne, 1982; Byrne and Walker, 1982; Nabalek, 1983). It remains to be seen whether some form of multi-band compression will indeed provide significant improvements of speech intelligibility in the presence of competing noise for most hearing-impaired persons. Several multi-channel compression aids are now commercially available in BTE-type hearing aids (Goldberg, 1982; Moore and Glasberg, 1986; Kates, 1986).

(c) Adaptive high-pass filters

Another method of adapting to a changing noise environment is utilization of a high-pass filter with adapatively changing cut-off frequency depending on the amount of noise in the input signal

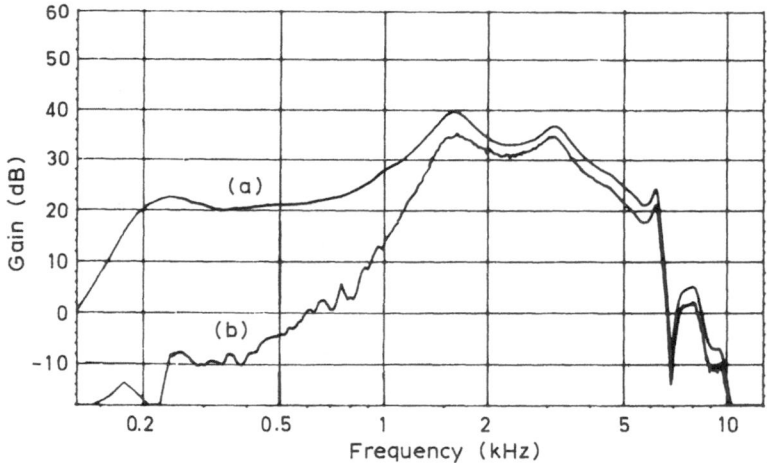

Figure 15.9 Change in frequency response of an ITE hearing aid containing an adaptive high-pass filter (Argosy Electronics Manhattan Circuit) on 2 cc coupler with input level of random noise having a flat spectrum varying between (a) 67 dB and (b) 87 dB total RMS SPL.

(Iwasaki, 1981; Kates, 1986; Preves and Sigelman, 1986; Sigelman and Preves, 1987). Adaptive high-pass filters have been implemented in ITE and even in ITC aids (Figure 15.9). Although this technique for low-frequency reduction is different in concept from the multi-band AGC approach, the effect on low-frequency response appears to be quite similar when the level of low-frequency noise is raised (compare Figure 15.8 with Figure 15.9). With either the multi-band-compression or adaptive high-pass-filter approach, the low-frequency gain of the hearing aid will be automatically reduced if the input signal contains sufficient low-frequency energy which is construed by the circuit to be noise.

15.6 EMPLOYING DIGITAL ELECTRONICS IN HEARING AIDS

(a) Improving signal-to-noise ratio with digital technology

Technological advances in other industries are providing the opportunity to have digital computers in hearing aids. A digital-computer-based adaptive noise-rejection circuit, the Zeta Noise Blocker (ZNB), is available in integrated circuit form for incorporation into head-worn aids

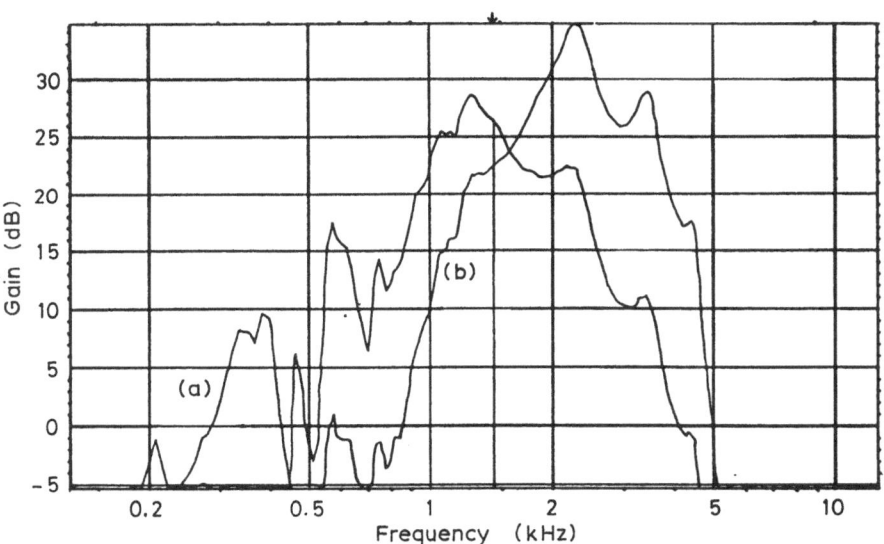

Figure 15.10 Change in frequency response of a postauricular hearing aid containing Zeta Noise Blocker (Maico SP335) resulting from input level of random noise having a flat spectrum varying between (a) 60 dB and (b) 80 dB total RMS SPL.

principally for the purpose of improving signal-to-noise ratio (Graupe, Beex and Causey, 1980). The computer in the ZNB separates speech from noise in several frequency bands by utilizing the temporal differences between the speech and the noise. The algorithm of the ZNB determines whether the energy level in a particular frequency band alters over successive one-third of a second intervals by more than a certain threshold. If so, it is assumed that the predominant signal in that frequency band is speech. If not, it is assumed that the predominant signal in that band is noise and the computer automatically reduces the gain for that band without changing the gain in other frequency bands. Figure 15.10 shows the frequency-response change of a BTE aid containing the ZNB resulting from raising the total RMS level of a continuous, flat spectrum input by 20 dB. Note that for the 60 dB SPL noise level, the low-frequency gain is greater and the high-frequency gain is less than for the 80 dB SPL noise input. Interestingly, little or no change in frequency response would have resulted had the higher level noise input been pulsed at a rate similar to that of the vocal cords turning on and off when producing speech vowels.

Both quantitative and anecdotal results examining the benefits of the ZNB in competing noise are mixed. Two studies, the first using a non-integrated circuit prototype of the device packaged in a large box, and the second using the actual integrated circuit in a hearing aid, found significant improvement for the majority of persons using the filter (Stein and Dempsey-Hart, 1984; Wolinsky, 1986). However, another study (Larsen, 1986) also implemented with the ZNB in integrated-circuit form, did not find significant improvement using a speech-reception threshold in noise protocol (Plomp, 1978; Van Tasell and Yanz, 1987). Thus, it remains to be seen whether the ZNB will provide significant improvement in speech intelligibility when used in competing noise situations.

(b) Programmable hearing aids with digital memory

Providing hearing aids with programmable capability allows the gain, frequency response and saturation sound-pressure level to be easily varied by dispensers over a wide electroacoustic performance selection range. This feature has significant implications for those ITE and ITC hearing aids that do not contain trimmer potentiometers for varying parameters such as low-frequency response and peak-clipping level. These trimmer-less, fixed performance hearing aids would have to be returned to the manufacturer to modify their electroacoustic characteristics unless sufficient variation could be achieved by modifying the earmould. Indeed, trimmer potentiometers in hearing aids

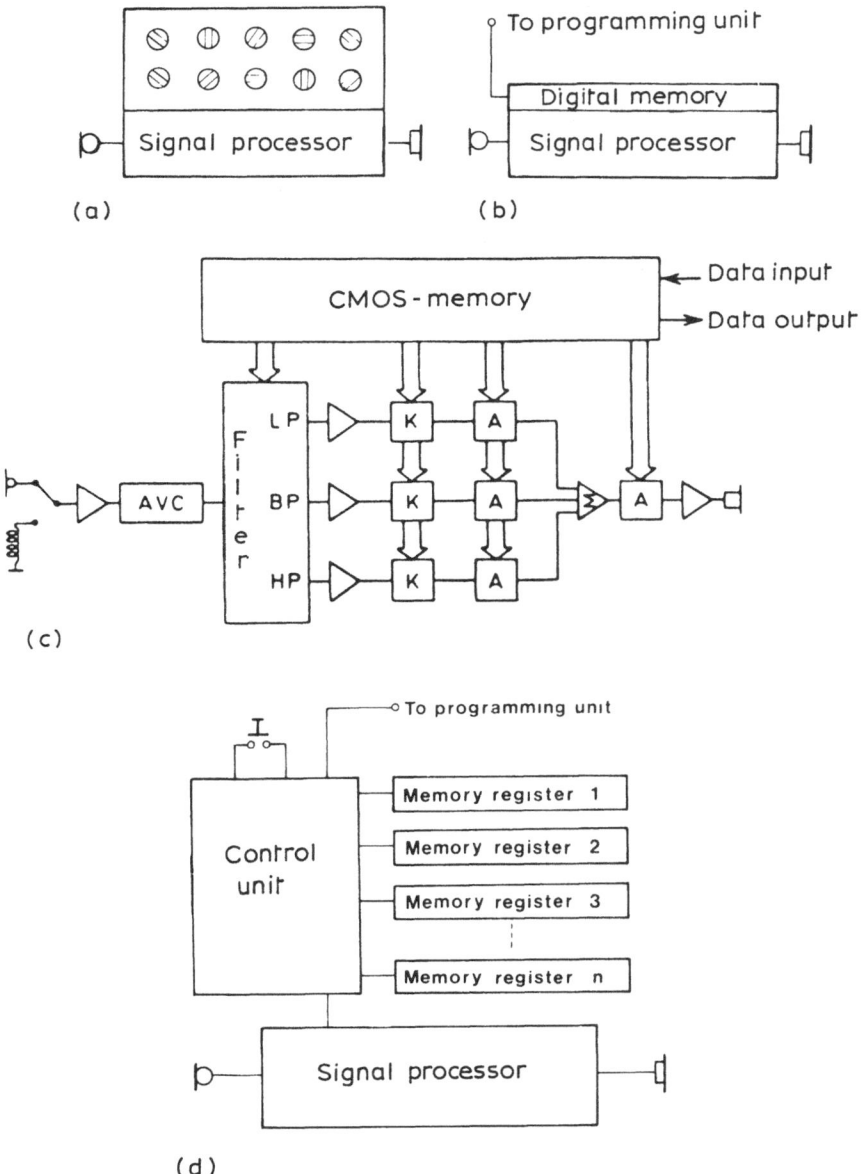

Figure 15.11 Block diagrams of programmable hearing aid with digital memory. (a) Conventional hearing-aid achieving 'programmability' with many mechanical trimmer potentiometers; (b) as (a) with trimmers replaced with digital memory and a programming unit; (c) 3-channel hearing aid with AGC and CMOS digital memory; (d) several memory registers shown for selection of different frequency responses by hearing-aid wearer for different listening environments. (Reprinted with permission of Mangold and Leijon, Hearing Instruments and Scandinavian Audiology).

could be replaced by programmability. Hand in hand with programmability is the requirement that the hearing aid be able to store the
programmed parameters. A programmable three-frequency band-
compression hearing aid has been proposed that would allow the
wearer to select from several frequency responses stored in an
electrically erasable programmable read-only memory (EEPROM),
depending on environmental listening situations (Mangold and Leijon,
1979; 1981). These authors note that the programmable aid is actually a
master hearing aid because of the wide range of electroacoustic
performance variation that can be achieved. The programmable feature
may be useful for assisting new hearing-aid wearers to adjust to
amplification and to optimize fittings for fluctuating hearing losses,
because the aid could be easily reprogrammed by the professional. A
block diagram for this system is shown in Figure 15.11. When
programming the aid, attention would be paid to the wearer's equal-
loudness contours in each of the three compression-frequency bands.

(c) Frequency-response shaping

One of the advantages of incorporating digital technology into hearing
aids is the ability to implement unusual frequency responses that are
virtually impossible to obtain with current analogue technology. These
unusual responses may include small bumps in gain at particular
frequencies (or notches in the frequency response) for the specific
purpose of compensating for a particular abnormality in a pathological
auditory system. An example of a notch filter actually implemented by a
digital hearing aid is shown in Figure 15.12(a). Figure 15.12(b) shows a
simulation of the filter which was performed by a computer prior to
actually implementing the filter. This electroacoustic response might be
useful for those persons having a 'cookie-bite' audiogram – good
hearing in the mid-frequencies and significant hearing loss at higher
and lower frequencies as shown in Figure 15.12(c). This notched response is difficult to achieve with currently available analogue electronics for hearing-aid amplifiers but can be achieved using specially
designed earmoulds or earhooks (McCrae, 1982; Killion and Wilson,
1985).

The digital hearing aid that produced the notched-frequency response
in Figure 15.12(a) and 15.12(b) utilizes the Texas Instruments 320 series
digital filter and was implemented as a laboratory exercise in a large box
because of its excessively large physical size and high current drain
(about 500 milliamps at 5 volts), which contrasts sharply with the 1
milliamp at 1.3 volts consumed by today's typical analogue-hearing-aid
circuitry (Nielsen, 1986).

The ZNB gets around the high-current requirement by utilizing

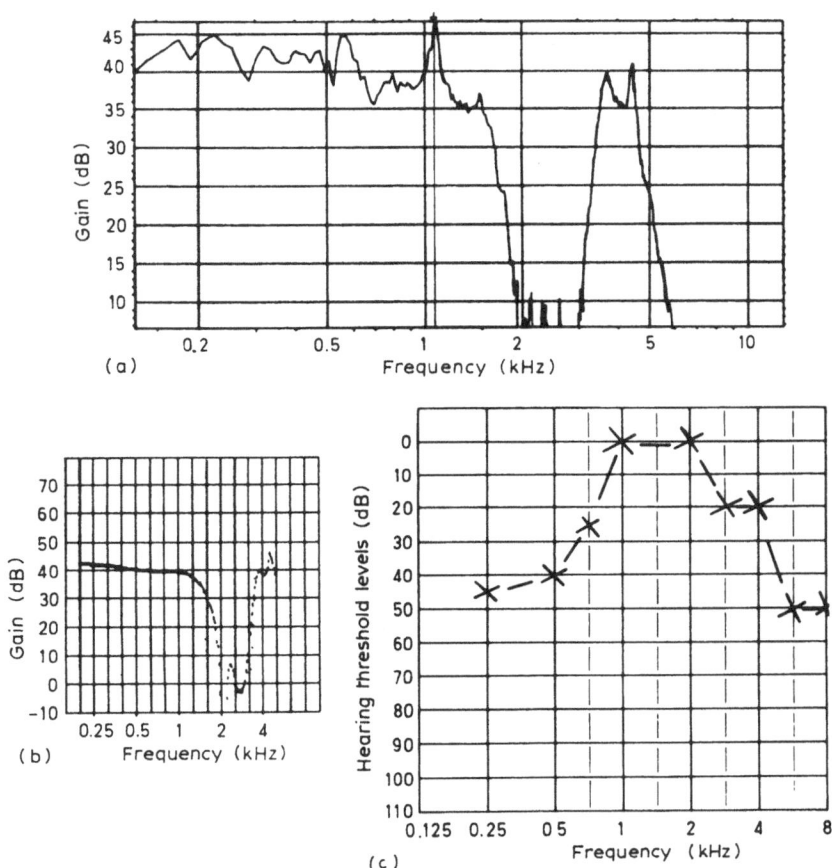

Figure 15.12 Frequency response shaping possible with a digital hearing aid. (a) Notched frequency response of a hearing aid in a 2 cc coupler produced by a Texas Instruments TMS 320 digital filter; (b) simulation of notched response whose actual response produced by a digital filter in a hearing aid is shown in Figure 15.12(a); (c) example of an audiometric configuration for which the notched frequency response shown in Figure 15.12(a) may be helpful.

extremely low-current digital logic and by leaving the audio signal in analogue form thus avoiding the need for analogue-to-digital and digital-to-analogue converters.

15.7 THE PACKAGING PROBLEM

In order to pack such sophisticated digital signal-processing devices into head-worn, cosmetically attractive hearing aids, considerable funds need to be devoted to improving the existing microcircuit packaging technology. This requirement includes the ability to integrate on a single chip both analogue and digital CMOS (complementary metal oxide semiconductor) circuitry that will perform adequately with the 1.3 volt batteries available for hearing aids, as well as the ability to package the external discrete components necessary, such as capacitors, in a microminiature volume. Custom (not off-the-shelf) standard types, CMOS circuits or microprocessors that will work at the end-of-battery condition (1 volt) may be produced for our special signal-processing applications, small enough to fit into totally head-worn hearing-aid cases. The Zeta Noise Blocker CMOS chip, which has an on-board voltage multiplier, is an example of this.

Another alternative would be to develop new higher voltage subminiature batteries that would better support existing state-of-the-art semiconductor technologies and existing size–shape restrictions of hearing aids. All of these efforts involve advancing the basic technology of semiconductor and battery packaging.

The hearing-aid industry is not flush with research and development funds to develop new basic technologies with which to solve these problems. On the contrary, there is only limited R & D funding available from most hearing-aid manufacturers. Consequently, technological developments from other related industries, which are applicable to the needs of the hearing-aid industry, must be used.

Once the penalty for increased hardware size and cost has been paid, digital filtering may be able to provide much more flexibility in signal-processing applications than analogue filtering. Adaptive algorithms may be implemented to shape the frequency response automatically to compensate for changes in environmental noise and to reject acoustical feedback oscillation. Additionally, digital storage of frequency responses will enable the hearing-aid wearer to manually select from dozens of frequency-response shapes as various listening occasions demand.

REFERENCES

Abramovitz, R. (1980) Frequency shaping and multiband compression in hearing aids. *J. Commun. Dis.*, **13**, 483–8.

Barfod, J. (1976) Multi-channel compression hearing aids. Report 11, The Acoustics Lab., Tech. Univ. of Denmark.

Beex, A. (1980) Moving-average notchfilter, US Patent 4 232 192.

Bennett, M., Srikandan, S. and Browne, L. (1980) A controlled feedback hearing aid. *Hear. Aid J.*, **12**, December, 42–3.

Berger, K. and Hagberg, E. (1982) Hearing aid attitudes and hearing aid usage. *Monographs in Contemporary Audiology*, **3** (4), 10.

Berger, K., Abel, D., Hagberg, E., Puzz, L., Varavvas, D. and Weldele, F. (1982) Successes and problems of hearing aid users. *Hear. Aid J.*, **14**, 26–30.

Berland, O. and Nielsen, T. (1968) Sound pressure generated in the human external ear by a free sound field, Oticon Laboratories, October, Copenhagen, Denmark.

Boner, C.P. and Boner, C.R. (1965) A procedure for controlling room-ring modes and feedback modes in sound systems with narrow-band filters. *J. Audio Eng. Soc.*, **13**, 4.

Braida, L., Durlach, N., De Gennaro, S., Peterson, P. and Bustamante, D. (1982) Review of recent research on multiband amplitude compression for the hearing impaired. Vanderbilt Hearing Aid Report (eds G. Studebaker and F. Bess), Upper Darby, Pa: 133–40.

Burchfield, S. (1970) Perception of amplitude compressed speech by persons exhibiting loudness recruitment, unpublished PhD dissertation, Michigan State Univ.

Burnett, E. and Schweitzer, H. (1977) Attack and release times of automatic-gain-control hearing aids. *J. Acoust. Soc. Amer.*, **62**, 784–6.

Byrne, D. and Walker, G. (1982) The effects of multichannel compression and expansion amplification on perceived quality of speech. *Aust. J. Audiol.*, **4**, (1), 1–8.

Caraway, B.J. and Carhart, R. (1967) Influence of compressor action on speech intelligibility. *J. Acoust. Soc. Amer.*, **41**, 1424–33.

Cranmer, K. (1983) Hearing-aid dispensing – 1983. *Hear. Instrum.*, **34** (5), 11.

Cranmer, K. (1987) Hearing-aid dispensing – 1987. *Hear. Instrum.*, **38** (5), 18.

Drysdale, A. and Gregory, R. (1979) Speech recognition with dynamic range reduction: field tests. *Brit. J. Audiol.*, **13**, 1–6.

Egolf, D. (1982) Review of the acoustic feedback literature from a control systems point of view, The Vanderbilt Hearing Aid Report (eds G. Studebaker and F. Bess), Upper Darby, Pa., 94–103.

FTC (1985) Federal Trade Commission Final Report on the Consumer Survey of the Hearing Aid Industry, Chap. 1, Hearing Industries Assn., Executive Summary, HIA, Washington, DC.

Freedman, S. (1970) The role of the pinna in speech intelligibility, *Final report for contract no. F44620-69-C-0064*, Lab. for Res. in Neuropsychology, Inc., Boston, MA.

Giolas, T., Owens, E., Lamb, S. and Schubert, E. (1979) Hearing performance inventory. *J. Speech Hear. Dis.*, **44**, 169–75.

Goldberg, H. (1982) Signal processors: application to the hearing-impaired. *Hear. Aid J.*, April, 23–7.

Graupe, D., Beex, A. and Causey, D. (1980) ARMA filter and method for designing the same, US Patent, 4 188 667.

HIA (1984) Hearing Industries Assn. Market Survey, special membership meeting, St. Louis, MO., October.

Iwasaki, S. (1981) Automatic noise suppression in hearing aids. *Hear. Aid J.*, **13**, 10–11.

Jervall, L., Almqvist, B., Ovegard, A. and Arlinger, S. (1983) Clinical trial of in-the-ear hearing aids. *Scand. Audiol.*, **12**, 1.

Johansson, B. (1973) The hearing aid as a technical audiological problem. *Scand. Audiol.*, suppl. 3, 55–76.

Kates, J. (1986) Signal processing for hearing aids. *Hear. Instrum.*, **37** (2), 19–22.

Killion, M. (1980) Earmould options for wideband hearing aids, Industrial Research Products, Inc., Elk Grove Village, Il.

Killion, M. and Wilson, D. (1985) Response-modifying earhooks for special fitting problems. *Audecibel*, **34** (4), 28–30.

Krebs, D. (1964) Considerations in the design and use of hearing aids. *Audecibel*, **13**, 90–5.

Larsen, S. (1986) MA thesis, Dept. of Communication and Speech Disorders, University of Minnesota.

Laurence, R., Moore, B. and Glasberg, B. (1983) A comparison of behind-the-ear high-fidelity linear hearing aids and two-channel compression aids, in the laboratory and in everyday life. *Brit. J. Audiol.*, **17**, 31–48.

Licklider, J. and Pollack, I. (1948) Effects of differentiation, integration and infinite peak clipping upon the intelligibility of speech. *J. Acoust. Soc. Amer.*, **20**, 42.

Linear Technology (1983) *Band Limiting Signal Processing Amplifier*.

Lippmann, R., Braida, L. and Durlach, N. (1981) Study of multichannel amplitude compression and linear amplification for persons with sensori-neural hearing loss. *J. Acoust. Soc. Amer.*, **69**, 524–31.

Lynn, G. and Carhart, R. (1963) Influence of attack and release in compression amplification on understanding of speech by hypoacusics. *J. Speech Hear. Dis.*, **28** (2), 124–40.

Mangold, S. and Leijon, A. (1979) Programmable hearing aid with multichannel compression. *Scand. Audiol.*, **8**, 121–6.

Mangold, S. and Leijon, A. (1981) Multichannel compression in a portable programmable hearing aid, *Hear. Aid J.*, **34** (6), 29–32.

Mahon, W. (1987) 1987 US hearing-aid sales summary. *Hear. J.* **40** (12), 9–14.

Martin, E. and Picket, J. (1970) Sensorineural hearing loss and upward spread of masking. *J. Speech Hear. Res.*, **13**, 426–37.

Macrae, J. (1982) Acoustic notch filters for hearing aids. *Aust. J. Audiol.*, **4**, 33–9.

Moore, B. and Glasberg, B. (1986) A comparison of two-channel and single-channel compression hearing aids. *Audiology*, **25**, 210–26.

Murphy, L. (1981) An investigation of the use of behind-the-ear and in-the-ear hearing aids with a geriatric population. *Hear. J.*, **34**, 4, 7, 38–41.

Nabalek, A. (1982) Temporal distortions and noise considerations in The Vanderbilt Hearing-Aid Report (eds G. Studebaker and F. Bess), Upper Darby, Pa., 51–9.

Nabelek, I. (1983) Performance of hearing-impaired listeners under various types of amplitude compression. *J. Acoust. Soc. Amer.*, **74** (3), 776–91.

Nielsen, B. (1986) Digital hearing aids; where are they? *Hear. Instrum.*, **37** (2), 6, 45.

Nielsen, T. (1979) Technical progress and requirements for hearing aids, Oticon Library, Pub. 909 04611/2–79.

O'Loughlin, B. (1980) Evaluation of a three channel compression amplification system on hearing-impaired children. *Aust. J. Audiol.*, **2**, 1–9.

Plomp, R. (1978) Auditory handicap of hearing impairment and the limited benefit of hearing aids. *J. Acoust. Soc. Amer.*, **63**, 533–49.

Preves, D. (1982) The potential of computers and signal processing for hearing aids. *Hear. Instrum.*, **33**, 15–16.

Preves, D. (1983) Signal processing methods for reducing acoustical feedback oscillation in hearing aid fittings. *Audecibel*, **32**, 10–14.

Preves, D. (1984a) Hearing aid signal processing for noise and nonsense syllables. Paper presented at 107th meeting of Acoust. Soc. of Amer., Norfolk, Va.

Preves, D. (1984b) Acoustic feedback rejection in hearing aid fittings. Paper presented at XVII International Congress of Audiology, Santa Barbara, Ca.

Preves, D. (1985) Evaluation of phase compensation for enhancing the signal processing capabilities of hearing aids *in situ*, PhD thesis, Univ. of Minnesota.

Preves, D., Ruzicka, J. and Peterson, E. (1985) Maximizing ITE and ITC fitting potential. *Hear. Instrum.*, **4**, 30.

Preves, D. and Sigelman, J. (1986) A new signal processor for ITE hearing aid fittings. *Hear. Instrum.*, **37** (10), 52–60.

Preves, D. and Sigelman, J. and Le May, P. (1986) A feedback stabilizing circuit for hearing aids. *Hear. Instrum.*, **37** (4), 34–41.

Randolph, K., Gierela, V. and Ross, M. (1977) Hearing aid microphone location and speech discrimination: hearing-impaired adults, pres. at the American Speech and Hear. Conv., Chicago, Il.

Rutherford, C. (1957) Instantaneous speech compressor. *Electronics*, **30**, 168–9.

Scharf, B. (1978) Comparison of normal and impaired hearing II. Frequency analysis, speech perception in Sensorineural hearing impairment and hearing aids (eds Ludvigsen and Barfod), *Scand. Audiol.*, Suppl. 6, 90–3.

Schroeder, M. (1961) Improvement of acoustic feedback stability by frequency shifting. *J. Acoust. Soc. Amer.*, **33**, 1718–24.

Schweitzer, H. and Causey, D. (1977) The relative importance of recovery time in compression hearing aids. *Audiology*, **16**, 61–72.

Shaw, E. (1966) Earcanal pressure generated by a free sound field. *J. Acoust. Soc. Amer.*, **39** (3), 465–70.

Sigelman, J. and Preves, D. (1987) Argosy Manhattan Circuit field trials. *Hear. J.*, **40** (4), 24–9.

Skadegard, J. (1985) Hearing-aid megatrends. *Hear. J.*, **38**, 12, 14–19.

Stein, L. and Dempsey-Hart, D. (1984) Listener-assessed intelligibility of a hearing aid self-adaptive noise filter. *Ear Hear.*, **4**, 199–204.

Studebaker, G. and Zachman, T. (1970) Investigation of the acoustics of earmould vents. *J. Acoust. Soc. Amer.*, **47**, 4, 2: 1107–14.

Sung, R. and Sung, G. (1982) Compression amplification: its effect on speech intelligibility in noise. *Hear. Aid J.*, **35** (11), 20–4.

Surr, R., Schuchman, G. and Montgomery, A. (1978) Factors influencing use of hearing aids. *Arch. Otolaryngol.*, **104**, 732–6.

Thomas, I. and Ohley, W. (1972) Intelligibility enhancement through spectral

258 Future trends

weighting. *Proc. Conf. on Speech Comm. and Proc.*, IEEE Cat. 72, CHO 596–7 AE, 360–3.

Thomas, I. and Niederjohn, R. (1970) The intelligibility of filtered-clipped speech in noise. *J. Audio. Eng. Soc.*, **18** (3), 299–302.

Thomas, I. and Pfannebecker, G. (1974) Effects of spectral weighting of speech in hearing-impaired subjects. *J. Audio. Eng. Soc.*, **22**, 690–4.

Thomas, I. and Sparks, D. (1971) Discrimination of filtered/clipped speech by hearing-impaired subjects. *J. Acoust. Soc. Amer.*, **49**, 1881–7.

Troscianko, T. and Gregory, R. (1984) An assessment of two amplitude-compression hearing aid systems, especially in high ambient noise. *Brit. J. of Audiol.*, **18**, 89–96.

Tyler, R., Baker, L. and Armstrong-Bednall, G. (1983) Difficulties experienced by hearing-aid candidates and hearing-aid users. *Brit. J. Audiol.*, **16**, 191–201.

Van Tasell, D.J. and Yanz, J.L. (1987) Speech recognition thresholding noise: effects of hearing loss, frequency response, and speech materials. *J. Speech Hear. Res.*, **30**, 377–86.

Veit, I. (1981) Ways and means of reducing feedback tendencies in hearing aids. *Audiological Acoustics*, **20**, 176–84.

Vargo, S. (1972) Compression amplification and hearing aids. Maico Audiol. Lib. Series, XII, 2.

Villchur, E. (1973) Signal processing to improve speech intelligibility in perceptive deafness. *J. Acoust. Soc. of Amer.*, **53** (6), 1646–57.

Walker, G. and Byrne, D. (1982) The effects of multi-band compression and expansion on speech reception. Paper presented at Amer. Speech and Lang. Conv., Detroit, Mi.

Walker, G. and Dillon, H. (1982) Compression in hearing aids: an analysis, a review and some recommendations. *National Acoust. Lab. report 90*, Canberrra Reprographics, Fyshwick, ACT 2609.

Wiener, F. and Ross, D. (1946) The pressure distribution in the auditory canal in a progressive sound field. *J. Acoust. Soc. Amer.*, **18** (2), 401–7.

Wiener, F. (1947) On the diffraction of a progressive sound wave by the human head. *J. Acoust. Soc. Amer.*, **19** (1), 143–6.

Wolinsky, S. (1986) Clinical assessment of a self-adaptive noise filtering system. *Hear. J.*, **39** (10), 29–32.

Yanick, P. (1973) Improvement in speech discrimination with compression vs. linear amplification. *J. Aud. Res.*, **13**, 333–8.

Yanick, P. (1975) Discrimination in the presence of competition with an AVC versus DRC hearing aid. *J. Amer. Aud. Soc.*, **1**, 169–72.

Yanick, P. (1976) Effects of signal processing on the intelligibility of speech in noise for subjects possessing sensorineural hearing loss. *J. Amer. Aud. Soc.*, **1**, 229–38.

Yanick, P. (1977) Transient distortion and hearing aid circuits. *Hear. Instrum.*, **28** (1), 8–9.

Young, L. and Goodman, J. (1977) The effects of peak clipping on speech intelligibility in the presence of a competing message. Paper 6.10 presented at IEEE conv. on acoustics, speech and signal proc., Hartford, Conn.

AUTHOR INDEX

SUBJECT INDEX